I0819189

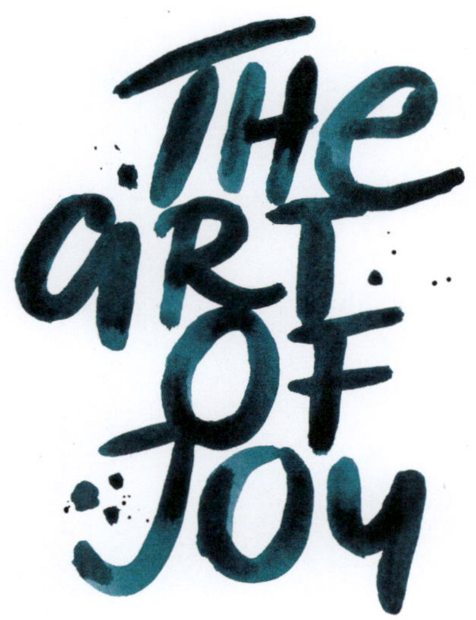
THE ART OF JOY

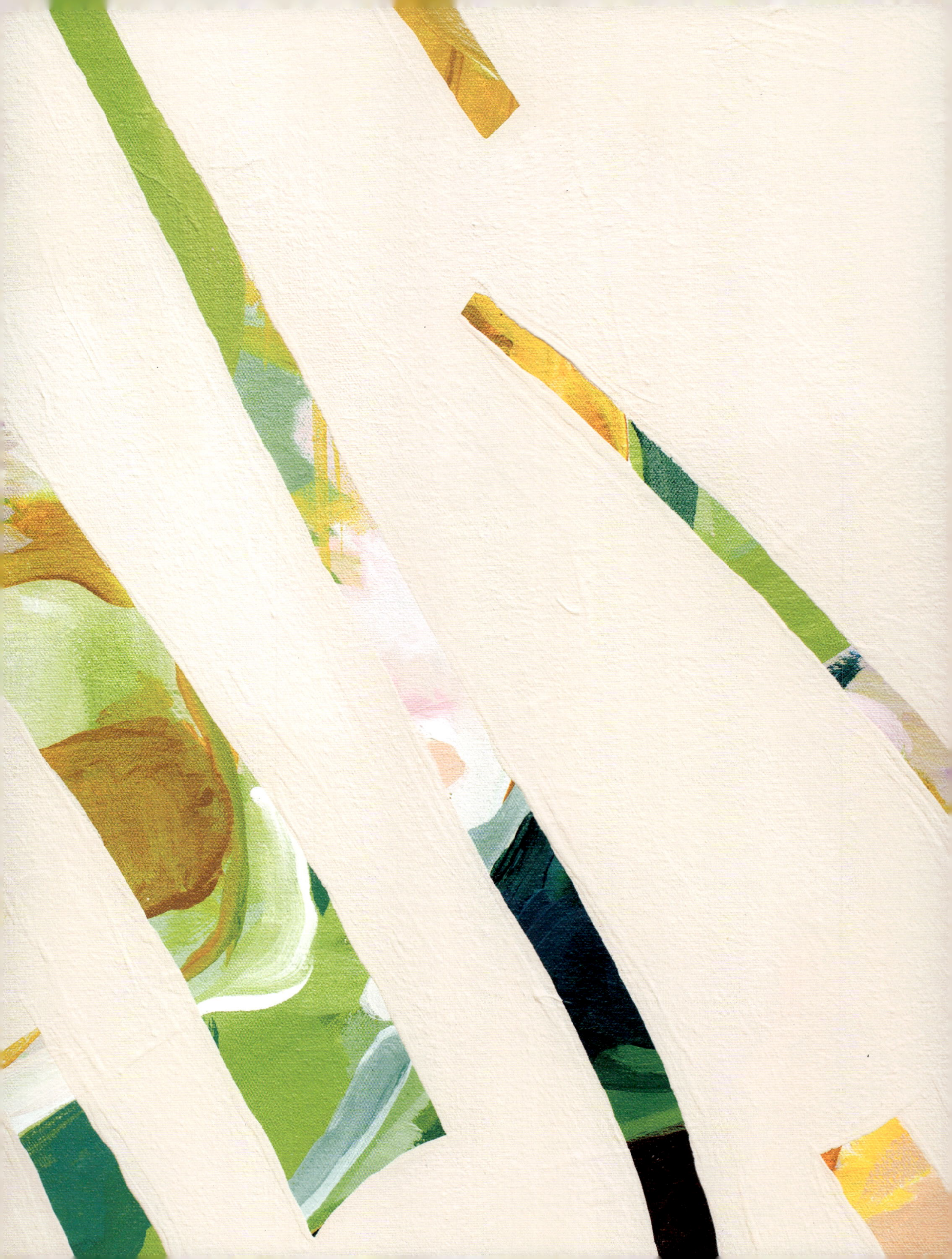

Jen Sievers

The Art of Joy

A creative guide to living a colourful, juicy life

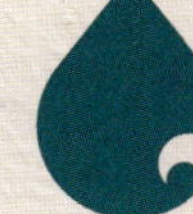

KOA PRESS

@jensievers_art

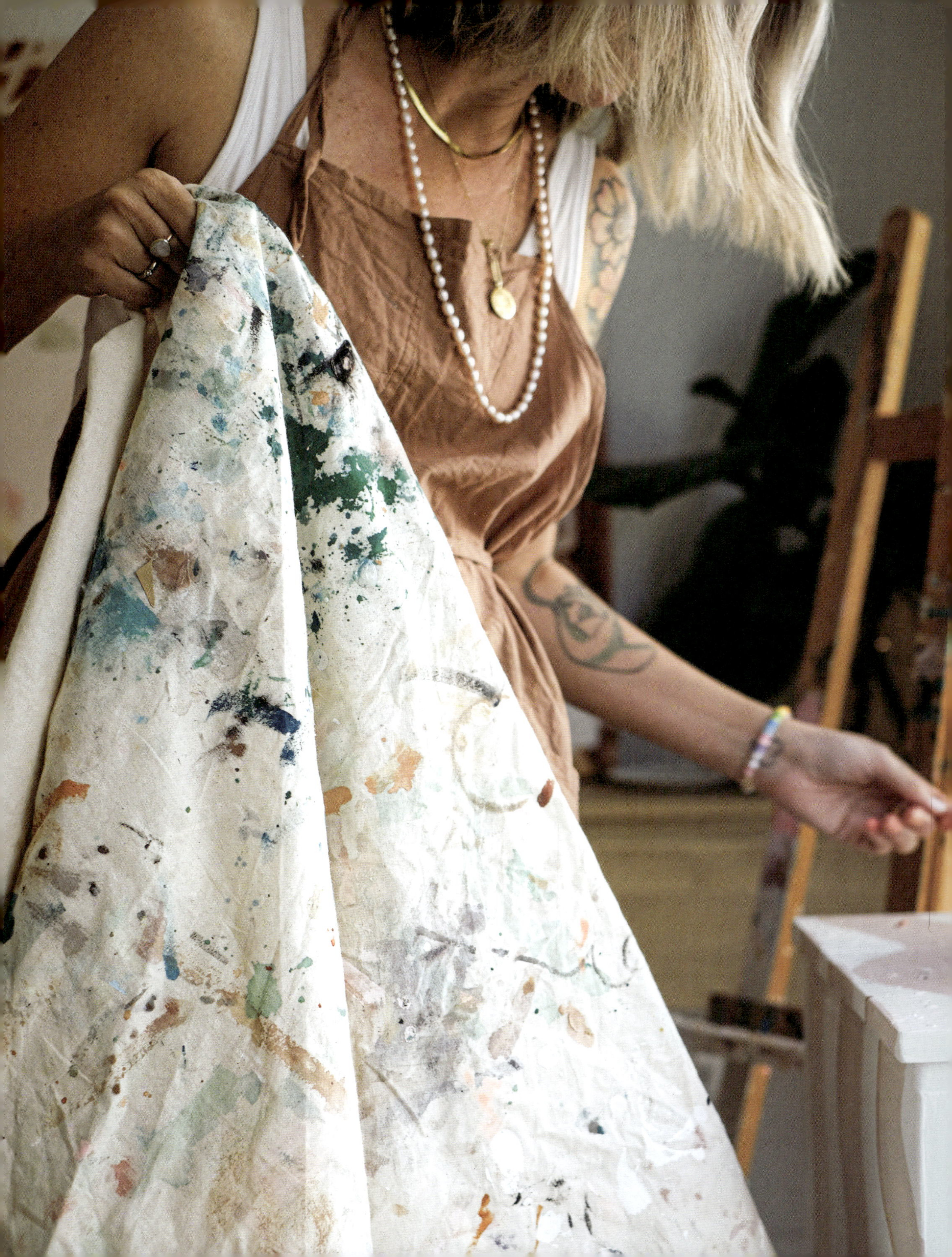

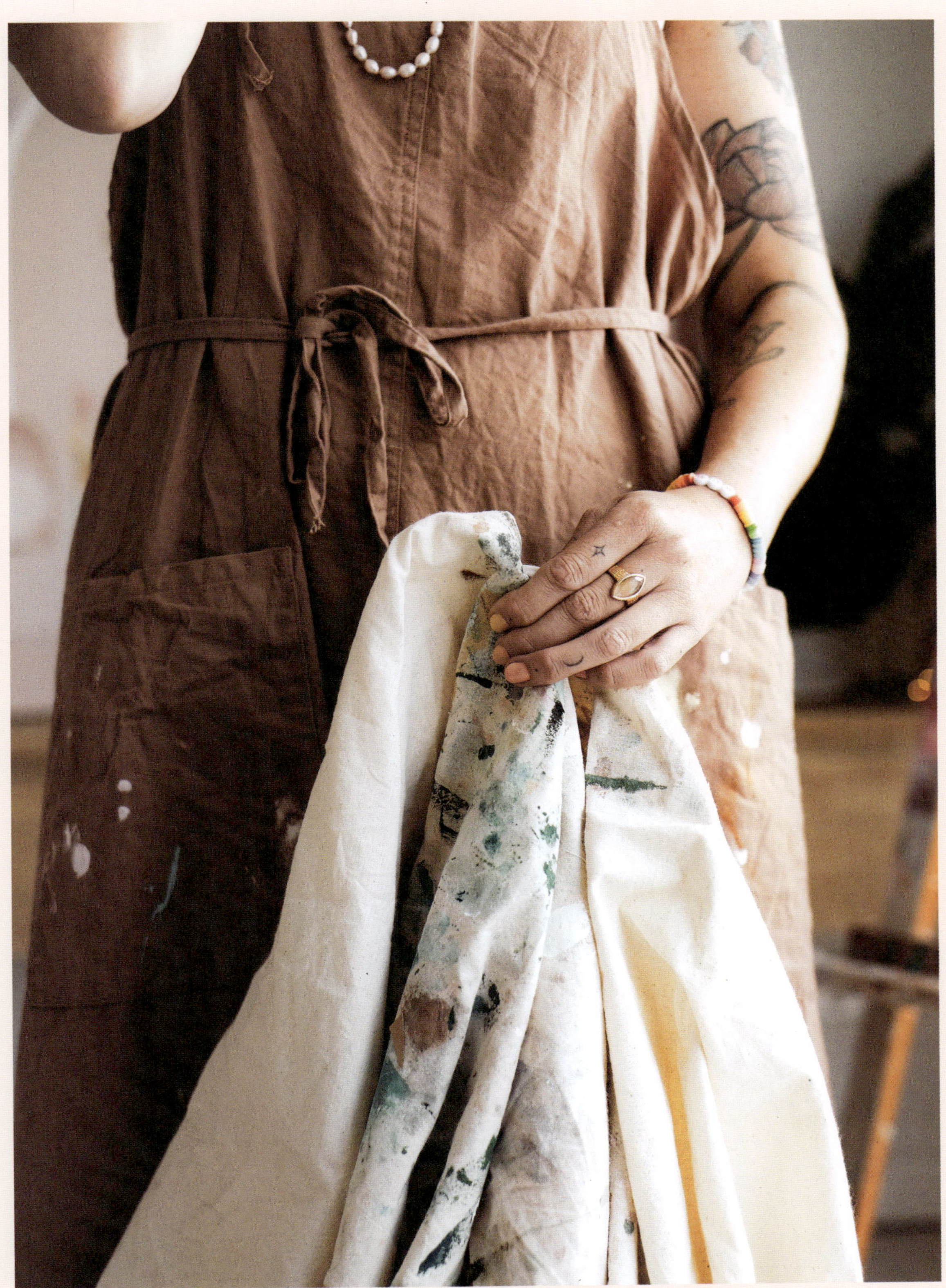

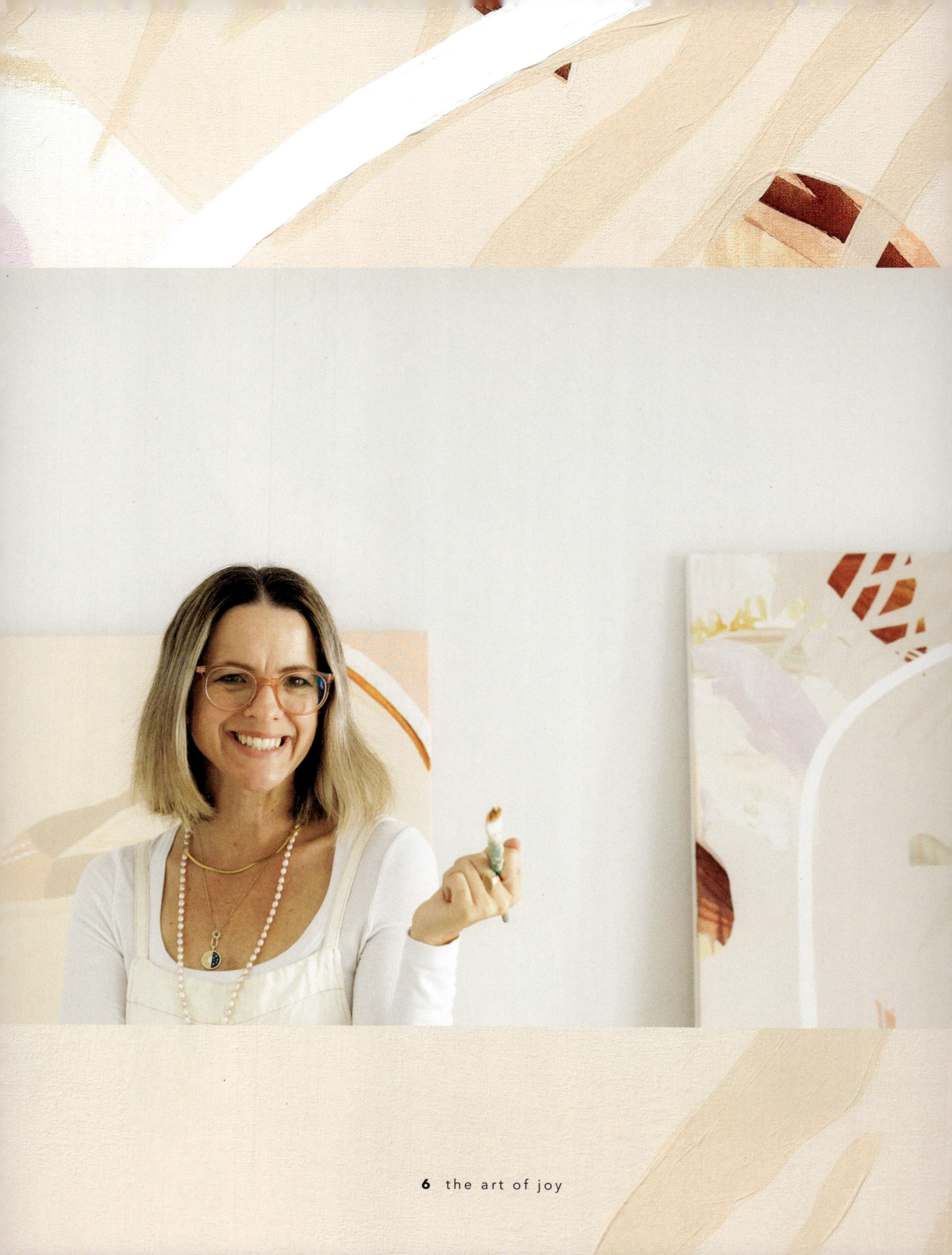

I'm here for a big life
A juicy life
A life with the volume turned up to 10
And music pulsing through my core.

I'm here for a fiercely kind life, a big-love life
A life where my heart beats loudly right out
of my chest and never hides.

I'm here for a weird life, an uncommon life
A life with stories my grandchildren
will never believe.

I'm here for a warm life, a velvet-soft life
A life of moments so tender I could weep.

I'm here for a full life, a real life
A life in full colour, with all the trims
and extra sprinkles.

I'm here for the wild life, the every-moment life
Every day here. Every second
A possibility for more.

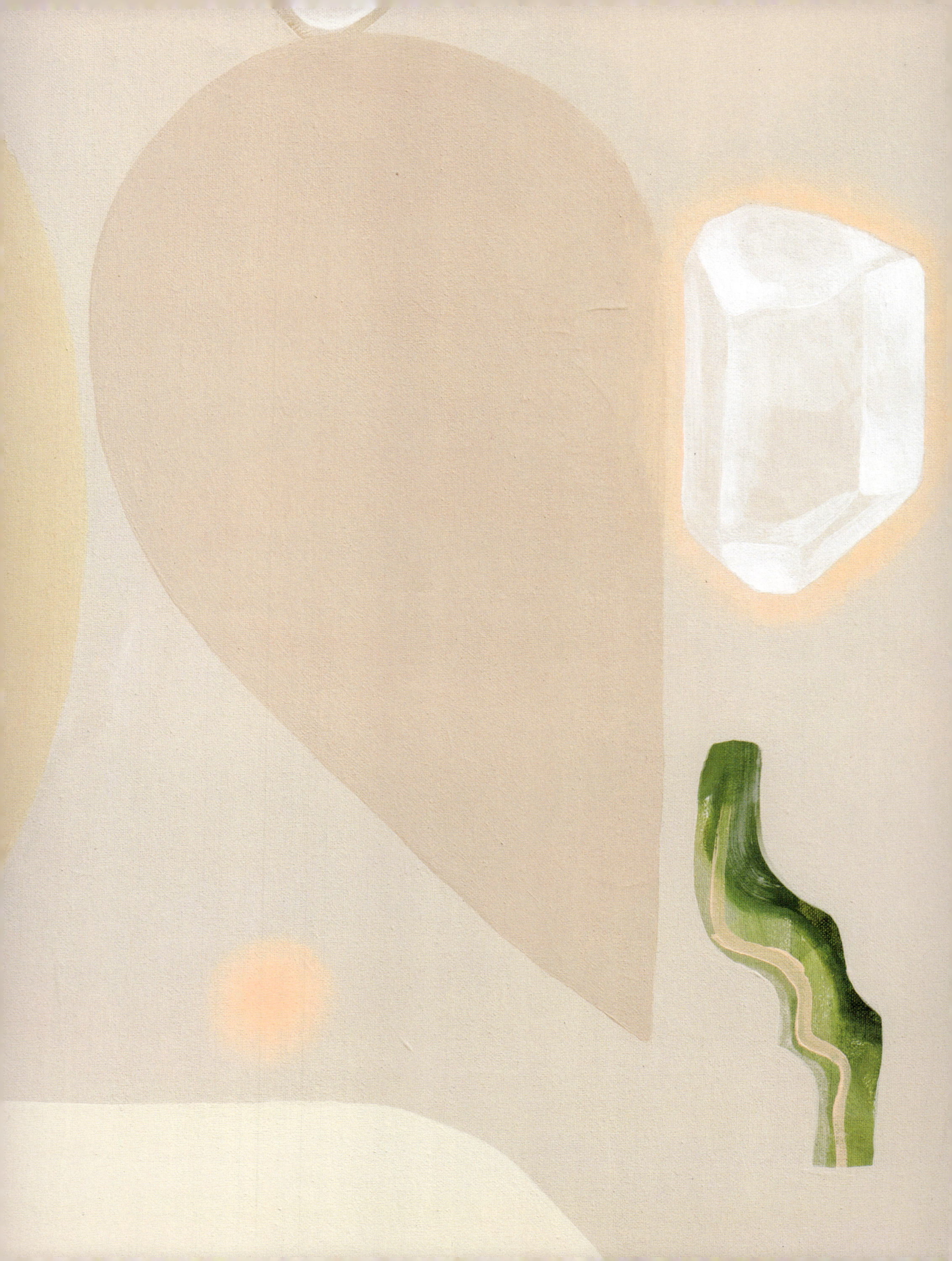

CONTENTS

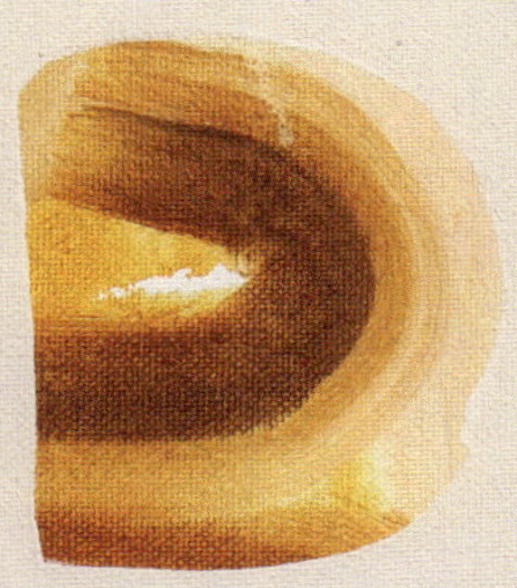

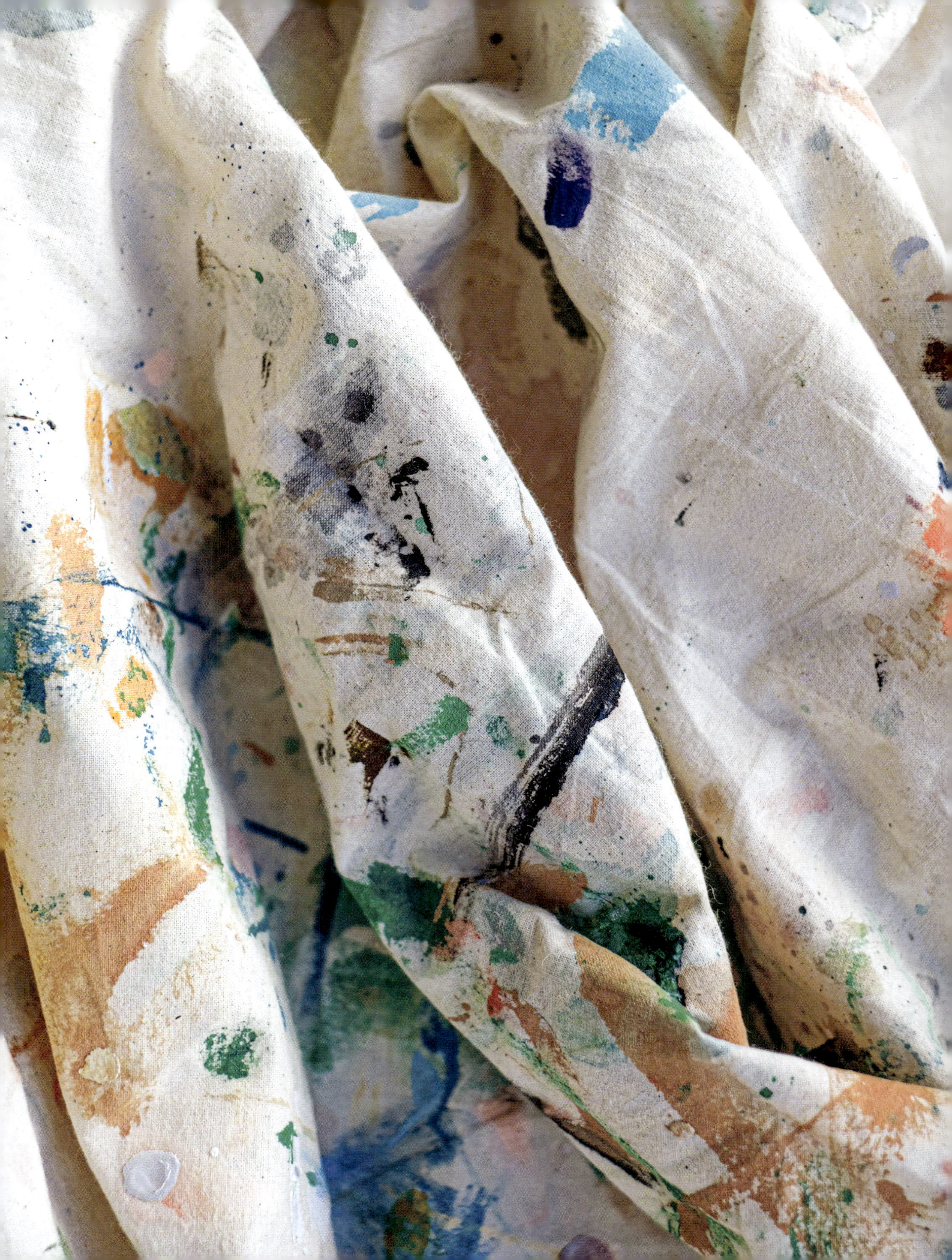

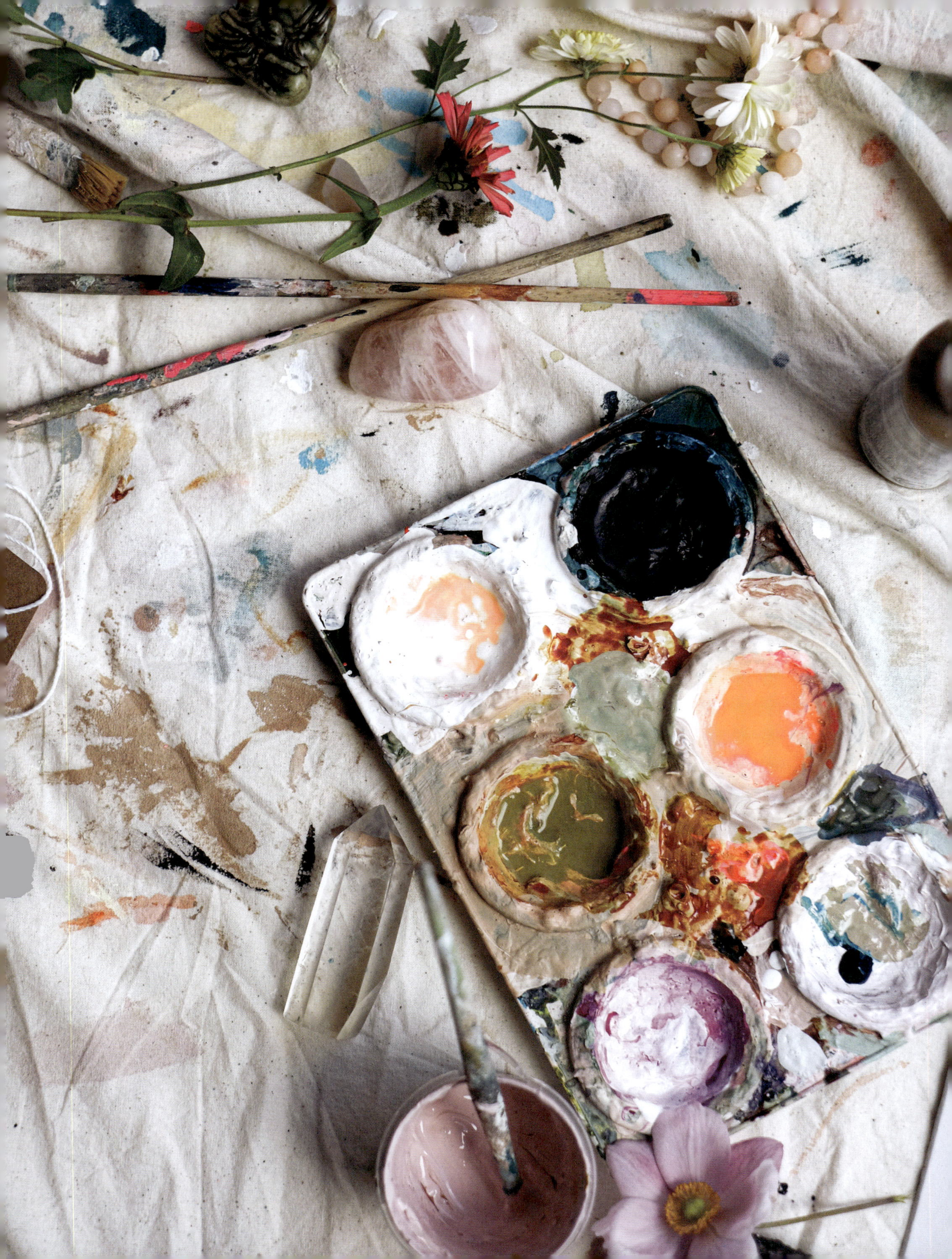

Welcome

I've heard it said that our natural human state is joy. That underneath all our worry, conditioning, to-do lists and real and imagined responsibilities we pile on top of ourselves, we do, in fact, have joy at our essence. And I believe this. I believe that each one of us, at our essence, is joyful.

In childhood, this joy is obvious: it's right there on the surface – easily accessible to us in any moment. As we grow, though, too many of us become disconnected from our sense of self, and consequently, our joyful essence. One by one, we set aside the interests, hobbies, friendships and activities that bring us happiness in the pursuit of reaching those adult milestones. Without meaning to, we resign ourselves to living an average life, only to wake up one day and realise that the mundane has devoured all of the magic, leaving us feeling hollow and bored.

This is a tragedy because we haven't been put in this world to just 'get by'; we are here to experience everything that life has to offer: the good, the bad and the juicy. It's true that life is filled with daily inconveniences and tough challenges, but it's also bursting with beauty and joy. For me, the art of joy is accepting that life is filled with equal parts incredible beauty and unbearable pain, and learning to hold both.

The art of joy is the process of peeling back those heavy layers and engaging in the world in a way that brings us back to the present and continuous flow of joy that moves inside us. By opening ourselves to more moments of curiosity, happiness, connection, and wonder again, we can realise our potential and begin to walk a bigger, more meaningful path.

I like to start every big project with an intention, and this book is no different. Here, my intention is to ignite a spark that helps you tune into those moments of wonder, delight and happiness. I hope the tips, suggestions and practices here will allow you to reconnect with the deep sense of joy you (hopefully) knew as a child. This isn't a book that will solve all your problems, but I do hope it will help put some of those problems in perspective, and give you the tools to tackle them more easily.

In the spring of 2015, during a challenging time in my life, joy called to me in a quiet moment and I listened. I had no idea that following that thread of curiosity would lead me to an entirely new career and life, but it did. I gave in to my child-like self that afternoon, and continued to nurture that side of me in the months and years that followed. Today it's in full bloom, and my life is full of creativity and connection, and, as a result of that, joy.

Jen xx

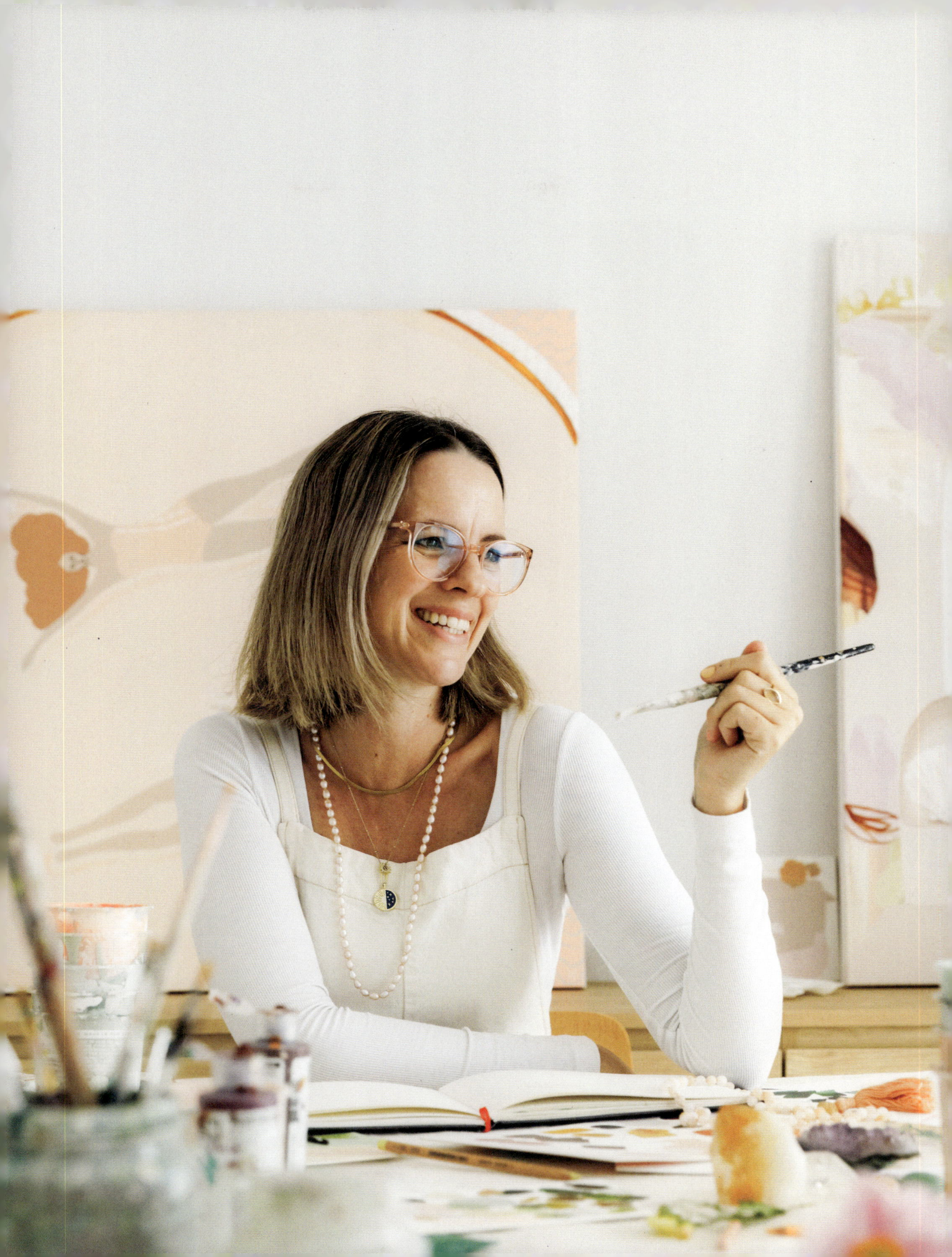

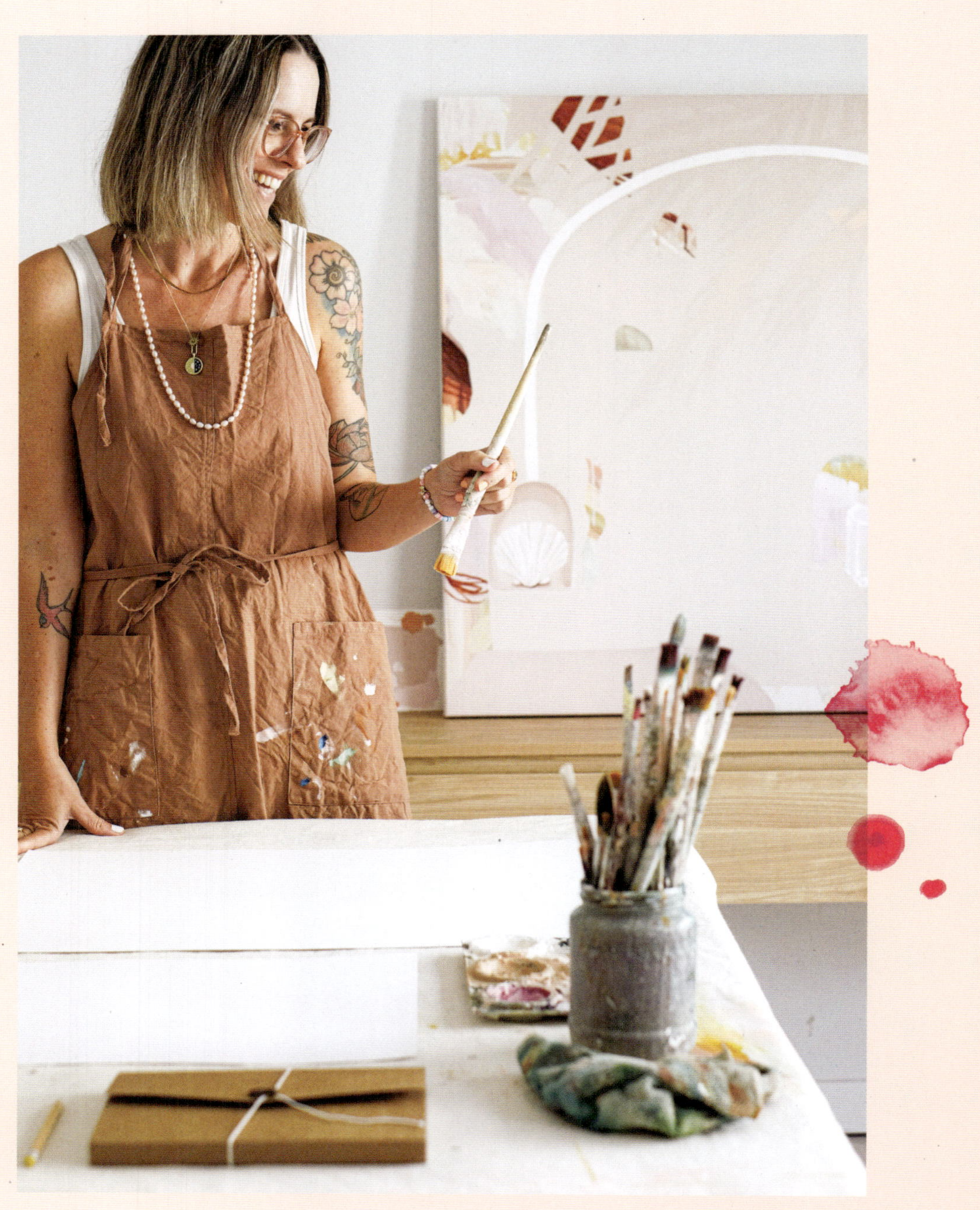

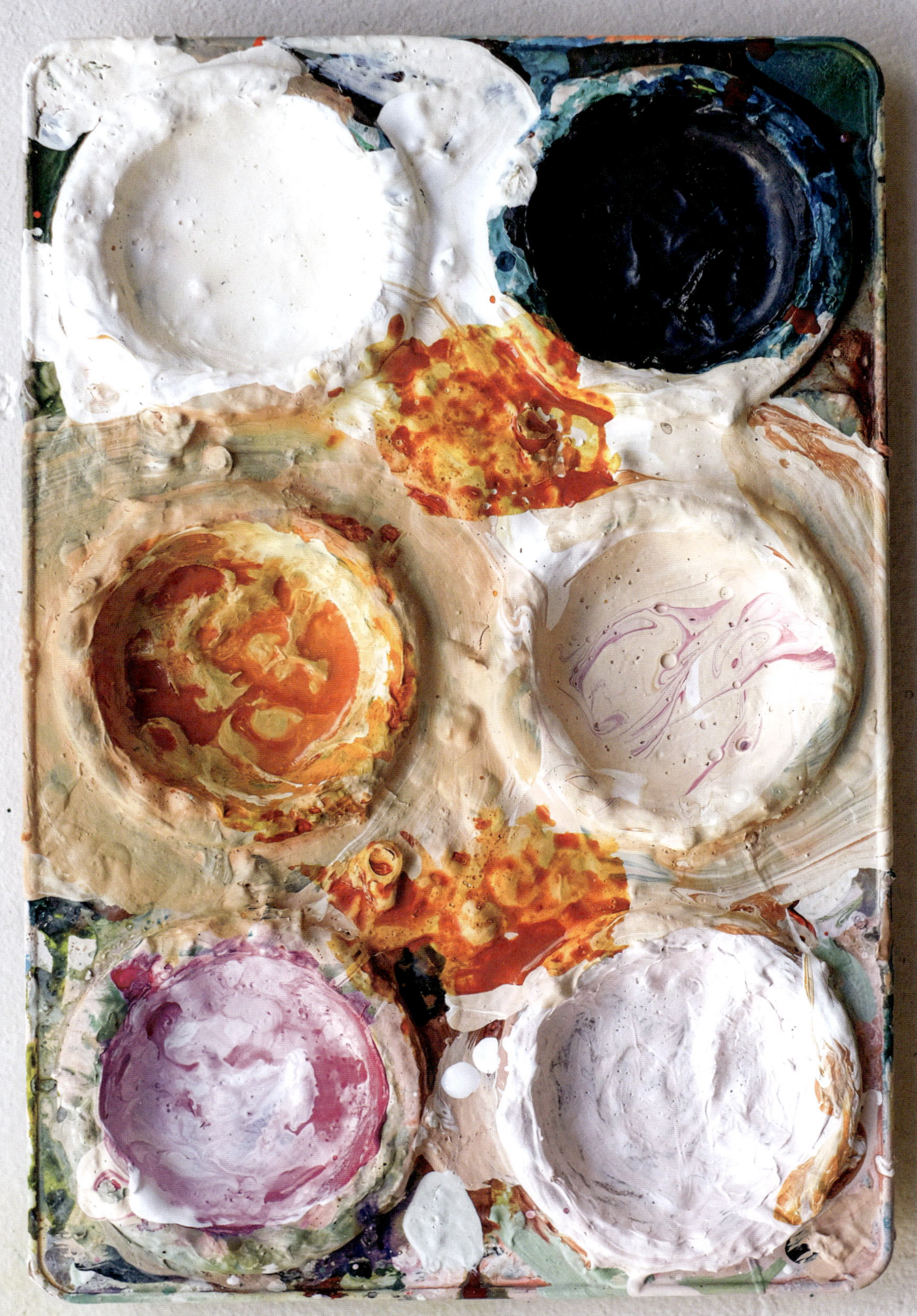

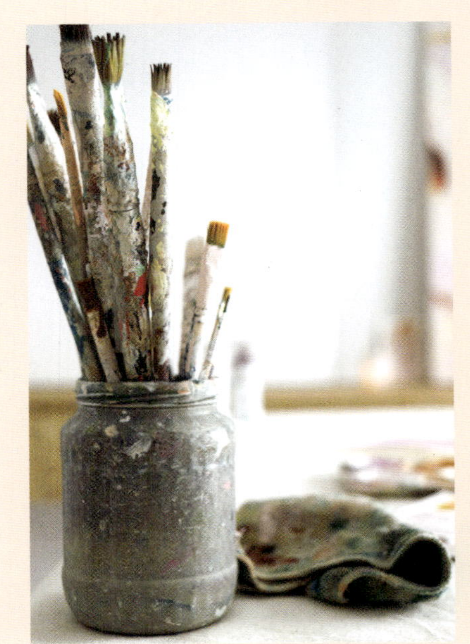

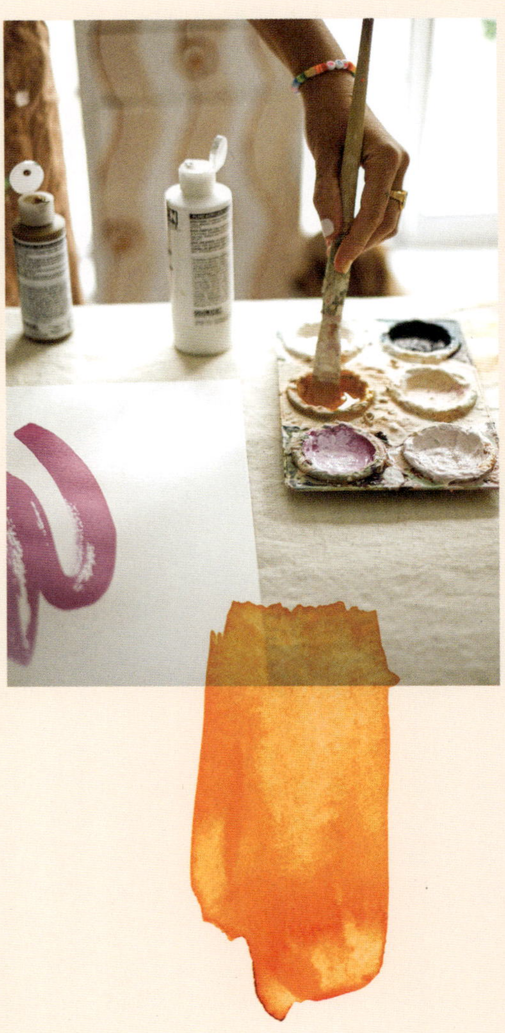

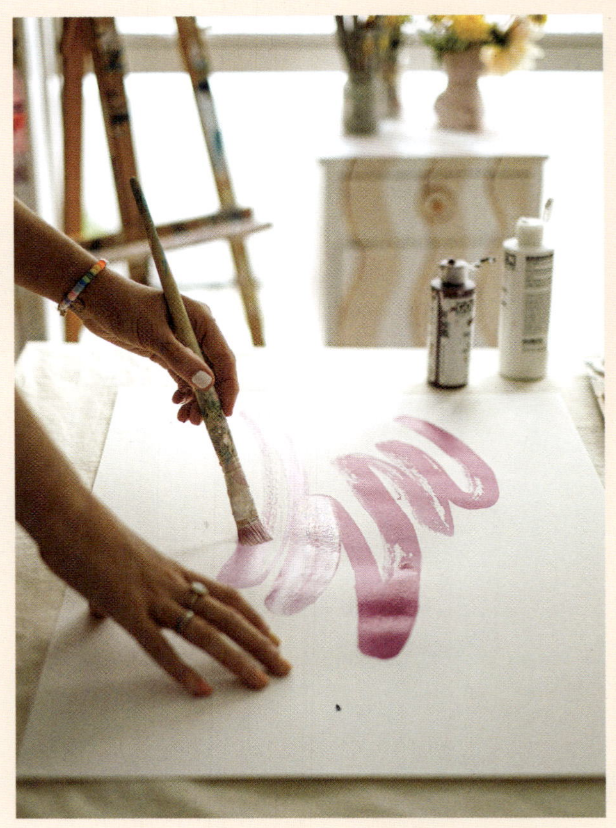

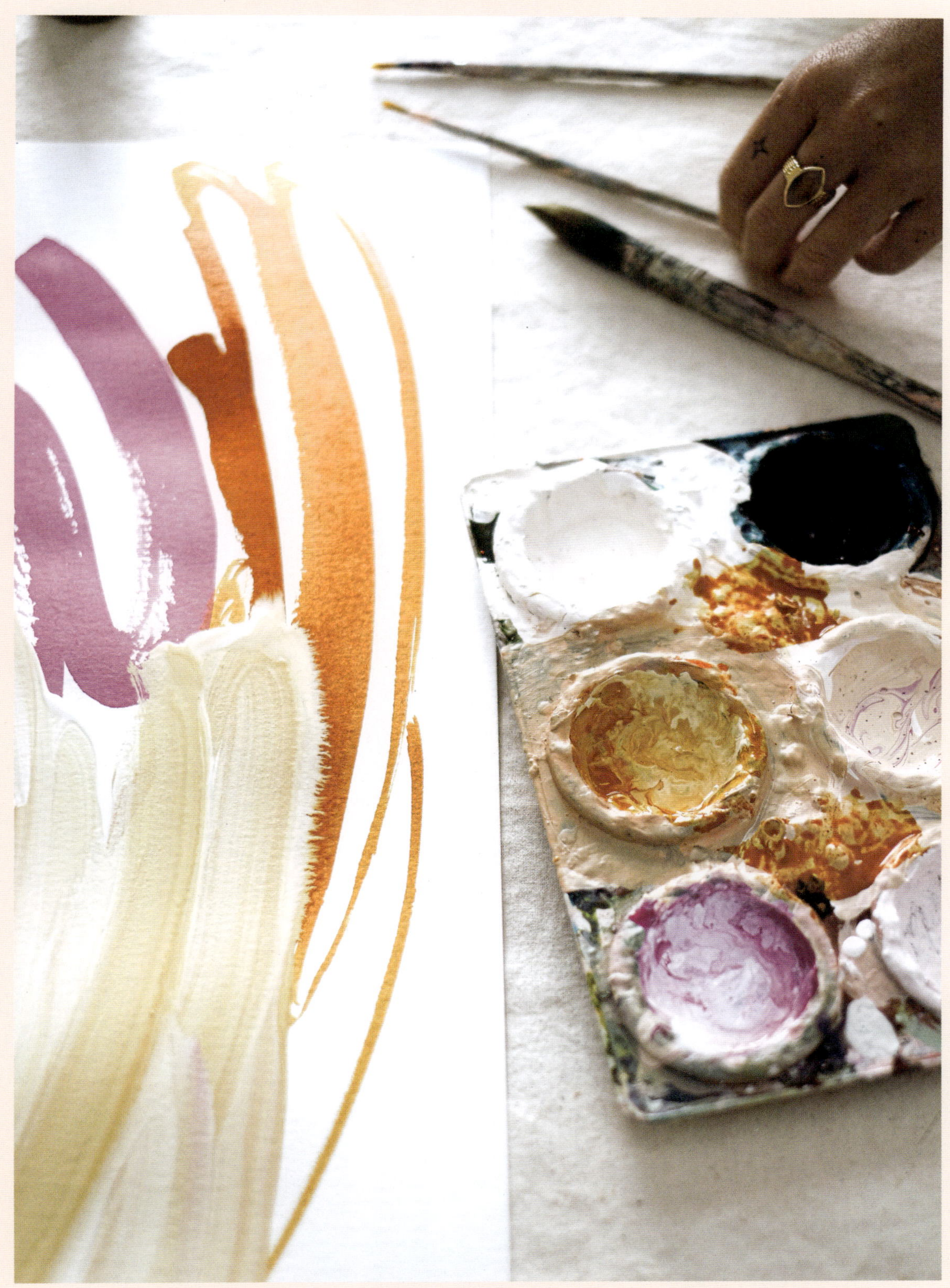

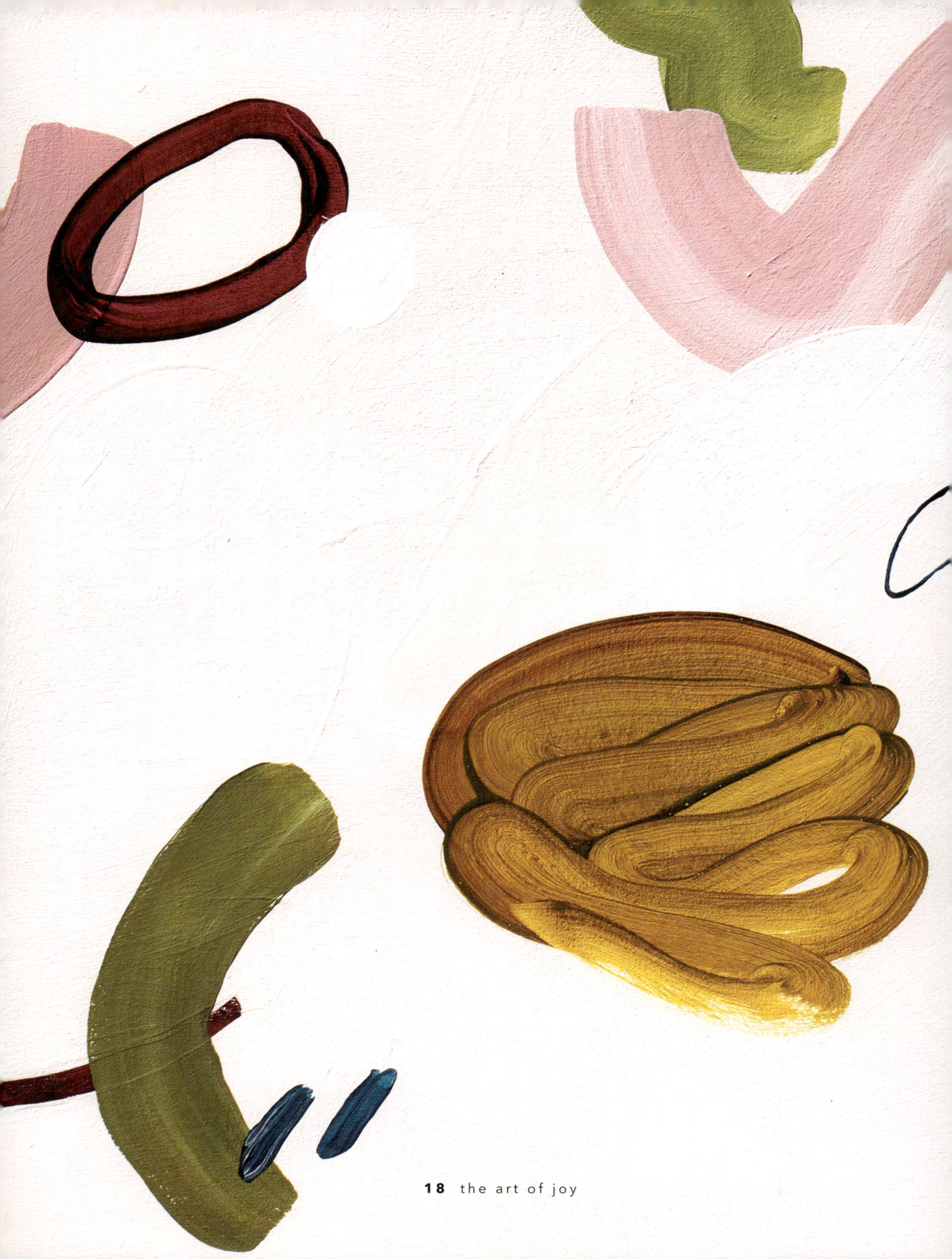

chapter one

Joy: What Is It?

First, let's make sure we are on the same page.

Have you ever stopped to think about joy? What is it, really? And how do you know if you're feeling it or experiencing it? If we're going to go on this adventure together, it's a good idea to agree on what we're seeking, and where we're heading.

Joy isn't about feeling happy every minute of the day. It's deeper and more sustainable than that; it's an ever-present internal reservoir to draw from. It's a quiet, powerful pulse deep in your chest.

Joy is cultivated by aligning with your true self, nurturing your spirit, and consistently making choices that grow your inner sense of presence and contentment. It feels like ease and authenticity – a reliable source of strength, no matter what's happening externally.

Happiness, in contrast, is fleeting and tied to specific moments or achievements. It comes quickly, but can vanish just as fast. Sometimes happiness and joy intertwine and appear together, amplifying one another. In these moments, the brightness of happiness meets the steady strength of joy, creating an experience that's both vibrant and deeply nourishing.

When you engage in practices that fuel joy, you're building a foundation that supports you through life's ups and downs with resilience and grace. But too often, we miss the opportunities to tap into joy that are right in front of us. There is wonder at every corner, hiding in plain sight, and this book has been written to help you find it.

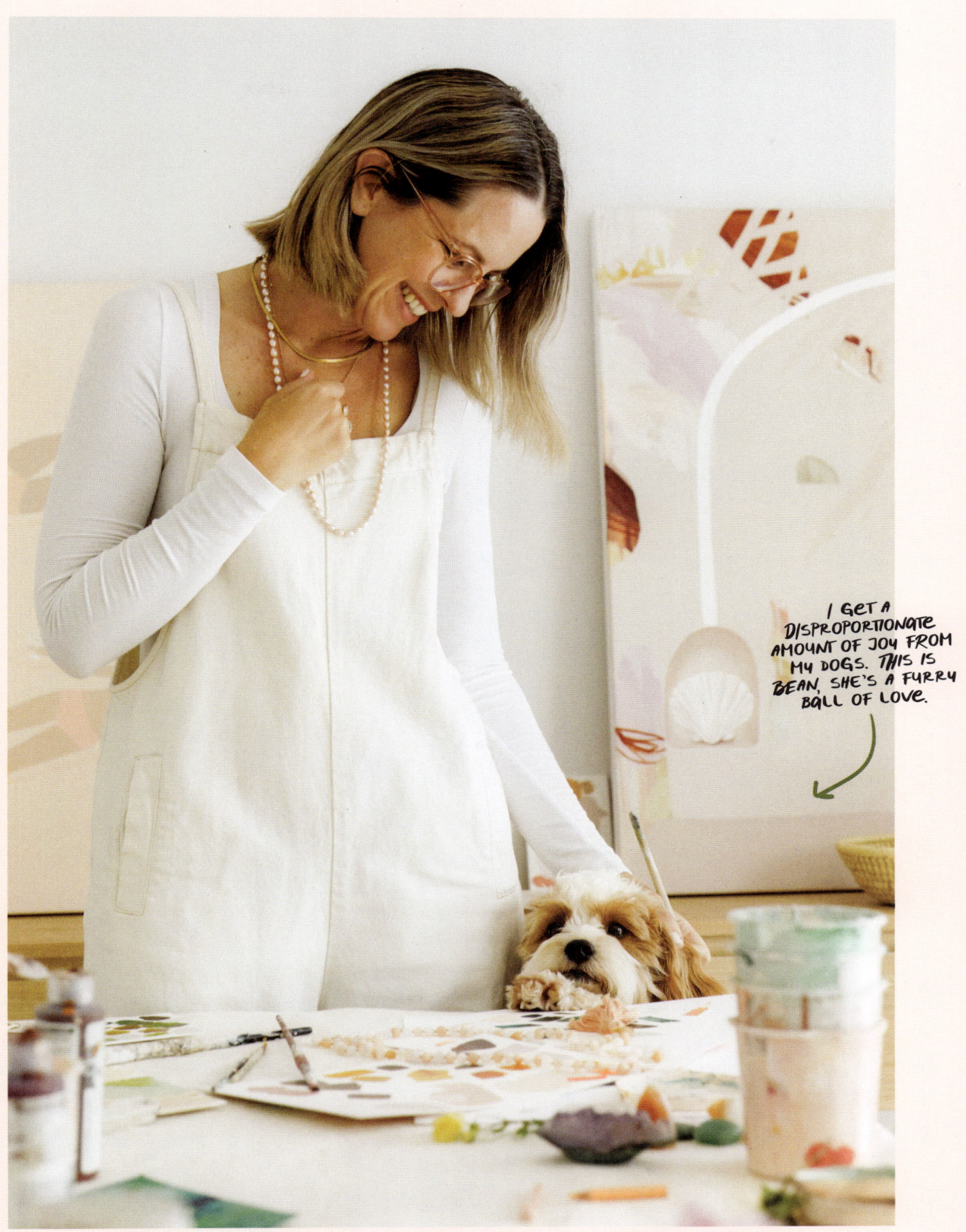
I GET A DISPROPORTIONATE AMOUNT OF JOY FROM MY DOGS. THIS IS BEAN, SHE'S A FURRY BALL OF LOVE.

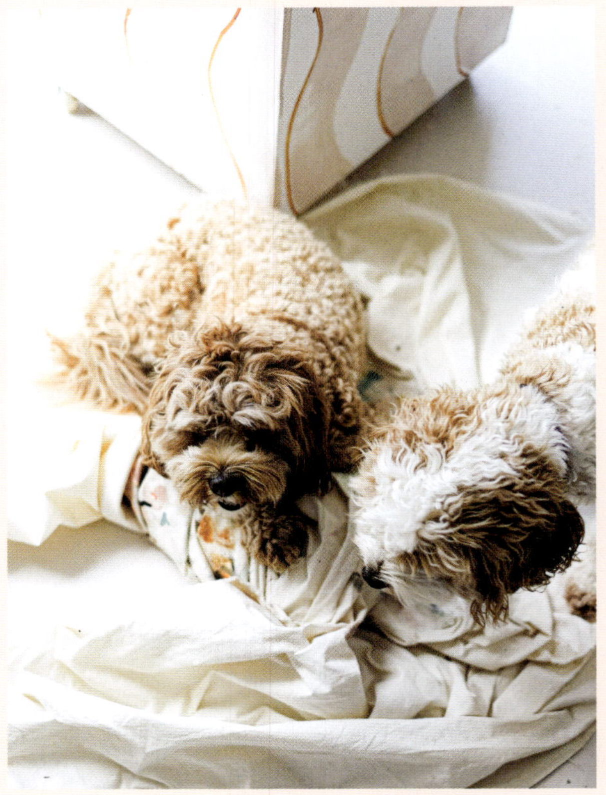

FIND JOY IN TINY MOMENTS - LIKE PEACHES AND BEAN MAKING A NEST ON A DROP SHEET.

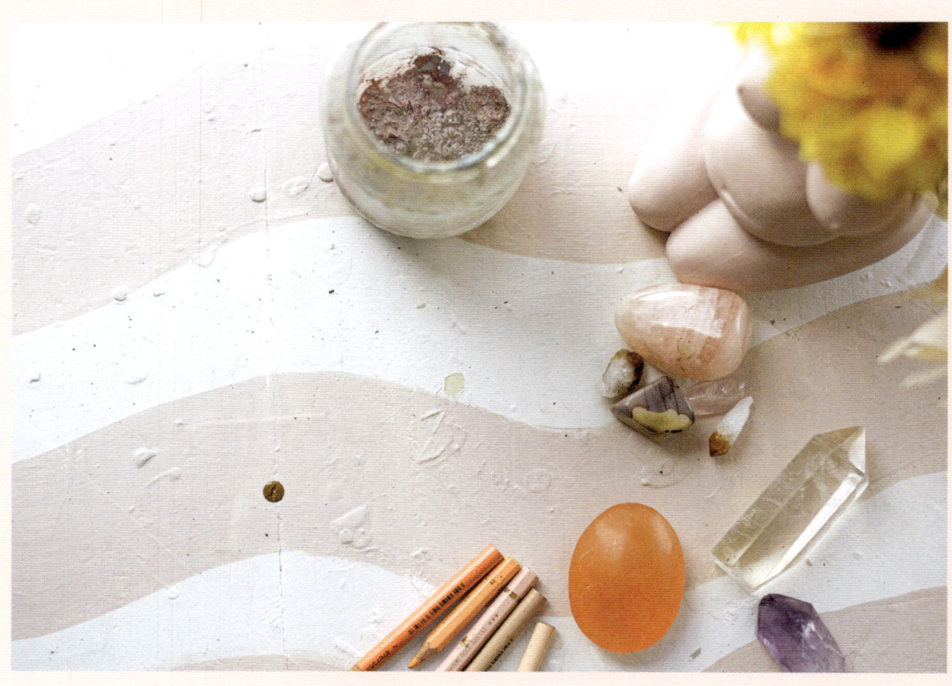

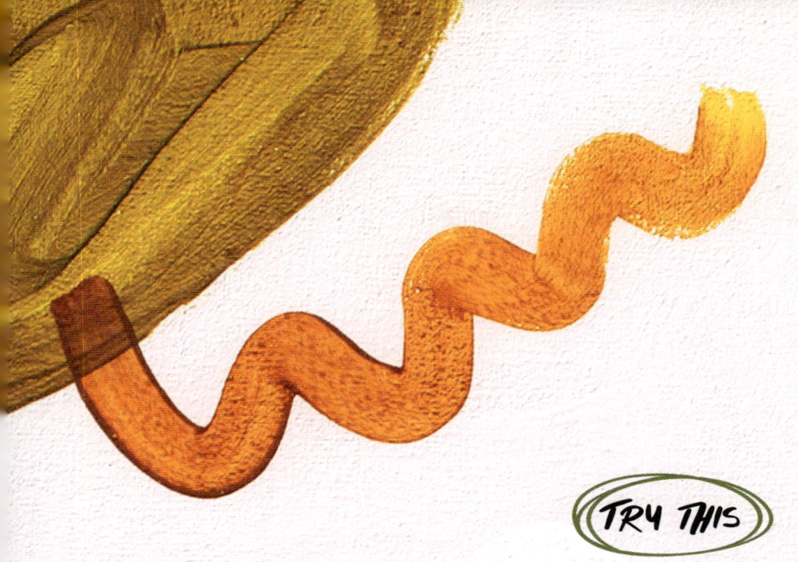

TRY THIS

Joy feels like ...

Sit quietly for a few seconds, close your eyes if you like, and recall a moment from your life that fills you with a sense of joy.

I'm imagining Bean, one of my cavoodles, first thing in the morning when she realises we're both awake, alive and in the same place. Her little tail (actually, her entire body) starts wagging as she plods up the bed towards me before plastering my face and ears with her slobbery kisses. I laugh, trying hard not to let her actually lick my face, and snuggle into her warm fur.

Imagine your moment, and don't feel bad if it doesn't involve your child or partner – no guilt allowed. It can be frivolous, life-changing or anything in between. While you bask in the feelings it brings up for you, notice where it lights up in your body. What type of physical sensations does it spark?

For me, it shows up as a warmth around my solar plexus, belly and chest. This leads to a sense of openheartedness that makes the world feel expansive, accepting and benevolent. It feels like a warm hug from within. Whatever sensations arise in you, that is the feeling you are seeking throughout this process. That state of joy – however it shows up for you – is the destination.

To better understand this feeling of joy, it might be helpful to contrast it with a memory at the opposite end of the spectrum. Picture a moment of fear, anger, or shame, and notice how that sparks sensations of contracting, coldness, feeling uncomfortable or prickly, as if the world is not a safe and welcoming place. Recognising this contrast helps to highlight the warmth and ease of joy even more clearly.

Big joy and little joys

We might assume that the state of joy always accompanies a colossal glitter bomb of good news and excitement. As a culture, we default to linking the experience of joy to life's big moments: the birth of a child, a wedding, a festival, or a memorable trip. But this view of joy is limiting because it can be found in so many small moments, too. The surest way to experience more of it is to actively choose and practise an openness to finding it.

Expanding our definition of joy to include quieter moments found in our seemingly dull day-to-day lives creates a much more enriching, juicy, joy-filled life. I find it helps to divide the broader concept of JOY into Big Joy and Little Joys. If we rely on only Big Joy to fill our joy bucket, it's limited to special occasions and remarkable days and we are more likely to believe that the ordinary is just that – ordinary! My life changed dramatically for the better after embracing the many Little Joys embedded in my days rather than waiting around for the big ones. Most of us are already good at noticing the Big Joy moments, so instead, we're going to focus on improving the skills to detect and nourish the smaller ones.

Just like an art practice, the process of training our brains to notice these moments when they occur takes consistent effort. The word 'effort' probably makes this process sound complicated and unpleasant, but, like painting, practising joy is incredibly enjoyable! Each tiny step that builds your practice is a joy in itself, so you're winning all the way.

I can pinpoint the rather unremarkable moment that I learned this lesson. I was 16, and had spent months in the throes of a teenage angst-fest. Most of my days were spent feeling misunderstood and churning out an endless stream of long-winded, awful poetry. Happiness, joy, and connection seemed like something other people felt.

But then my twin brother said something in passing one afternoon that changed my perspective. While shopping, he mentioned how easy it was to make other people smile (my

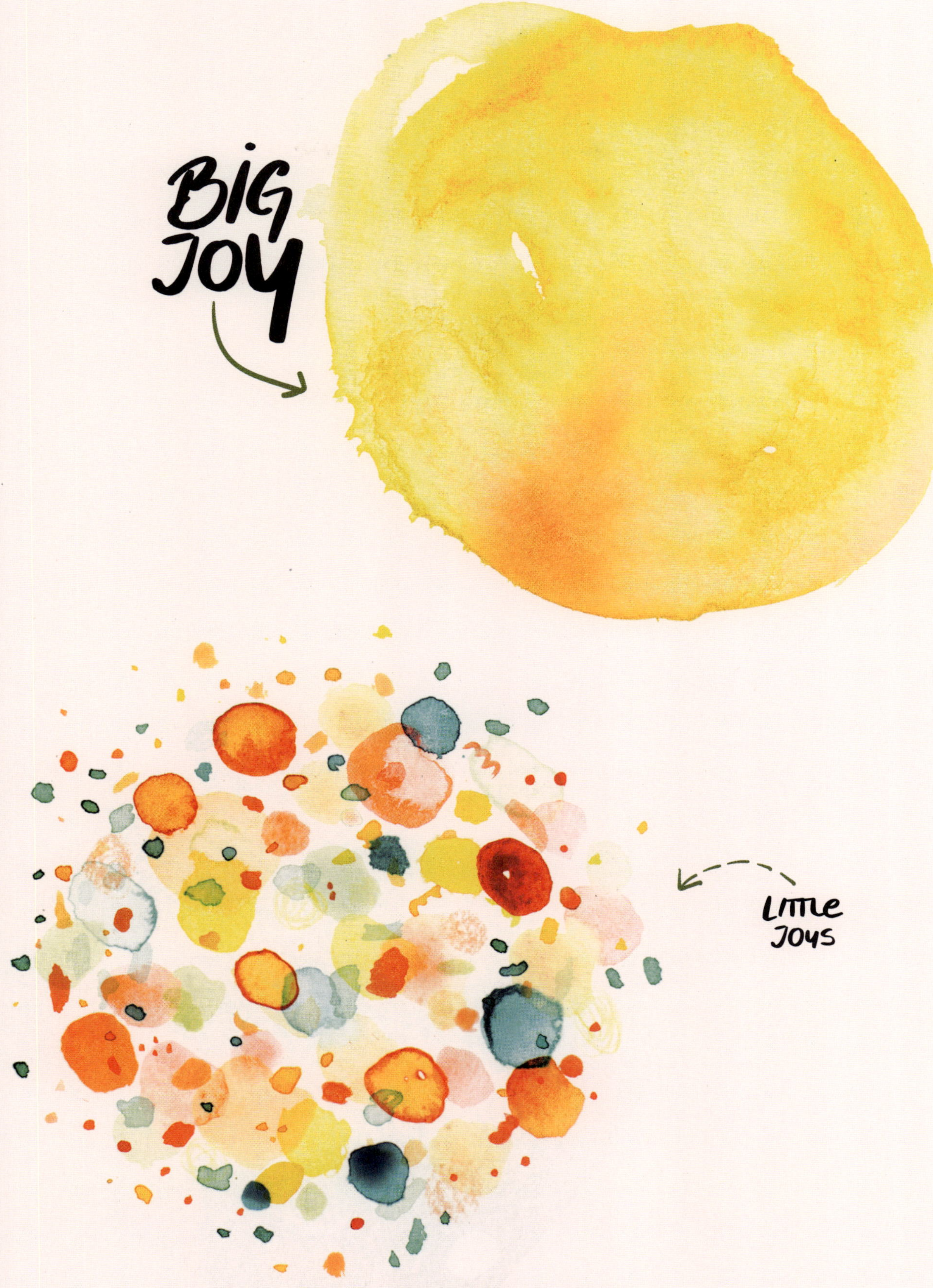
BIG JOY
LITTLE JOYS

brother is very funny). The lady working the checkout seemed disinterested and a bit down, so he said something funny, and immediately, her face lit up. This small, seemingly insignificant moment stuck with me because I experienced on a cellular level the lesson that happiness is a choice, and that being kind to another person is one of the quickest ways to access that happiness yourself.

Since then, my life has been a joyfest. That's not to say I've been continually happy – I haven't. Like everyone, I've been through awful situations that have knocked me, quite hard, off my joy train. One of the most painful was the sudden death of my sister in a car accident when we were both in our thirties – something I would never wish on anyone. Then, a few years later I was diagnosed with breast cancer, and not long after that I left my marriage. You'll read later that each of these events – although devastating at the time – held their own blessings.

All feelings should be felt

All feelings – joy and pain – are important, and glossing over hard emotions to remain joyful isn't healthy. Instead, I strive to find, experience and pour out as much joy as possible in my day-to-day life, regardless of whether those days are average, awful or beautiful. If I'm stuck in traffic, washing the dishes or dealing with difficult people, I can generally preserve my sense of joy. I carry it with me, and if I go within myself, I can access it most of the time. With time and practice I've learned how (mostly) not to get unnecessarily tangled up in all the extra drama that we constantly search for. I want to help you do the same.

I once read that joy doesn't have to make sense. If it comes at you – feel it. Don't spend energy investigating why you're feeling it. That process will likely just kill the feeling completely. I wish I could remember where I read this or who wrote it, because it's great advice. So my suggestion for you today is to accept that joy can just come out of nowhere. Step one to experiencing more joy, is to allow it in whenever and however it comes your way. Don't question. Don't overthink. Just go with it.

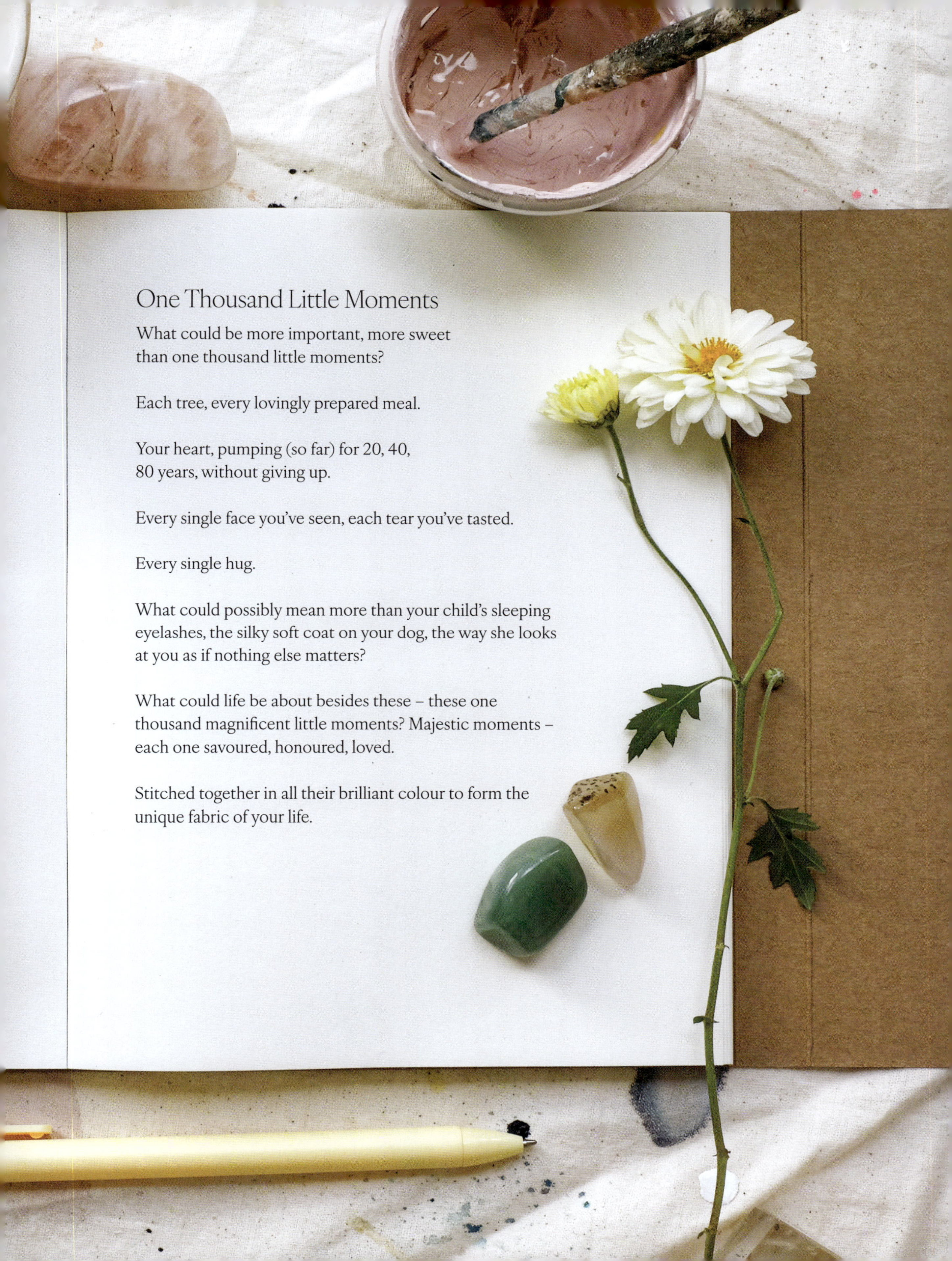

One Thousand Little Moments

What could be more important, more sweet
than one thousand little moments?

Each tree, every lovingly prepared meal.

Your heart, pumping (so far) for 20, 40,
80 years, without giving up.

Every single face you've seen, each tear you've tasted.

Every single hug.

What could possibly mean more than your child's sleeping
eyelashes, the silky soft coat on your dog, the way she looks
at you as if nothing else matters?

What could life be about besides these – these one
thousand magnificent little moments? Majestic moments –
each one savoured, honoured, loved.

Stitched together in all their brilliant colour to form the
unique fabric of your life.

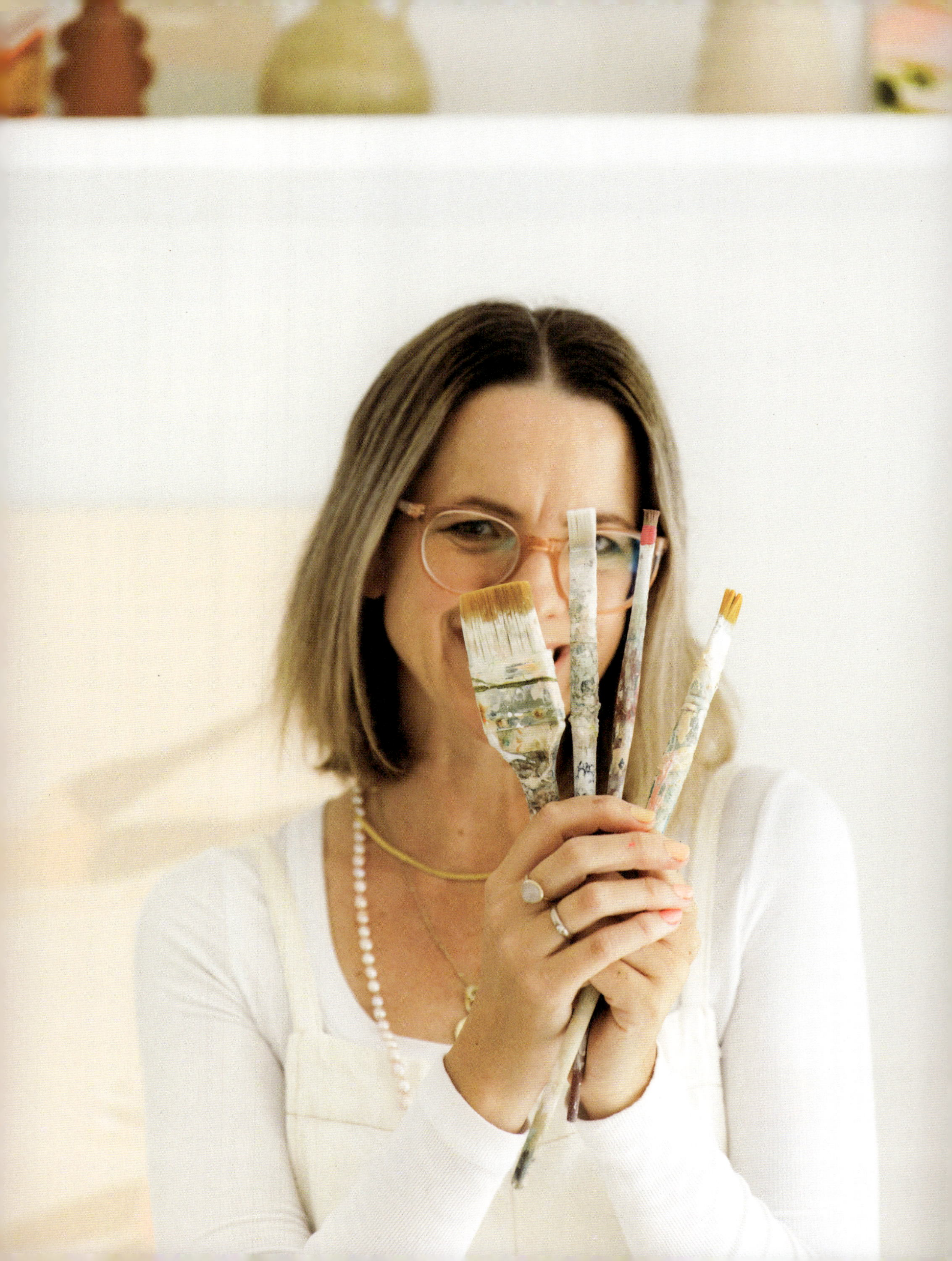

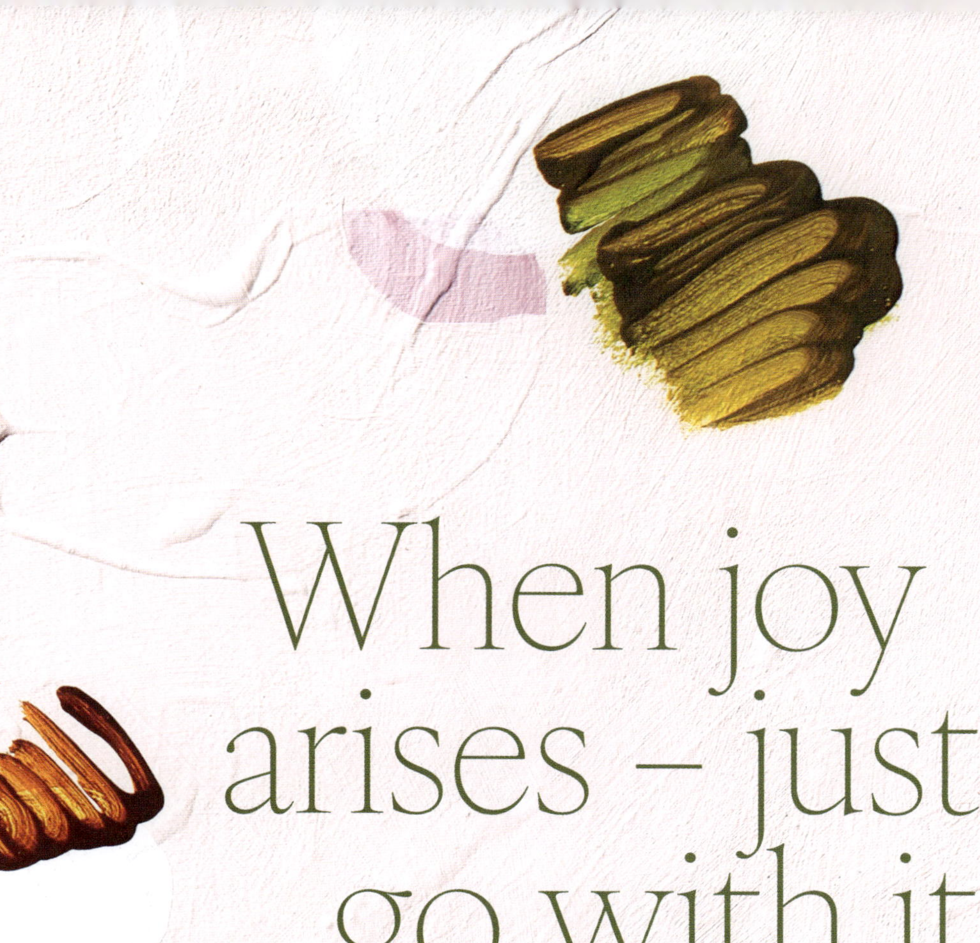

When joy arises – just go with it; it doesn't need a reason.

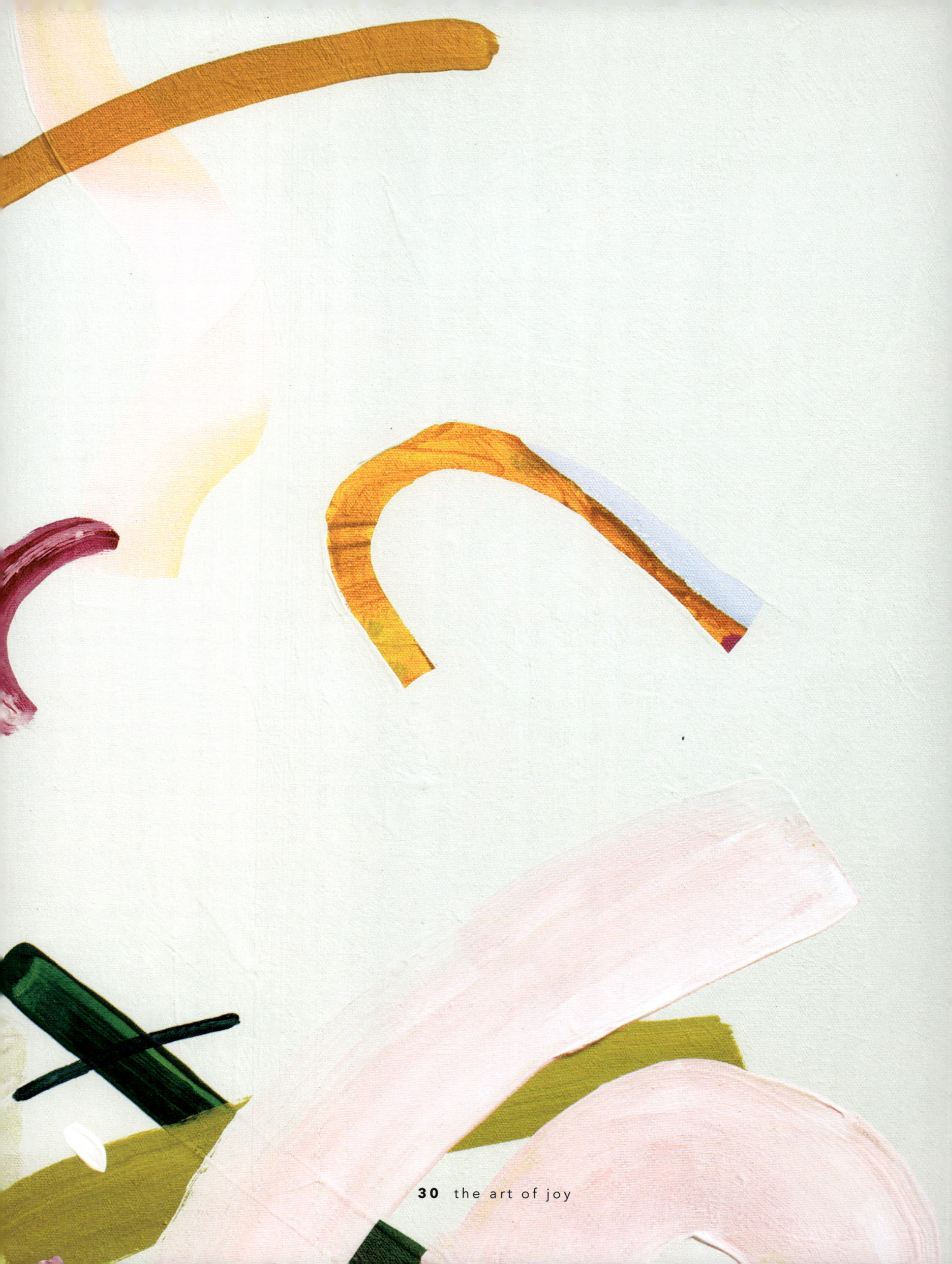

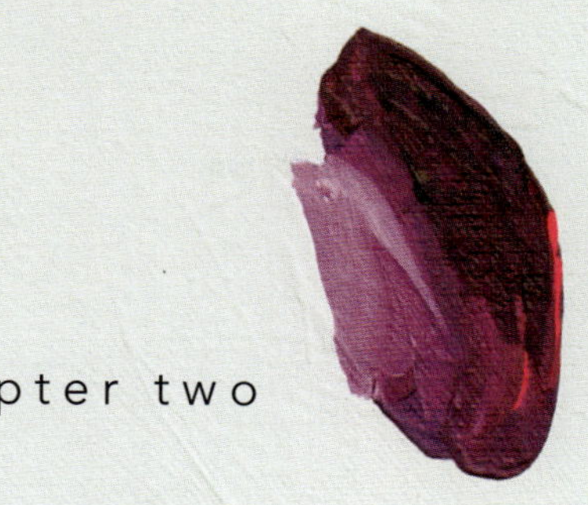

chapter two

A More Joyful Path

Tools to help you tap into meaning and purpose in your life.

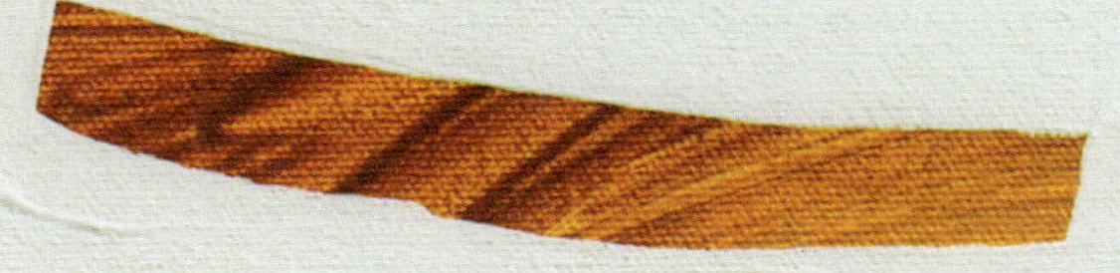

We are all born with something special in us, or rather, many extraordinary things! We contain multitudes of treasures to enrich our own lives and share with the world. Somehow, these pieces of treasure are often buried along the way. They're hidden under expectations, limiting beliefs, practicalities and difficulties. Our role in this game is to find the treasure. And please don't think that you're the one and only person on this planet who was born without them. We *all* have them. If you don't think you're included in this, it just means they're buried a little deeper. What if your life were an internal treasure hunt? How would you go about finding your unique gifts, abilities and quirks?

The first thing to do is to connect with what brings you joy. Luckily, if you've been trying out any of the practices in this book, you might be realising what your joy triggers are. I believe that the universe uses joy as a signpost to our purpose. Isn't that a wonderful thought?

Purpose often hides in our interests

Things don't always add up immediately. For example, your love for forest walks might not feel purposeful right away, but taking more walks in nature could incite new thoughts or ideas that eventually lead towards purpose. In her excellent book about creativity, *Big Magic*, writer Elizabeth Gilbert (of *Eat, Pray, Love* fame) writes about using curiosity as a method to find your way to a fuller, more creative life. Curiosity feels easier than purpose, and it's a stepping stone towards it. If you notice yourself thinking, *What if …* or *I wonder why …* lean in a little closer and explore that thought. There might be something in it. Curiosity, like joy, is a marker on the path to your most authentic life.

Don't question why you're suddenly curious about how slime mould could engineer the network of the Japanese subway system in a fraction of the time of actual human engineers. If you have a strange and exciting curiosity, follow it. Read about it, or go down a YouTube or podcast rabbit hole. You never know where it might lead. That's how I started painting again and how I came to write this book.

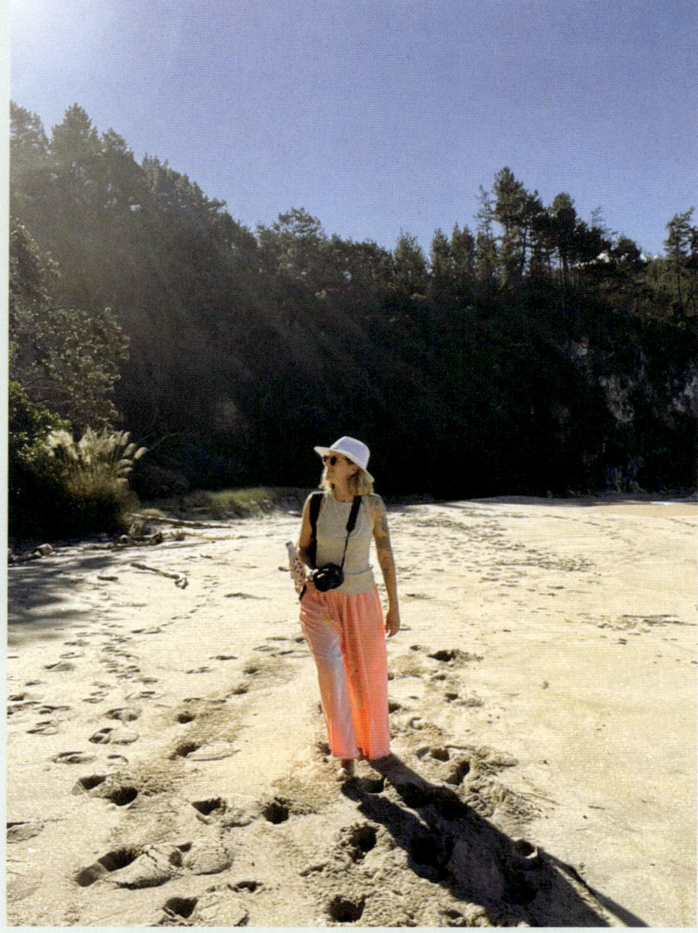

CONNECTING TO INSPIRATION IS EASIER IN THE MAGIC OF NATURE.

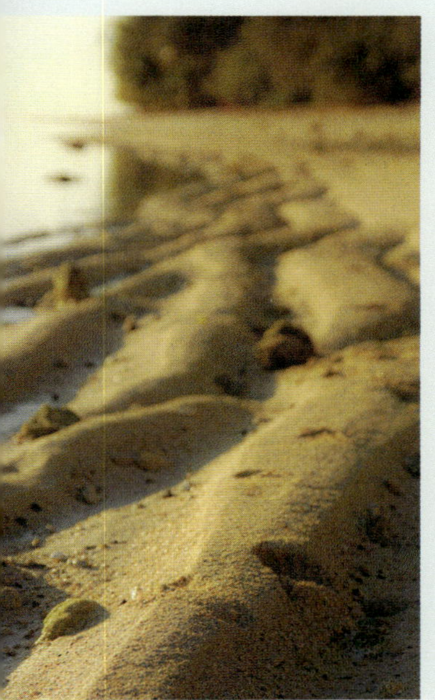

Intuition is a doorway to a juicier life

Before writing this chapter, I went for a walk. At the start of it, I had a quick internal conversation with the Universe or 'Love' (more about this on page 100), asking it to send me the inspiration or information I'd need to sit down and write. While walking, I pictured light or energy flowing into my body as I breathed in, and my energy field expanding as I breathed out. Standard Sunday morning walk stuff. It may sound a little strange, but I see my intuition – my connection to wisdom – as one of the most essential tools in my creative toolkit.

I first explored the idea of creative intuition while reading *Big Magic*. In it, Liz Gilbert writes about how she believes creative inspiration comes from somewhere outside of us: from a larger consciousness that we can tune into and receive.

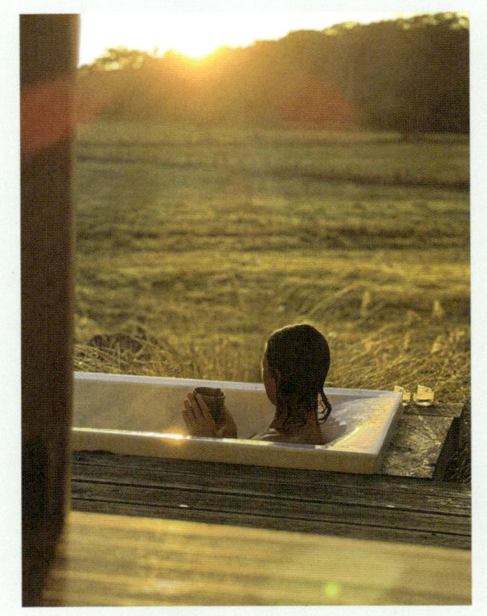

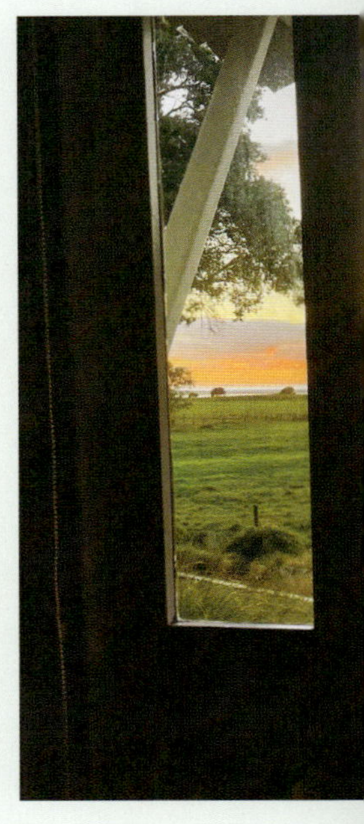

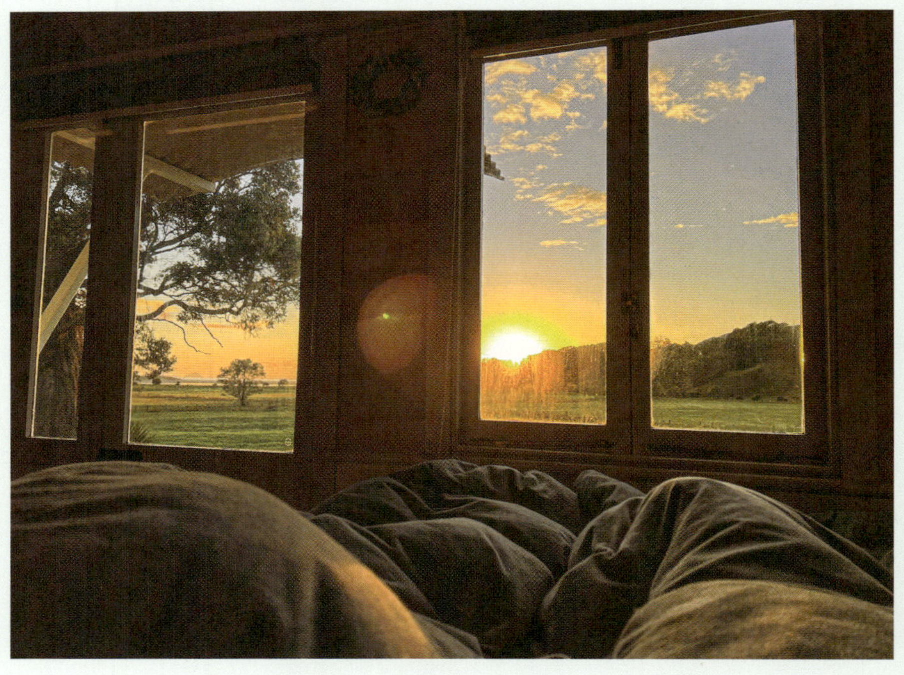

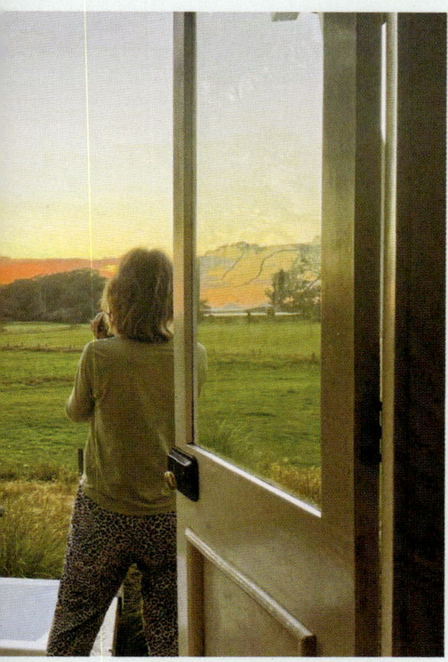

GETTING OUT OF THE CITY, BEING SOMEWHERE QUIET, LEAVES SPACE FOR INSPIRATION.

For centuries, creatives have referenced the idea of the muse – an external force (or forces) that sends ideas to be expressed in the world via humans. For the ancient Greeks, these heavenly muses usually took the form of beautiful women who'd whisper ideas into the ears of musicians, writers, artists and scientists.

Anyone involved in consistent creative practice who stops to think about and notice it, would probably agree that there's something in this idea. Maybe not the otherworldly beautiful women part – but the whispers. If you learn to tune into your intuition, it becomes very clear and easy to recognise an intuitive 'hit'. And when you do, it opens up a world of excitement and possibility you couldn't access before.

Imagine that there are millions of ideas out there floating around, trying to find the right person to birth them. They look around for people who seem motivated, excitable, and with the correct life experience to execute them – then they arrive in their minds as if out of nowhere. If the creative mind receiving the idea tunes into it, it will often act with urgency to start executing the idea. If the idea is ignored or started and then forgotten, it packs up and moves on to the next suitable candidate.

Intuitive ideas often present as curiosity, often in something you've never considered. Follow the breadcrumbs of curiosity to see where they take you. I get these hits quite regularly with my art. Sometimes, they're little hunches about what step to take next in a painting or what scene to paint. Other times, they literally land in my brain as a fully baked idea. Steaming hot and wrapped up in a pretty ribbon, ready to go. Those are the best, but often the scariest kind – because I feel compelled to take them seriously.

The idea for this book came to me as an intuitive hit one Saturday night while watching a documentary. It tumbled into my brain as a vision of me stepping into a spotlight to do a public talk. Then, moments later, the theme of the talk popped

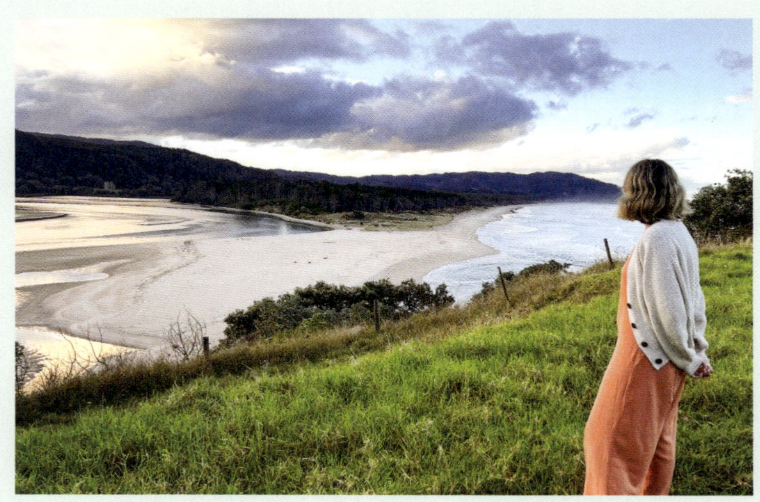

into my head, followed by the book I was going to write to get to that point. It unfolded in seconds, all in reverse. I felt the importance of the message and quickly wrote some notes into my phone – chapter headings that formed the basis of a book. Granted, it's been quite some time, and the idea has evolved, but that spark is what put me on this path. It was the catalyst I needed to get me going.

In *Big Magic*, Liz writes about a poet, Ruth Stone. When Ruth was growing up in rural Virginia, she'd often be out working in the fields when inspiration would suddenly sweep towards her out of nowhere. She described this as a poem surging toward her across the landscape – roaring like a powerful, unstoppable wind. It was so strong she could feel it vibrating the earth beneath her feet. When that happened, she knew there was only one thing to do: run! She'd sprint as fast as she could back to her house, chased by this invisible force, hoping desperately to reach pencil and paper in time. If she was quick enough, she'd catch the poem, capturing its magic onto the page.

This idea about creativity doesn't give us a free ride or a ticket out of the slog of the creative process. Intuitive ideas seem to flock to those who can be trusted to bring them to life. The hard-working, curious types who want to see what happens if they listen to the call. I'm speaking about this from a creative point of view because this makes the most sense to my own life and experience. But I'm certain that it applies to all aspects of life. Tuning in to intuitive information can enrich anything, from parenting to running a small business or being a high-powered chief executive.

How to recognise intuition

I've learned to notice the difference in feeling and tone between my own thoughts and ideas that have come from somewhere bigger. A few things that make intuitive hits stand out for me:

1

They sound louder in my mind than my regular thoughts, and often feel more urgent.

2

They often seem a bit random and leave me with a sense of 'Where did that come from?'

3

They arrive fully formed or close to it, and there's a feeling of having to capture them as they come into my mind.

4

I notice shivers, tingles, excitement, or a physical gut feeling.

5

Occasionally, they hang around, replaying in my mind like a catchy pop song that won't go away.

6

Sometimes they're linked to synchronicities or coincidences as an extra nod to their importance.

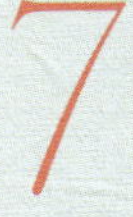

7

They come from a place of excitement and joy – a high energy rather than a low or fearful one.

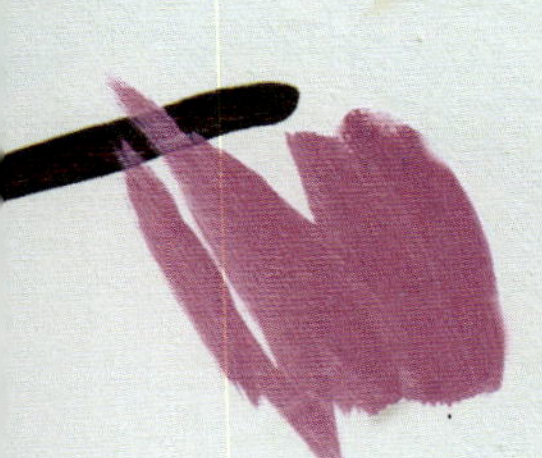

Tapping into your intuition

Knowing how to tune into that inner wisdom will set you on your way to a fulfilling life aligned with your purpose. Learning how to tune in is easier than you might think, and there are many ways we can strenghten this ability so it becomes more natural.

The best way to become aware of what intuition is trying to say is to quiet your mind regularly. On this page, I'm sharing a simple body-based technique, but there are several other approaches, including breathwork, journalling, meditating, or even just walking that are also great for this. Use your intuition to pick which method to explore. Which one feels right in your body when you read the options?

The aim is to take time out from trying to solve problems, and become aware of the stream of thoughts that flow through your mind (more on this in chapter eight). Becoming aware of your own internal chatter helps you to realise when the message comes through in a different tone, and when it doesn't feel like an everyday thought. Open yourself to messages that stand out more clearly or have a sense of excited urgency.

Our bodies are constantly giving us yes or no answers, but we've become experts at ignoring those. Becoming aware of these signals makes it easier to tune into that inner wisdom. One way I do this is by looking out for tingles: if a thought or idea elicits a tingle, that's my intuition giving me a strong 'yes'. For example, when searching for a landscape to paint, I'll scroll through photos quickly and mindlessly, paying attention to how my body feels. When my eye lands on an image that sends a shiver through my body, I know that's the one I should paint.

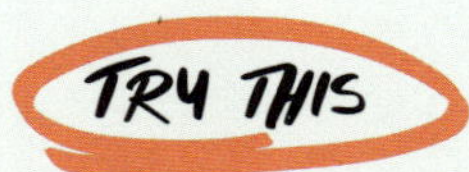

Ask your intuition a question or run through the various scenarios of a choice you've been deliberating. For example, take a few deep breaths and ask 'Should I apply for this job?' If your intuition is saying yes, you'll feel excited and joyful, with a sense of openness and expansiveness. If your intuition is saying no, you might notice a cold sensation or an unpleasant gut feeling suggesting it's not a good idea.

+

Intuition is like a muscle that needs to be developed. The more you consciously work on searching for those intuitive clues, the more easily you'll find them. Eventually, receiving those messages will become second nature, and following them will lead you down the most incredible path.

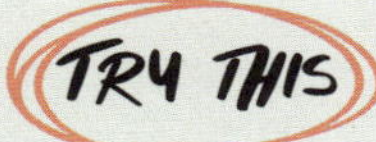

Access your inner knowing

This exercise comes from Glennon Doyle's *Untamed*, though iconic life coach Martha Beck also works with a similar concept. It's based on the theory that our bodies contain a wisdom often clouded and confused by our minds. Try this when you're making a decision. You can practise on small things that are quite clear-cut already to feel how it works. Then build up to bigger things.

1

Think of a decision you need to make – a this or that type of scenario. (E.g. should I quit my job? Should I go to that party?)

2

Picture making a choice, and then being in that scenario. Does it feel open and expansive, or does it feel closed and cold?

3

This feeling should show up in your body – usually around the middle of your torso or around your heart space.

Don't worry if you can't feel it at first. We have been so conditioned to make decisions with our minds that we sometimes struggle to feel our bodily knowing. It will get easier – practise with small things (like what to eat for lunch) and really quiet yourself to feel the difference between the open and closed feelings. Once you've tuned in, it becomes easier and more obvious to feel the answers.

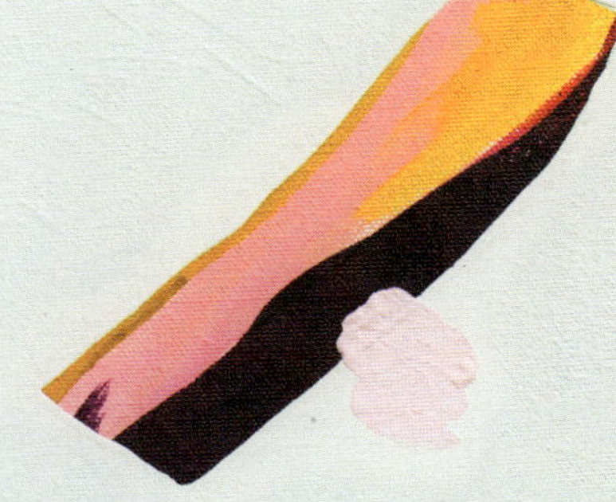

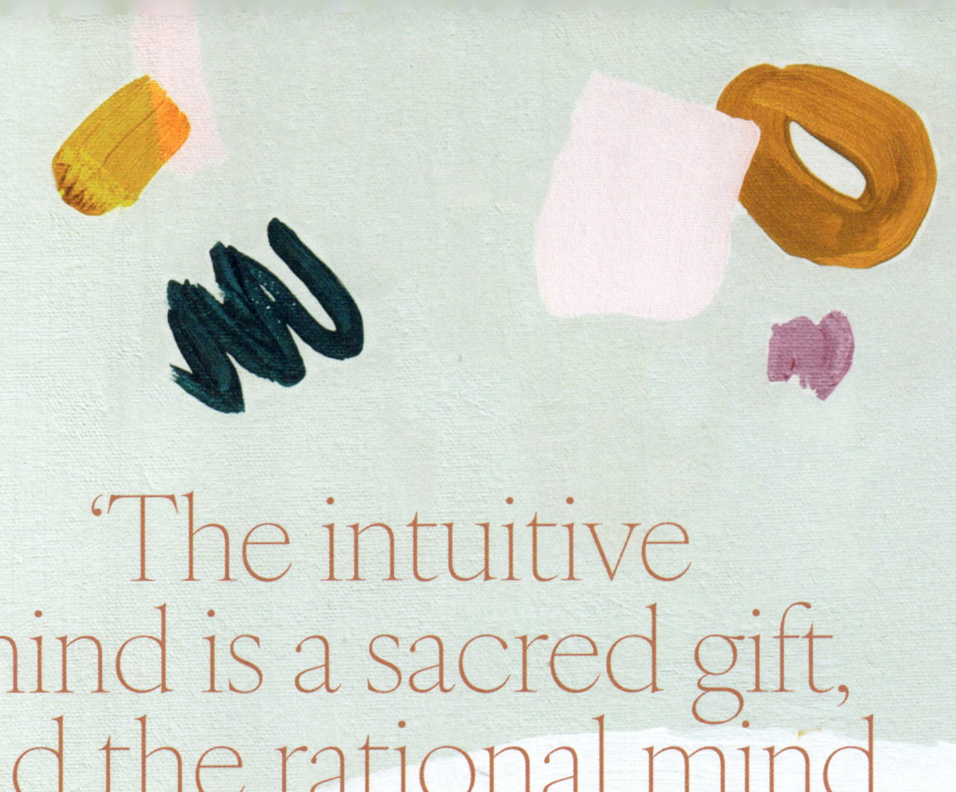

'The intuitive mind is a sacred gift, and the rational mind is a faithful servant. We have created a society that honours the servant and has forgotten the gift.'

– Albert Einstein

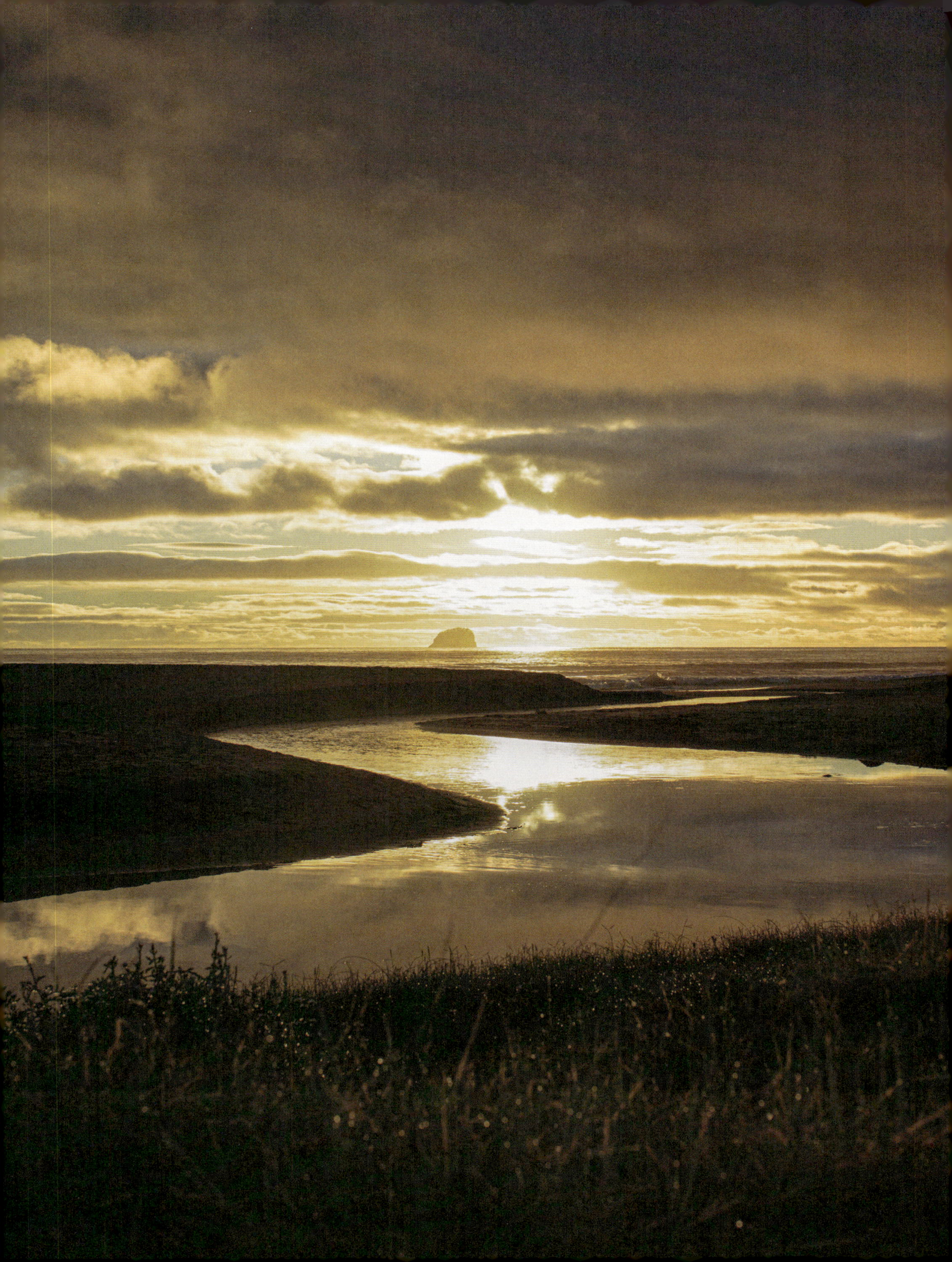

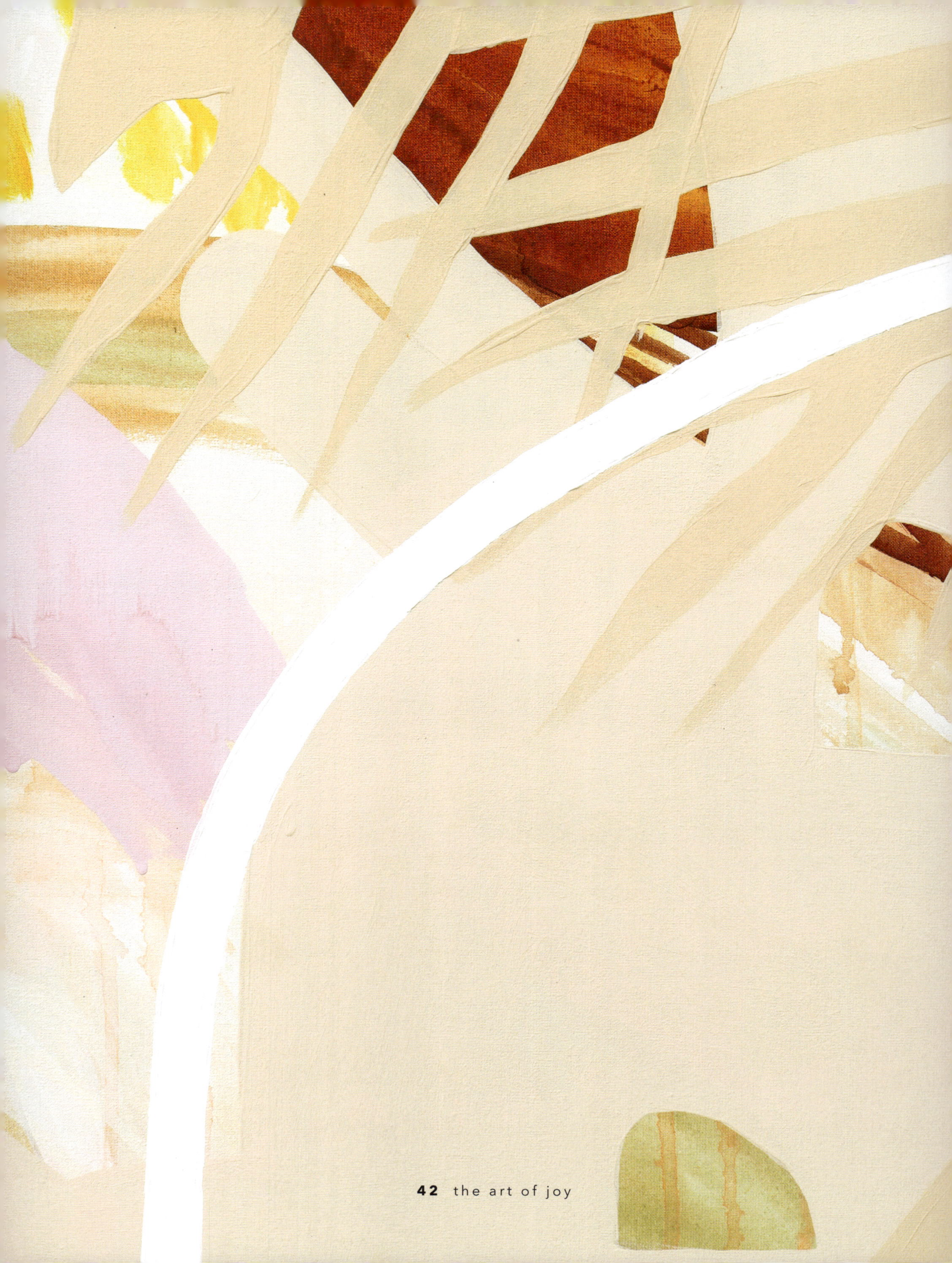

chapter three

FOLLOW THE FEELING

How listening to yourself can lead to a life beyond your imagination.

It's funny how – even with all our plotting, planning, dreaming and doing – we never know where life will lead us. In the spring of 2015, I was a first-time mum in her thirties on maternity leave, working four days a week in advertising. I'd spent my entire adult life working at ad agencies and design studios as a graphic designer and art director, and I adored my job. Agency life was intoxicating and adrenaline-filled, and I loved being surrounded by sharp, creative minds every day. For the longest time, my job had been my passion. I got paid to be creative. What could be better than that?

However, the shine of the industry dulled after returning from maternity leave. The job I'd always loved felt different. Time away and a new perspective on life highlighted how toxic life in advertising land was. Late nights (without overtime pay) were standard and expected, but that was no longer an option for me. Colleagues seemed less enthusiastic about my ideas now that I was 'a mum', and the pace I'd once found so intoxicating was souring into a relentless treadmill. I needed to get out.

By the time my daughter was two, I had lost myself between the constant demands of work and caring for her. My own needs and wants faded into the background, along with my personality and sense of self. This was an aspect of parenting I hadn't been warned about: that feeling that I was losing grip on who I was and what I stood for outside of being a mum. My daughter was my biggest priority, but despite all the love and beauty that comes with parenting, I felt a huge hole in my life. I was yearning for something, but I couldn't put my finger on what that was.

Fridays were now spent at home with my daughter and mum friends, and this slight shift in work-life balance was a tremendous gift and one that would reveal its actual value later down the track.

My pivotal 'fork-in-the-road' day came on one of my Fridays off. It was the start of spring, and the warm air was infused with a beautiful feeling of possibilities. After a coffee date with a friend, I went home and put my little one down for her nap. Suddenly, I had this overwhelming urge to paint, and this was strange

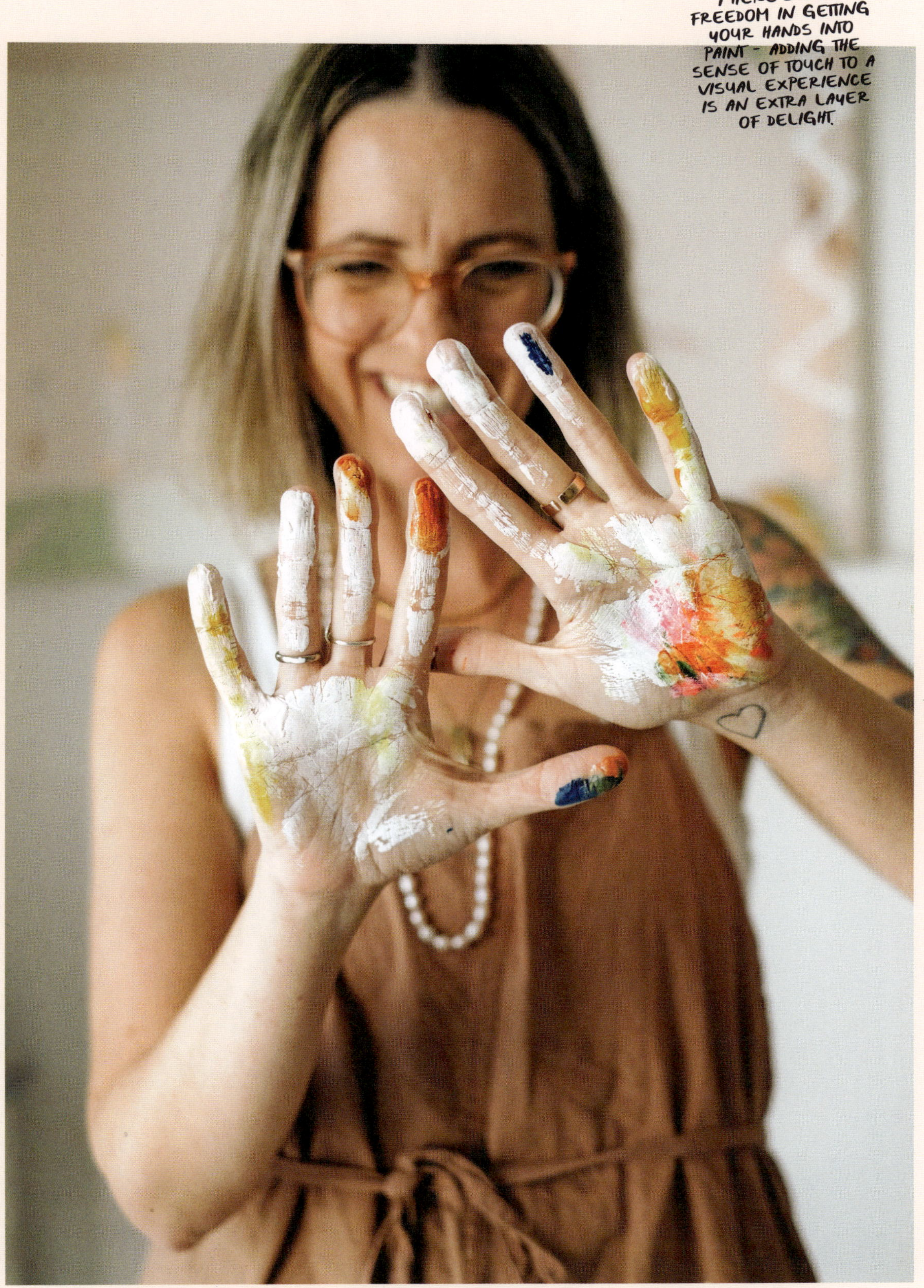
THERE'S SUCH
FREEDOM IN GETTING
YOUR HANDS INTO
PAINT - ADDING THE
SENSE OF TOUCH TO A
VISUAL EXPERIENCE
IS AN EXTRA LAYER
OF DELIGHT.

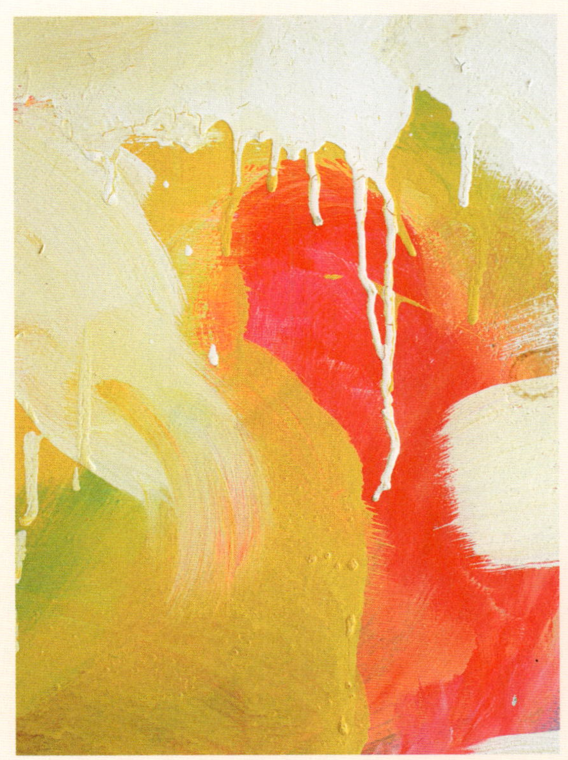

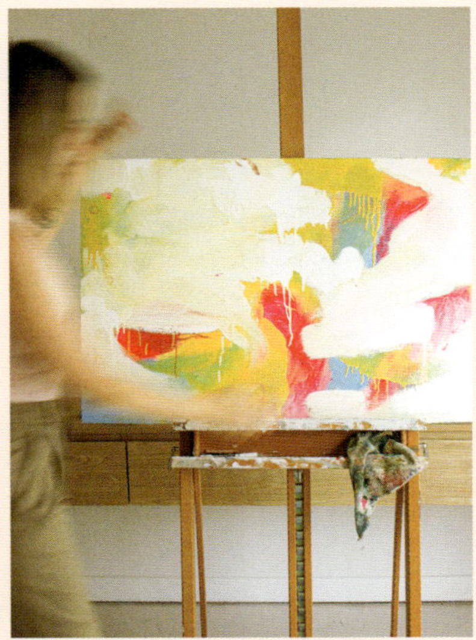

THIS IS 'INTRODUCTIONS', THE PAINTING I DID ON THAT PIVOTAL AFTERNOON. I'VE NEVER SOLD IT, I LOVE HAVING IT AROUND AS A REMINDER OF HOW IT ALL BEGAN.

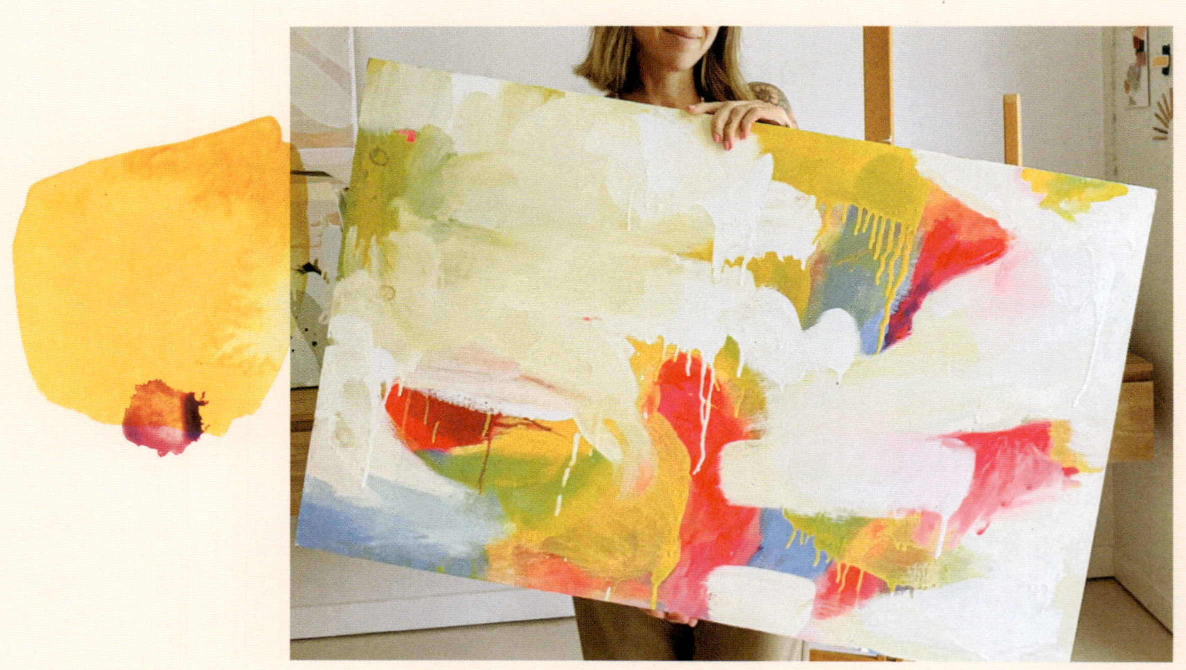

because I hadn't painted in many years. I'd dropped out of an art degree about 25 years earlier, so this urge came entirely out of the blue, but it came with such a burst of excitement that I couldn't ignore it. I cobbled together some equipment: a sheet of dusty plyboard from the garage, some sticky half-empty tins of house paint and tubes of plasticky craft paints from my daughter's supplies. Serendipitously, one of these tubes was filled with a fluorescent pink paint – a colour I fell in love with instantly and have used in almost every painting since that day. I sat in the sun on the back deck and splashed paint around the board in a very expressive abstract. The two hours that my daughter was asleep went by in seconds.

I started painting that day for the sheer joy of it, but by the time I had finished, I knew in my soul that I wanted to be an artist. I wanted to make this the focus of my life. It was like fate had delivered a fully baked idea; all I had to do was keep going until it happened. And that's precisely what I did. I kept going.

I worked at the advertising agency during the days and painted every evening after all the rituals of dinner, bathtime, and storytime were over. I painted on the weekends in little gaps of time. Amazingly, the exhaustion of parenting a tiny, strong-willed Leo disappeared when I was painting. Instead, I was filled with curiosity and excitement. Every brush stroke, every colour mixed, felt like an outpouring of pure joy.

The boss babe in me wanted to turn this new passion into a business, and eventually, I did. But even then, the motivation behind creating remained the sheer joy of it.

Over time, I became just as interested in my experience of this joy as I was in painting. The two became intertwined. I had always been a happy person – generally, my default mode was joy – but having this concentrated practice where it was so apparent made me curious about the concept of joy: what it is, why we experience it, how it affects us. The more I painted, the better I got, and that got me thinking: what if we applied this same type of practice to joy? Could we get better at tapping into joy, too?

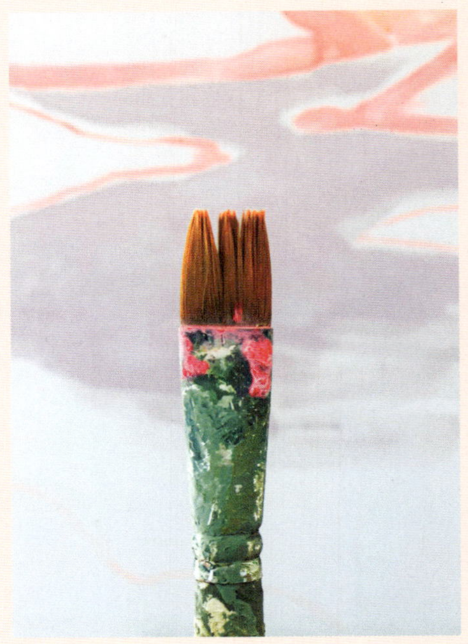

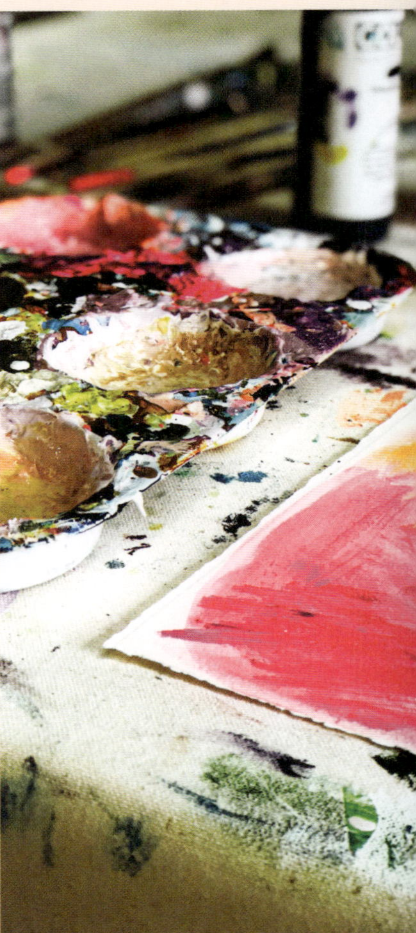

Start seeing your life as a work of art

When we're wrapped up in the necessary tasks involved with survival, such as working or caring for those who need us, we can lose our direction and forget to create our own beautiful life. This is why it helps to see your life as your biggest and best work of art.

Just as a physical work of art requires certain tools (i.e. a canvas, paint and brushes) and structural elements (composition, form and flow); responsibilities such as mortgage payments, shopping or cleaning can't be ignored when creating a life.

Provided that foundational structure is there – in art and life – we get to decide how to make it beautiful. What colours will we use? What sort of marks will our brushes make? How will we go about our daily tasks? In a worried haze of responsibilities, or awake to the beauty of life and finding ways of being that add to the artfulness of living and creating?

This is the life you have been given, and possibly the only life you'll get (although I, and so many others, believe there are more lives to come). So why not make it juicy? Why not fill it with joy whenever possible?

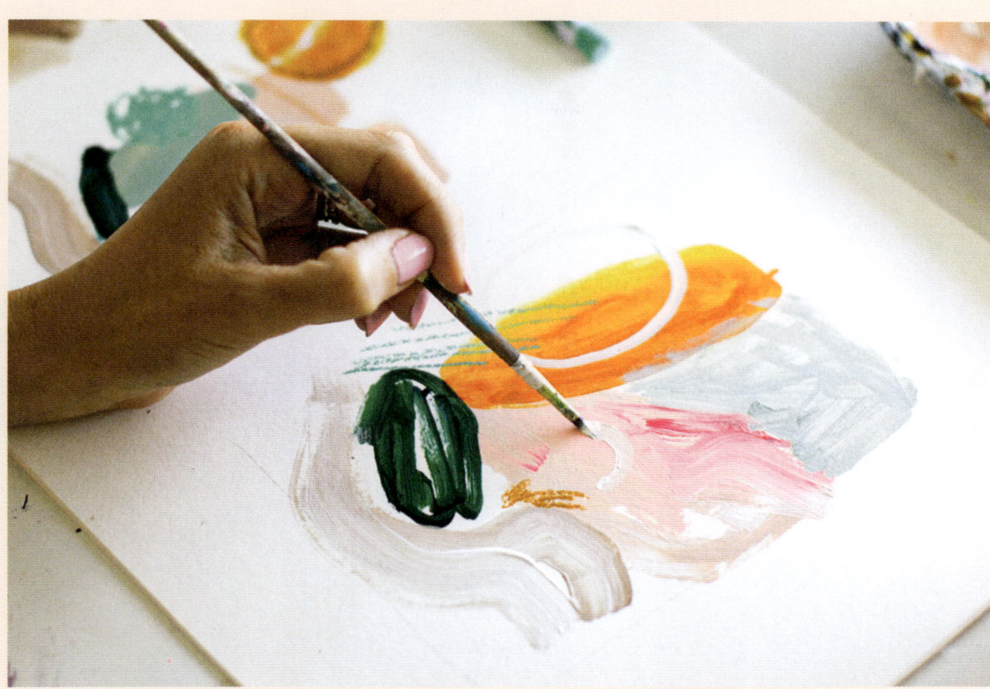

CAN WE STOP TO GIVE THANKS TO FLUORO PINK? IT IS THE EPITOME OF JOY.

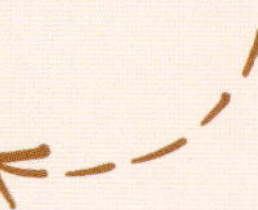

Introduce small joy practices into your day

When we collect moments of joy like an archaeologist, eventually, that collection adds up to a beautiful life. In the chapters that follow, I share my own joy practices, as well as many others to help you start your own collection of little joys.

As you read, pay attention to any exercises or ideas that stand out to you. Some might shine a bit brighter or jump off the page when you read them. Others might give you an excited feeling in your belly. Take note of this, because that's your curiosity showing you the way.

Building any new practice can feel complicated and intimidating, so I suggest picking one exercise to try each time you open this book, even if it's small. Tiny steps can add up to big changes. You definitely don't need to do every exercise in the book, but keep an open mind. It might be that certain practices serve you for a while, but then you need to move on to something else. If your experience is anything like mine, you may also find that your overall mindset changes after introducing a few of these practices into your day, and that adding other joyful practices comes naturally.

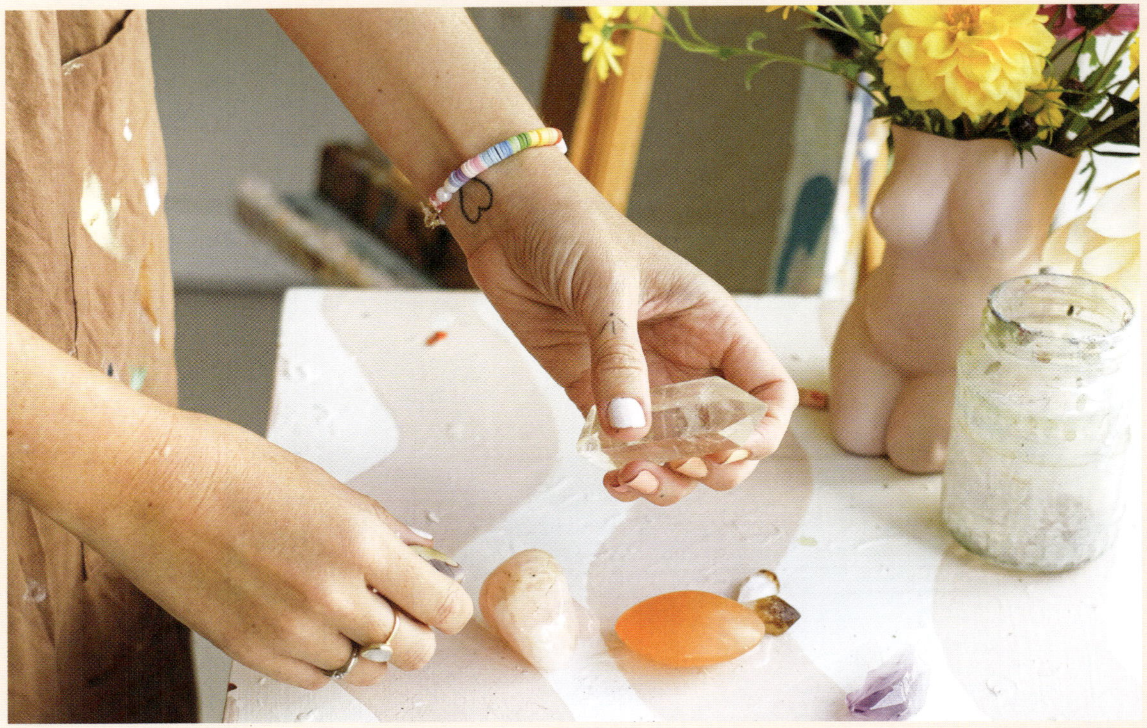

Make time for these new endeavours

Time is typically the first barrier that comes up when starting anything new, and lack of free time is a valid concern, particularly for those of us juggling multiple balls. Unfortunately, more time doesn't magically appear when we need it, so in order to do something new, we might need to go looking for the time we need, and carve it out intentionally. The best place to start is with blocks of time that can be easily reclaimed. For example, if scrolling through your phone takes 30 minutes of each morning, maybe cutting this by just 10 minutes might be enough to create space for a really meaningful practice.

Thankfully, most of the exercises in this book are more about shifting perspective than making a significant time commitment. You'll find many of the practices can be done in just a few minutes, and slot easily into your current routine. Of course, some practices will benefit you more if you can do slightly longer sessions, so if you have more time available, great! But if not, just do whatever you can. If you have children, it helps to involve them in your new practices, since they're often better at holding us accountable than we are ourselves, and those skills are a lovely gift to pass on to them.

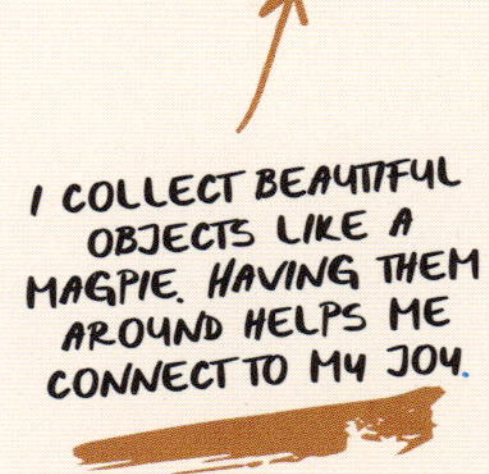

When we collect moments of joy like an archaeologist, eventually, that collection adds up to a beautiful life.

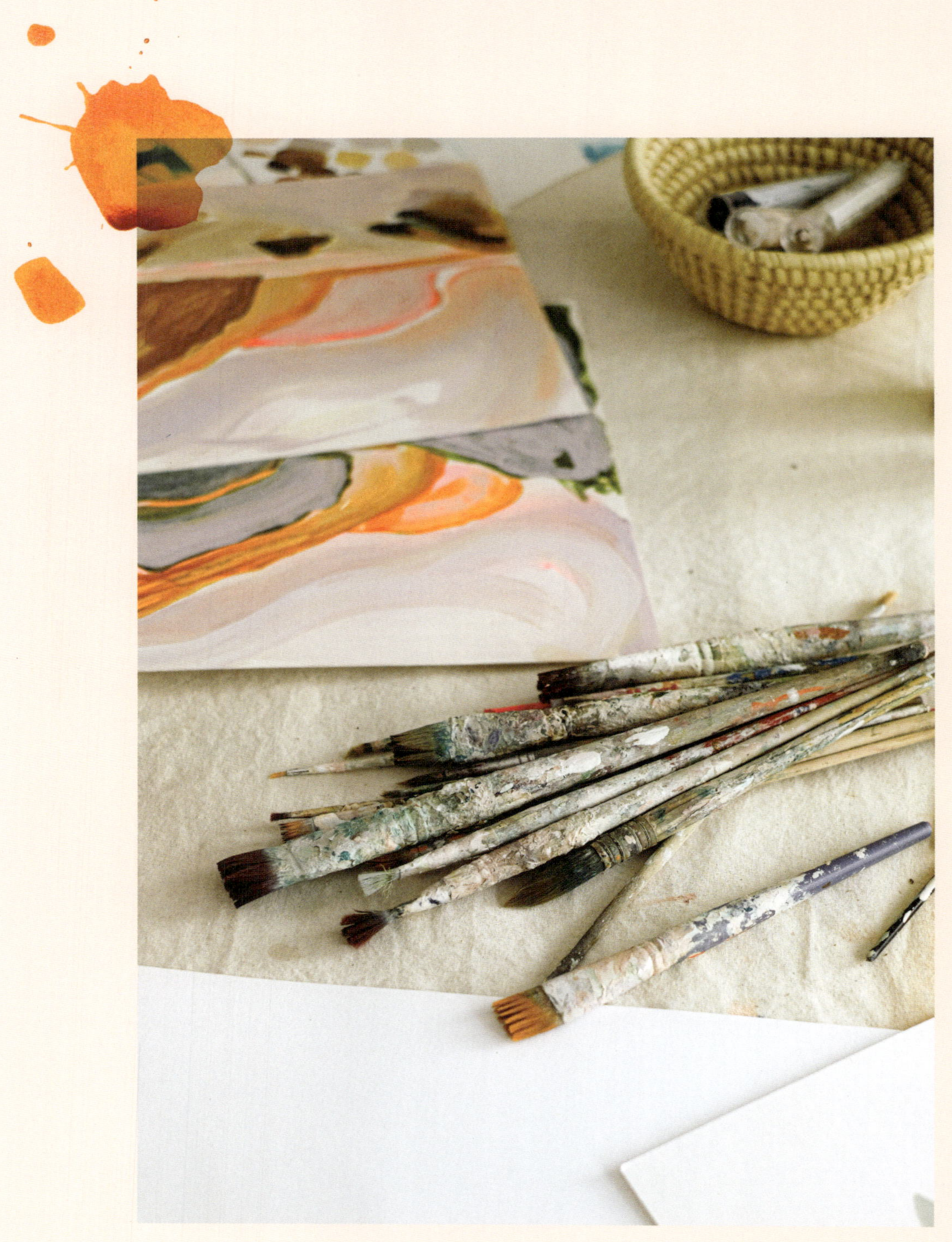

Even commuting can be joyful

Not long after I picked up my brushes again, I found a new job working in a marketing role at a childcare company. Not only did the slightly shorter hours mean I could focus more on my budding art business, but the company also stood for principles I believed in and gave me a chance to work with some phenomenal people. It was the perfect role. The only downside was the commute: on a good day, it was an hour's drive each way, and on a bad one, it was two. When there was heavy traffic on the way to work, I would go into somewhat of a panic. There's nothing like being stuck in the middle of a long line of cars in an already crammed-full life to make you feel claustrophobic and unhappy.

Around this time, an artist I admire posted an Instagram story about how enlightening she'd found an interview with Michael A. Singer, author of *The Untethered Soul*. Curious, I downloaded that podcast episode and pushed play on it as I started my commute home. I spent the next hour completely immersed in that conversation, and rather than feeling trapped and panicked during the drive, I felt excited, alive, and connected to the world.

After this, I threw myself into the light-filled rabbit hole of self-help podcasts. There were so many topics to explore, and each conversation felt like it had been sent to me at precisely the right time. I couldn't, and still can't, believe the wealth of information that is constantly delivered for free in such a soul-nourishing format.

This small discovery turned my car into an enriching 'life university' where I was expanding my knowledge and learning to live more fully. Being in my car became one of my favourite, most exciting parts of the day, and I realised that I'd unintentionally created a daily 'joy practice'.

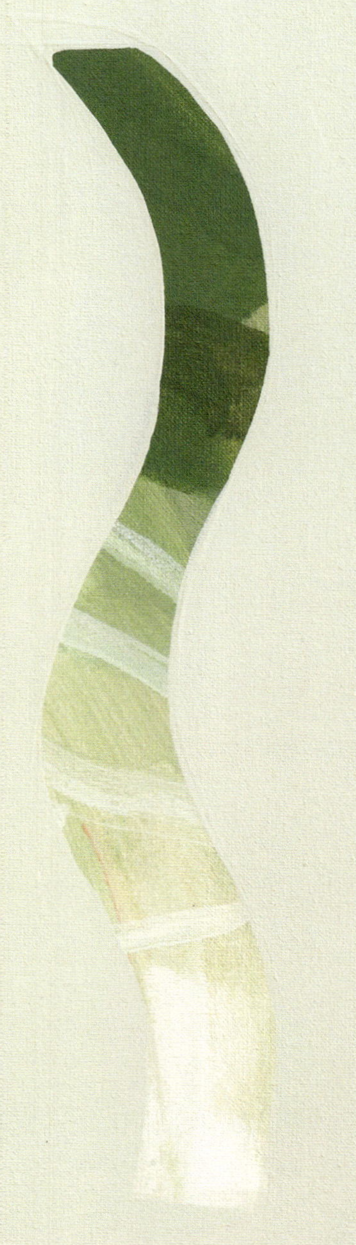

chapter four

Meet Your Brain

A quick introduction to the grey stuff.

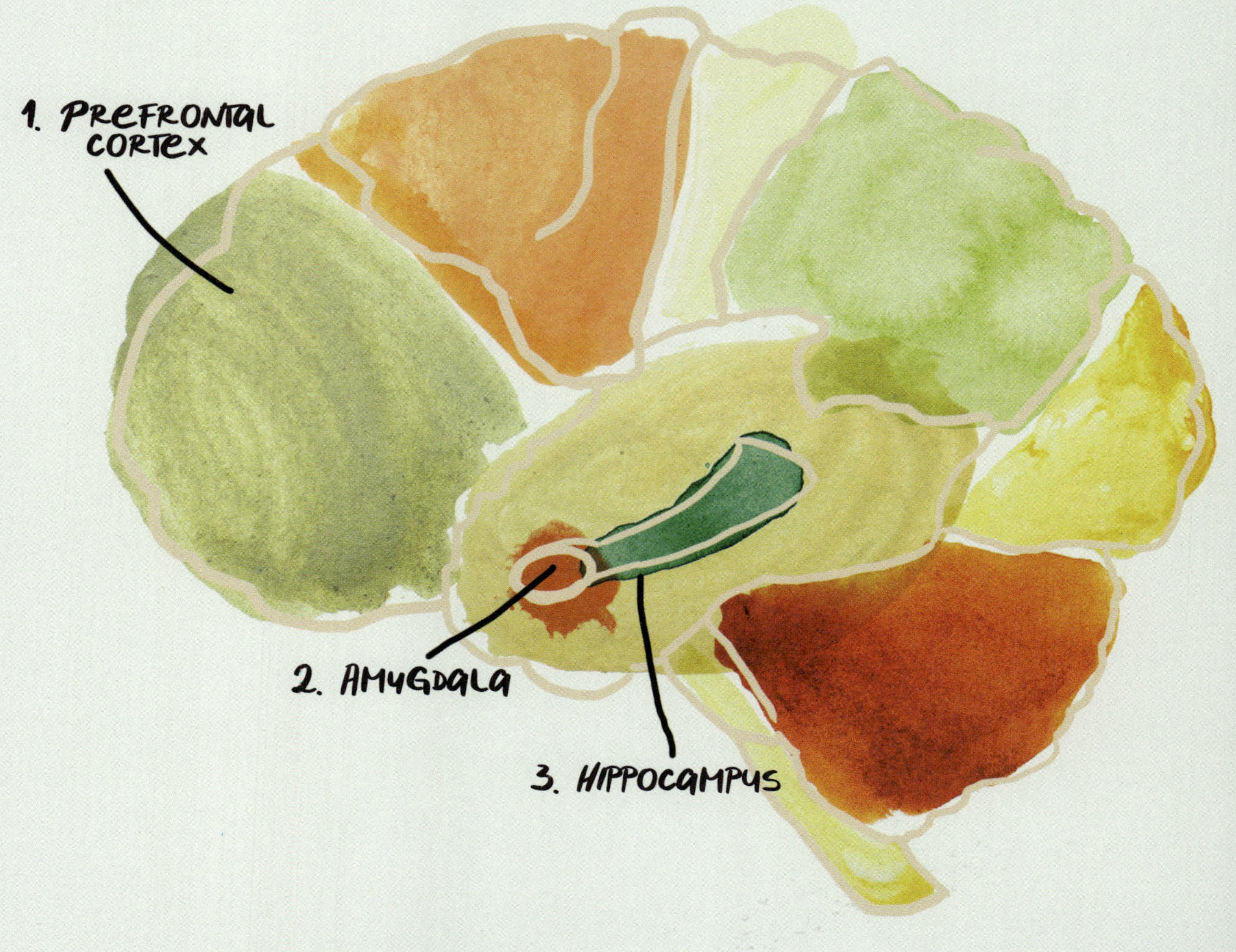

Often, we assume that the emotions we're feeling are based solely on the facts of the situation we're in, but that's not the whole story. The parts of the brain involved in creating emotion translate those facts based on past experiences and learned behaviours. Having a basic understanding of how your brain processes information, and then learning practical tools to help you regulate your brain, and therefore your emotions, can be incredibly empowering on your joy journey.

1 The prefrontal cortex

This is the brain's executive centre. This area sits behind our forehead and above the amygdala, and is instrumental in rational decision-making. The functionality of the prefrontal cortex is lessened when the amygdala is in distress, as this stops us from processing information effectively or accurately.

2 The amygdala

A little, almond-shaped structure plays the role of the brain's alert system. It evolved to protect us from immediate, life-threatening danger, and functions like a vigilant guard dog – scanning for threats and alerting us at the first whiff of danger. This type of alarm system is very useful if you're being chased by a tiger, but much less effective when a minor event such as an angry email gets misinterpreted as a severe threat.

From birth, the amygdala keeps track of your life experiences, etching negative ones a lot deeper in your mind than positive ones. It's known to plant negative self-talk seeds in our minds. Thoughts such as 'you aren't good enough', 'you are unlikeable', or 'you'll never match up to them' are deceptive messages, not reflections of reality. They're the by-products of an amygdala in overdrive. Our job is to soothe the amygdala, to prevent it from falsely perceiving danger at every turn – from turning a nasty email into a ferocious tiger, and joy can be a very effective way of doing this.

3 The hippocampus

The hippocampus is like the brain's memory bank – a library storing our life experiences so we can refer back to them later. It interacts closely with the prefrontal cortex, feeding it information to help us make clear, logical decisions. For the hippocampus to do its best work, the amygdala needs to be calm. Stress can make it difficult for the hippocampus to store or retrieve information clearly.

Joy practices (such as gratitude and mindfulness) pacify the amygdala, allowing it to stand down from its guard position. This relaxation facilitates the flow of information to the prefrontal cortex empowering us to make thoughtful, composed decisions. Additionally, a calm amygdala enhances the hippocampus's ability to archive and recall memories. Nurturing a calm and happy brain is not just a frivolous way of being happier – it is training our brain for better cognitive and emotional wellbeing.

Put simply, calming the amygdala helps us to make better decisions, and improves our memory.

Turns out you *can* teach an old dog new tricks

Up until the1960s, scientists believed that our brains stopped developing in adulthood. Since then, however, we've discovered that our brains never stop developing. We can learn new behaviours, skills and develop new thought patterns through practice and repetition at any point in our life. We aren't stuck with our default 'factory settings'; we can change them! We owe this continuous development to the neurons in our brains, which create pathways from one area to another.

Just like pathways in a forest, the paths in our brain become clearer and deeper the more they're used. The process of creating new paths is known as neuroplasticity. By introducing short, joy practices into our day, and repeating them often, we can create new paths and rewire our brains to be more positive and calmer. At first, these may feel like unfamiliar back roads, but with regular practise, they can become super-highways that we take automatically.

To create new, more positive neural pathways, we must cultivate mind strengths such as calmness, contentment and caring. As we build the pathways of these positive traits, our brains eventually change how they work. Our old habits of reacting quickly or letting our minds chatter negatively to us all day long, slowly get replaced and repaired.

What effect does joy have on the brain?

When you experience joy, your brain lights up in the prefrontal cortex and ventral striatum, which are linked to reward, motivation, learning, and decision-making. At the same time, your body releases a cascade of feel-good neurochemicals such as dopamine, oxytocin, and serotonin. These not only improve mood, but also help regulate stress and support better emotional balance.

Over time, regularly experiencing joy helps form and reinforce positive neural pathways. These 'joy circuits' make it easier for your brain to return to a calm state, stay open to new experiences, and regulate emotions more effectively. In short, joy builds brain resilience. It trains your nervous system to spend more time in the rest-and-digest state, and less time in fight-or-flight.

Joy is so much more than a moment of pleasure; it's a practice that rewires your brain for greater ease, connection, and wellbeing.

Just like pathways in a forest, the paths in our brain become clearer and deeper the more they're used.

The body–brain connection

So much of how we feel at any given moment depends on the state of our nervous system. We often assign unnecessary meaning, and weight, to feelings that a dysregulated nervous system can explain. I find the topic so fascinating, but I will only bore you with a little jargon. I find it useful to frame things, in my own experience, from the viewpoint of a nervous system that's either calm or activated, because the state we are in absolutely changes how we feel and how we function at any given moment.

Our autonomic nervous system consists of two separate systems: the sympathetic and parasympathetic.

1 **The sympathetic nervous system** controls our body's fight-or-flight response; it responds to danger (or the perception/thought of danger). When this system is engaged, our heart rate goes up, we experience breathlessness, our pupils dilate, and perspiration occurs. Clearly, this response is unpleasant, and it's not good for our health to be in this state for long periods of time.

2 **The parasympathetic nervous system** is sometimes called the rest-and-digest system. When this response is activated, our breathing slows, our heart rate drops to a normal level, and our blood pressure drops. Our body is then in a state suited to rest and recovery. Sounds good, doesn't it?

Unfortunately, many of us spend more time than necessary in fight-or-flight mode. The accumulation of daily stressors activate the same response that, in ancient times, caused our nervous system to evolve to make us run away from a ferocious tiger.

Being tired and burned out can put us in a state of overwhelm and make it impossible to think clearly or feel motivated. In that case, rest can be the best medicine. Find your favourite way to do this. I'm not a napper, so I prefer to hang out on the couch and watch a juicy TV series. Maybe resting for you is closing your eyes and listening to a podcast, reading a book in the sun or playing with your dog. The key is to notice when your body needs a rest, and prioritising that. If that isn't quite enough, there are several simple strategies we can use to move from fight-or-flight to rest-and-digest. These include breathing exercises, awe practices, and mindful moments. Many of the practices in this book can bring us back into our bodies and into the moment, thus activating the wonderful parasympathetic nervous system.

SYMPATHETIC

FIGHT-OR-FLIGHT

PARASYMPATHETIC

REST-AND-DIGEST

OUR AUTONOMIC NERVOUS SYSTEM

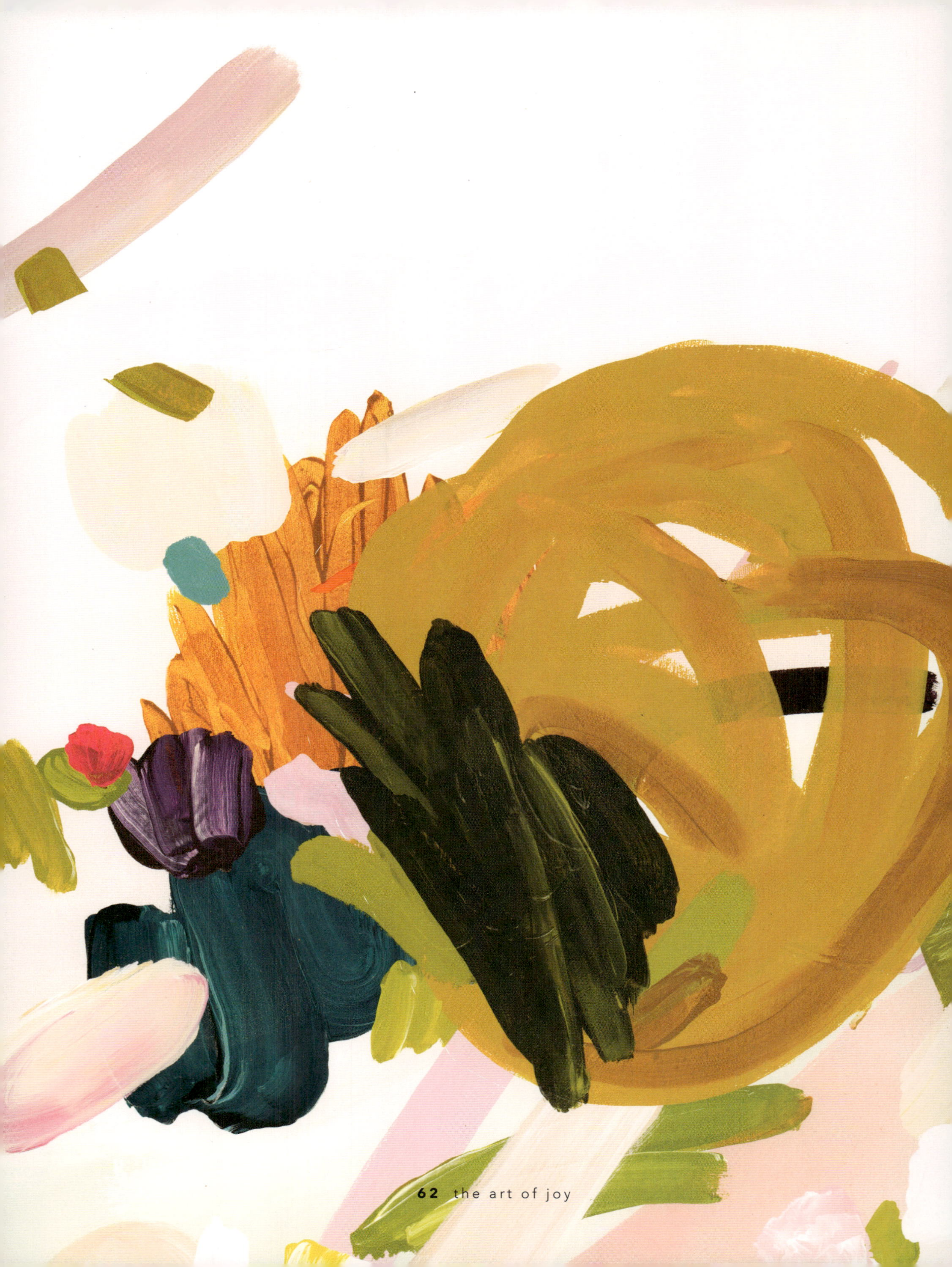

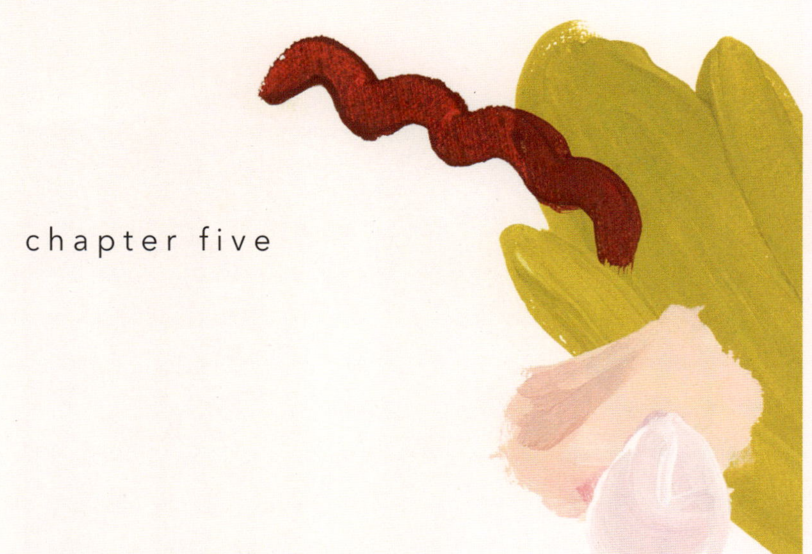

chapter five

GETTING UNSTUCK

State-changers – quick, joyful ways to get out of a funk and into a better mindset.

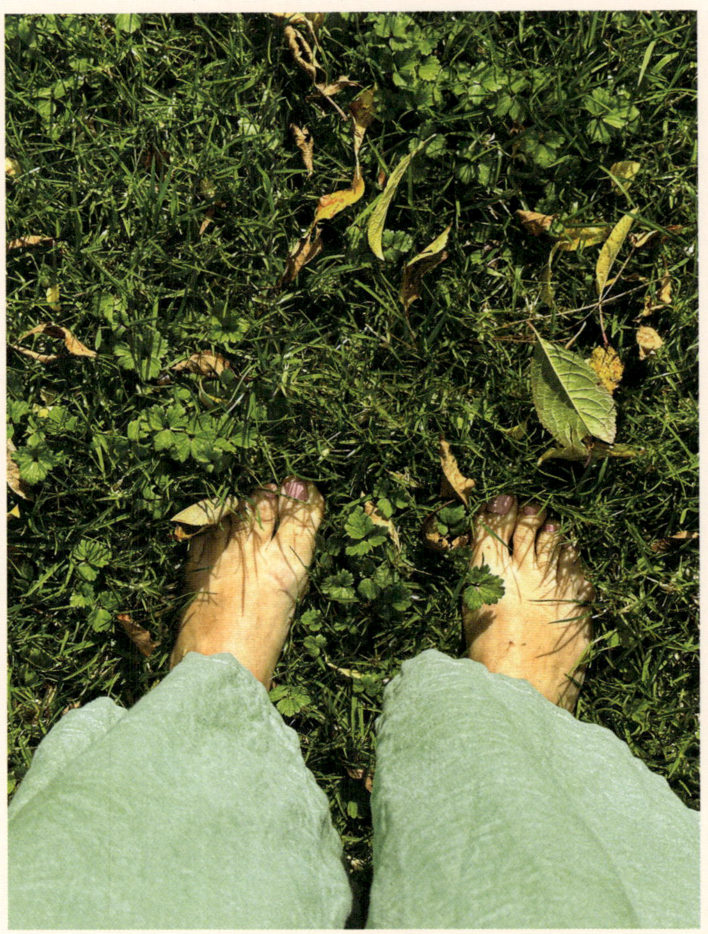

State-changer #1
Dose up on nature

Humans have only been living in buildings, disconnected from nature, for a tiny percentage of our existence. Every cell in our body has evolved to crave a connection to the natural world, and this is why getting a 'dose of green' offers us so much more than beauty. It can literally change our brain.

Research into the benefits of forest bathing and spending time in nature shows that even a few minutes outdoors can prompt feelings of awe, reduce stress hormones, boost mood, and increase clarity. Simple things such as gazing at trees, touching the earth, listening to birds calm the nervous system and activate the parasympathetic response. You don't need to go on a forest retreat to experience this shift.

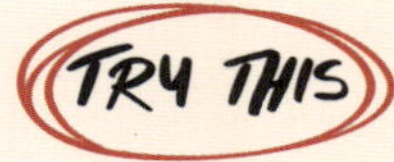

If you're near some grass, get your feet onto it! Walk outside, take your shoes off – don't worry if it's raining, just grab a coat. Wet grass can actually heighten the sensation and add a bit of fun. Stand or walk for a minute or two, focusing on what you're feeling rather than what you're thinking.

+

Notice the slightly prickly feel of the grass, the cool or warm air, maybe even the squish of mud or dew. Let yourself tune in to those sensations – your body waking up to where it is. Imagine the life in the soil, the roots beneath your feet, the oxygen in the air from the plants around you. You're part of all of it.

+

If you're at a beach, dip your feet in the water or, better still, jump in! Notice the temperature shift, feel the texture of sand or rock underfoot, and the sensation of water on your skin. Being in water reminds us that we're elemental creatures too. Let yourself be held by nature, even for a moment.

+

Return to your day with a renewed sense of wonder and connection Let this moment anchor you. You're not just passing through nature – you're part of it. The sense of awe and belonging you experience in these moments isn't fluffy or indulgent. It's powerful. And it's available to you anytime you step outside.

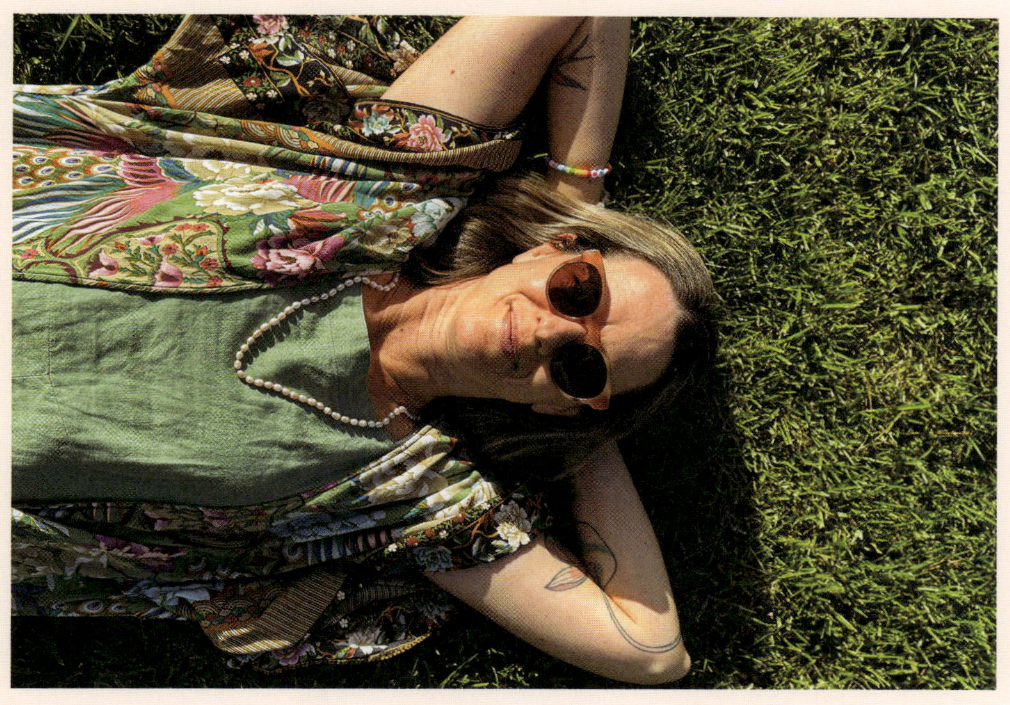

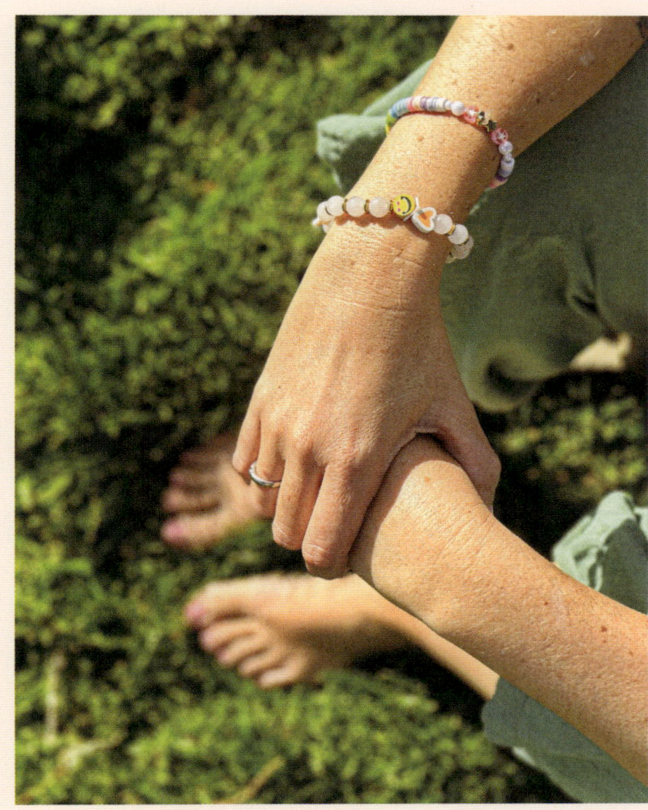

State-changer #2
Transient art

Best-selling author and life coach Martha Beck has spoken about the link between creativity and calm, and how creative acts can be a powerful way to interrupt anxiety and shift the nervous system into a more settled state. The reason this works is because when we make something – especially something low-stakes and hands-on – we move out of hypervigilance and into a state known as flow. We're not escaping the anxiety, but gently re-routing it. A small, natural art piece can become a quiet, meditative act. And if the wind scatters it later, that's a beautiful reminder that not everything is meant to last, or be meaningful.

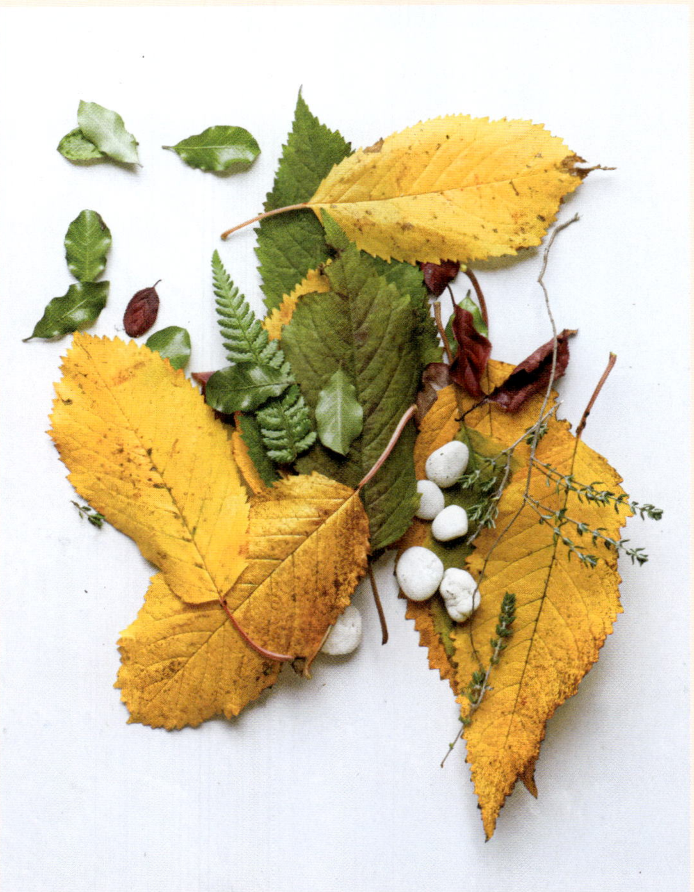

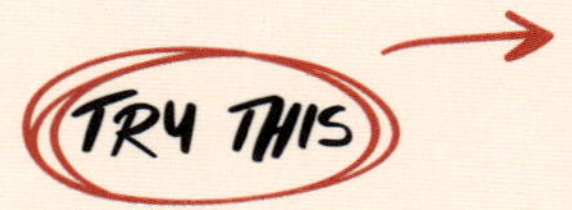

Head outside and collect natural items that catch your eye – leaves, stones, twigs, seed pods, petals. Let yourself be guided by curiosity, not outcome. Then, use these finds to create a piece of temporary art: a shape on the ground, a mandala on your doorstep, a leaf sculpture on a tree stump. This kind of transient creation isn't about making something to keep. It's about getting out of your head and into your body. As you notice textures, colours, and patterns, you'll start to slow down. Your focus will shift from anxious thought loops to the rhythm of your breath, the textures felt by your fingers, and the world in front of you.

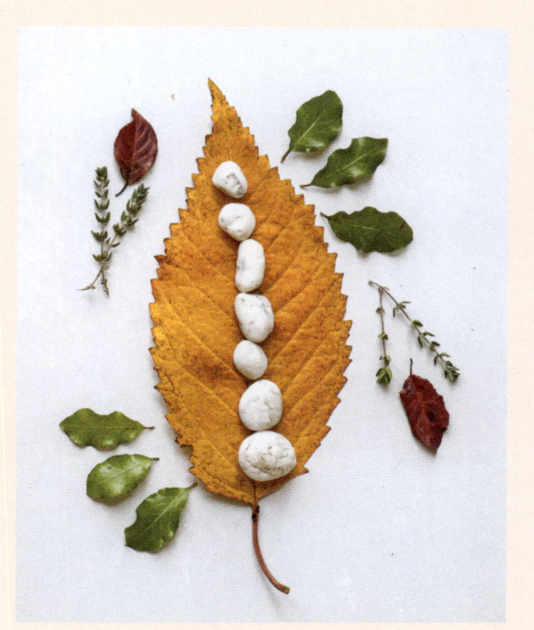

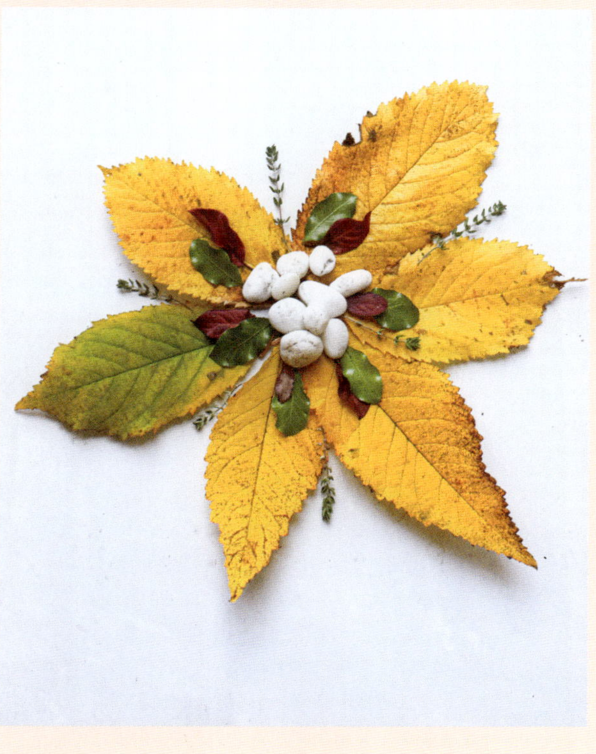

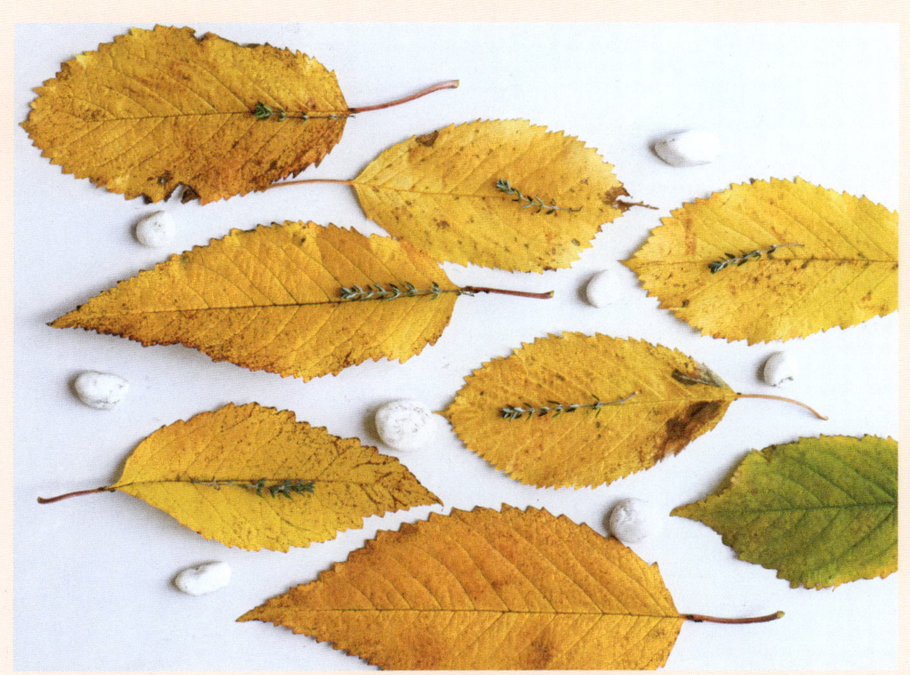

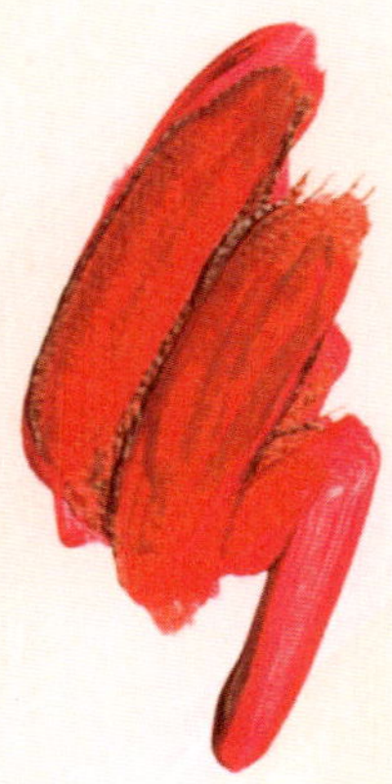

State-changer #3
Use your body

Shifting your attention from your mind to your body is one of the quickest ways to change your state. Movement sends signals through the nervous system that can help us feel calmer, more grounded, and more present. Whether it's dancing, shaking, baking, or singing at the top of your lungs, these small, physical acts help bring you back into your body – and back to the moment.

Dance

I'm a huge fan of music with very loud bass – the old nineties raver in me just can't resist. Maybe you prefer to sway like a willow to Fleetwood Mac or thrash your air guitar to some loud rock. The point is to get your body moving; it just takes one song (but there are no rules against more!) for a quick mood reset.

Make

Using your hands to bake, sculpt, or paint pulls you out of your head and into your senses. The act of shaping something physical is grounding and calming – especially when you let go of perfection. Messy, tactile play isn't just for kids; it's a powerful way to shift your state and feel more grounded.

Shake

Science backs shaking as an effective tool for changing states. Animals do this instinctively to release stress, think of ducks beating their wings after a squabble on a lake. Shaking is also a great exercise to do with kids who are overstimulated or upset because it activates the rest-and-digest nervous state, and signals to the body that it's time to relax. It's easy, quick, and can be done to music, with others, or alone in a bathroom cubicle on a bad day.

Sing

Turn on a tune. I have a playlist of some of my favourite songs to really belt it out to. You know, the ones that sound epic in the shower or in a car – and sing loudly! Put your heart into it and let the music move through you.

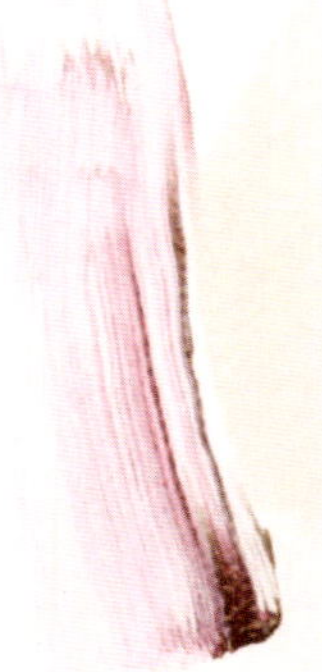

TRY THIS

SHAKE IT OFF!

1

Start by rolling your shoulders and moving your hips to loosen up – a bit like a snake.

2

Shake both hands in front of you for the count of eight.

3

Add in your feet and legs, one at a time, alternating between sides.

4

Now jiggle your knees, your waist and your butt – all while shaking the previous parts.

5

Gently, shake your head.

6

Keep this up for a minute or so, then stop and take four deep breaths.

7

Put both hands on your heart (this is also soothing for your nervous system) and finish with a smile. The act of smiling sends signals to the brain that we are safe, calm and happy.

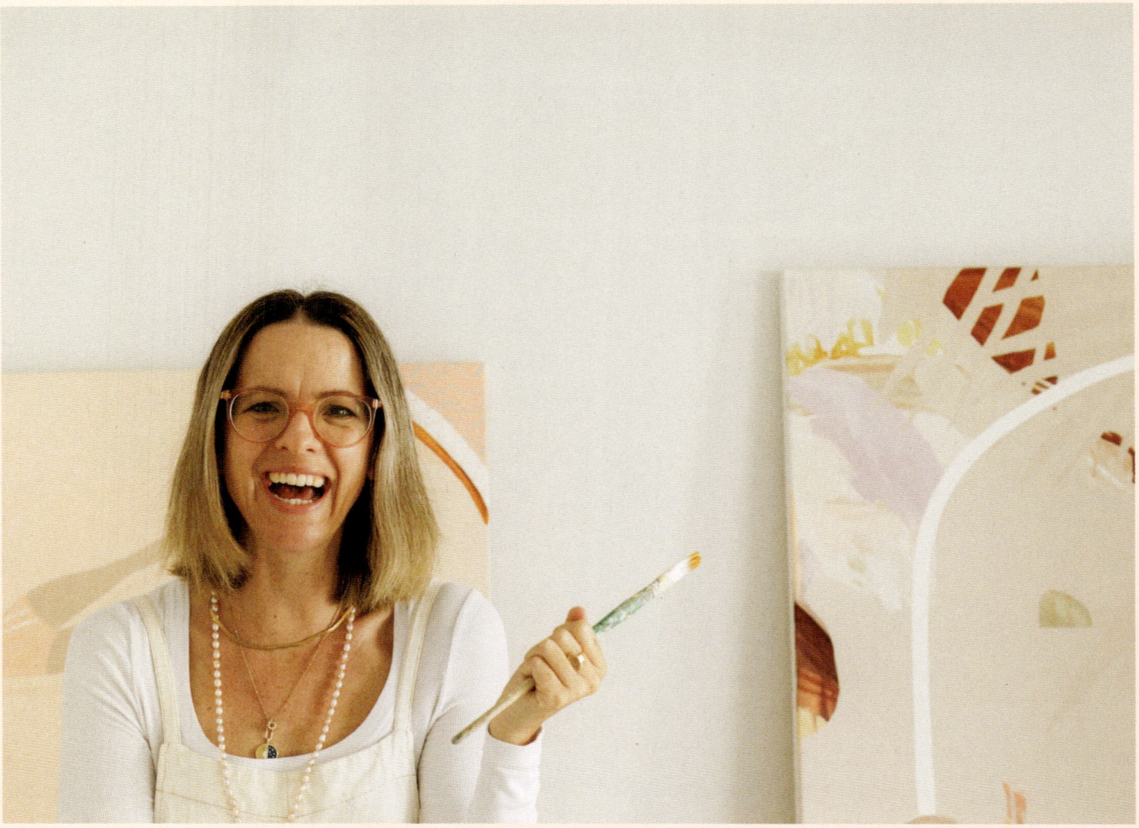

State-changer #4
Smile

Smiling can change our state in two ways: the first is that you see, feel or think of something that makes you happy, and your brain tells your facial muscles to smile. The second is that you intentionally smile for no reason, and when your brain registers the position of your facial muscles, it gets the message that you're happy, and generates feelings of genuine happiness. This works because the action of smiling is so closely intertwined with the feeling of joy, that your brain will switch gears to match your face. It feels like your eyes scan the room for something to smile about. Spoiler – there is usually something there. Life is good that way.

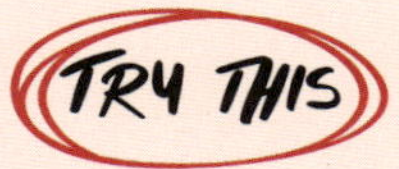

Smile for one minute while you do something that usually bores you, or even try it now. Set a timer on your phone and let it run visibly next to you, so you don't forget to keep smiling – check in with how you feel afterwards.

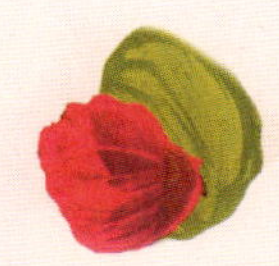

State-changer #5
Connect

Human connection is a powerful regulator for the nervous system. When we feel safe with others – through a hug, a kind word, or even eye contact – our bodies shift from stress into calm. This is because connection activates the parasympathetic nervous system, helping to lower cortisol, steady the heart rate, and release oxytocin (the 'love hormone'). This is why a hug can feel like medicine, and why a quick chat with someone you trust can change your whole day. These simple acts don't just help others feel better – they improve our own mood and sense of safety, too.

Hug someone

Ideally you would hug someone you care about, but even hugging yourself can have benefits. Make it meaningful: hug tight, be present and focus only on the hug. Hold it for at least 20 seconds to feel the full benefits on your nervous system.

Snuggle a pet

Cuddling a pet is one of the easiest ways to feel calm and connected. Stroking fur, hearing a purr, or just having a warm body nearby can regulate your nervous system and ease anxiety. Animals offer unconditional presence, and sometimes that's all we need.

Hold a hand

Human touch is deeply soothing. Holding hands – even briefly – can lower stress, reduce heart rate, and create a sense of shared safety. Whether it's your partner, child, or friend, let it be intentional and unhurried.

Phone a friend

Connection doesn't always need to be physical. A quick call with someone who gets you can have a huge impact. Hearing a familiar voice, feeling seen and heard, even through a screen, reminds your nervous system that you're not alone.

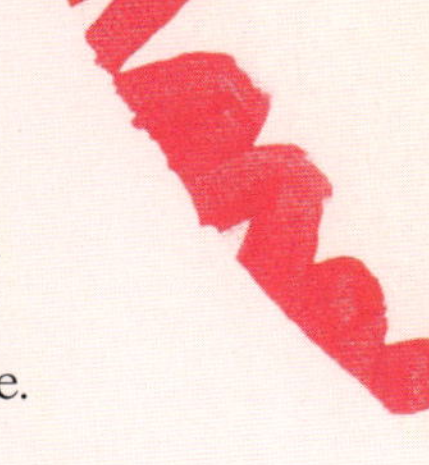

State-changer #6
Parasympathetic breathing

I promise this is a lot easier to do, than to pronounce. The concept is simple – if you spend longer on your out-breath than your in-breath, your body switches from the sympathetic to the parasympathetic nervous system, helping you feel calm and relaxed, and much more open to giving and receiving joy. This breathing technique signals to your brain that you're safe, prompting it to release tension and dial down stress hormones such as cortisol. Essentially, breathing is your body's natural way of shifting gears, and creating an ideal internal state for calmness, clarity, and joy.

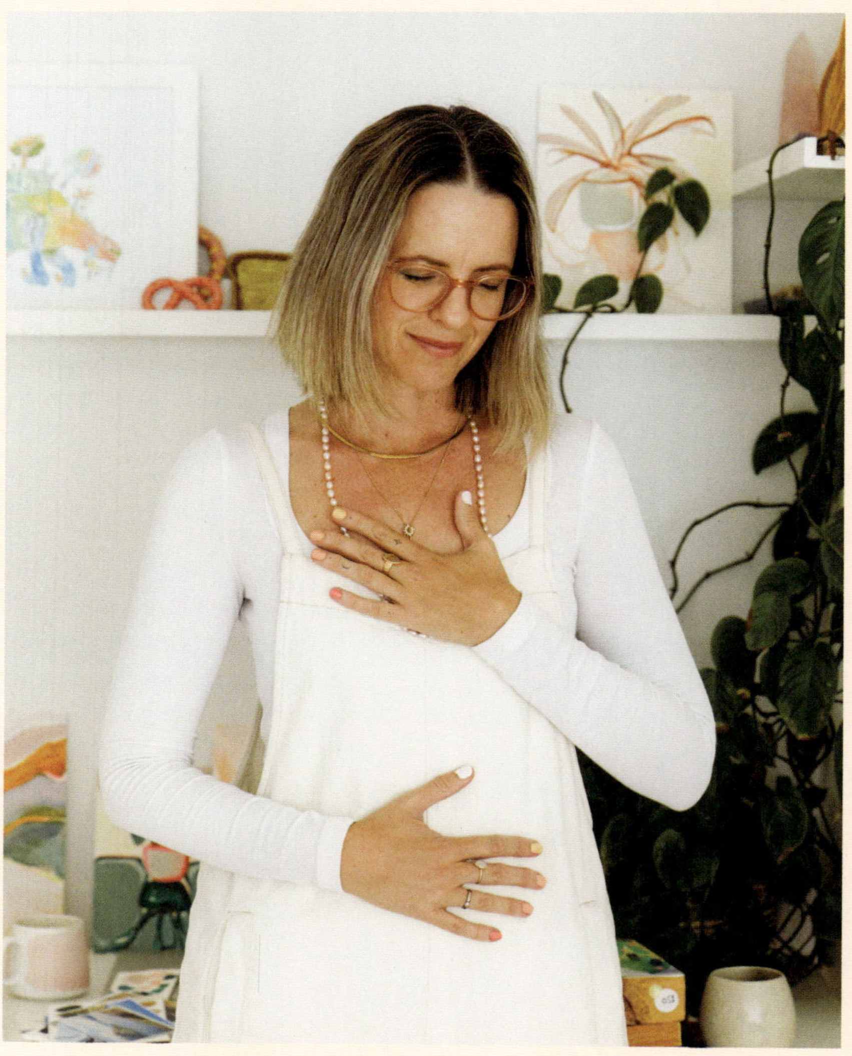

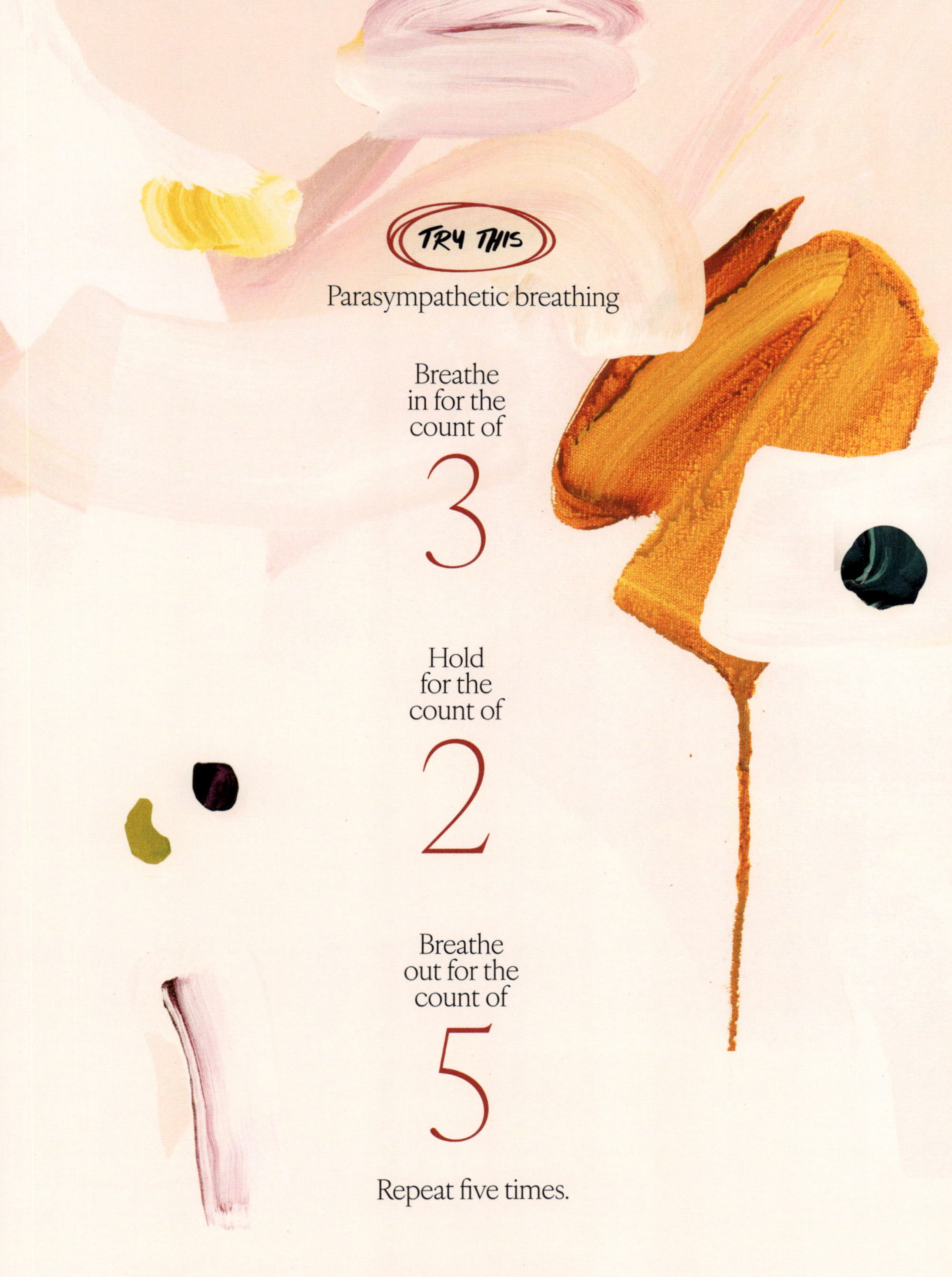

TRY THIS

Parasympathetic breathing

Breathe in for the count of

3

Hold for the count of

2

Breathe out for the count of

5

Repeat five times.

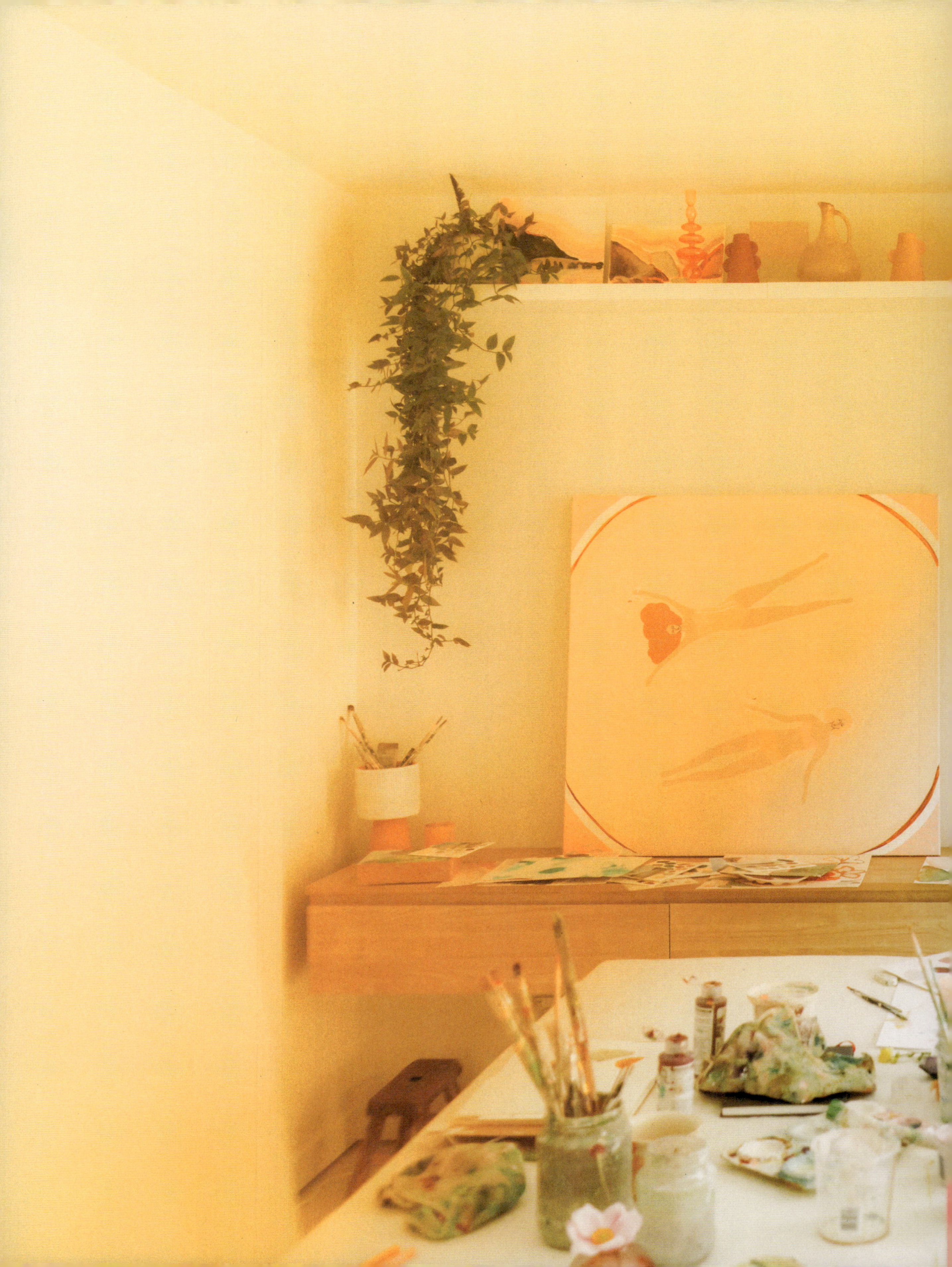

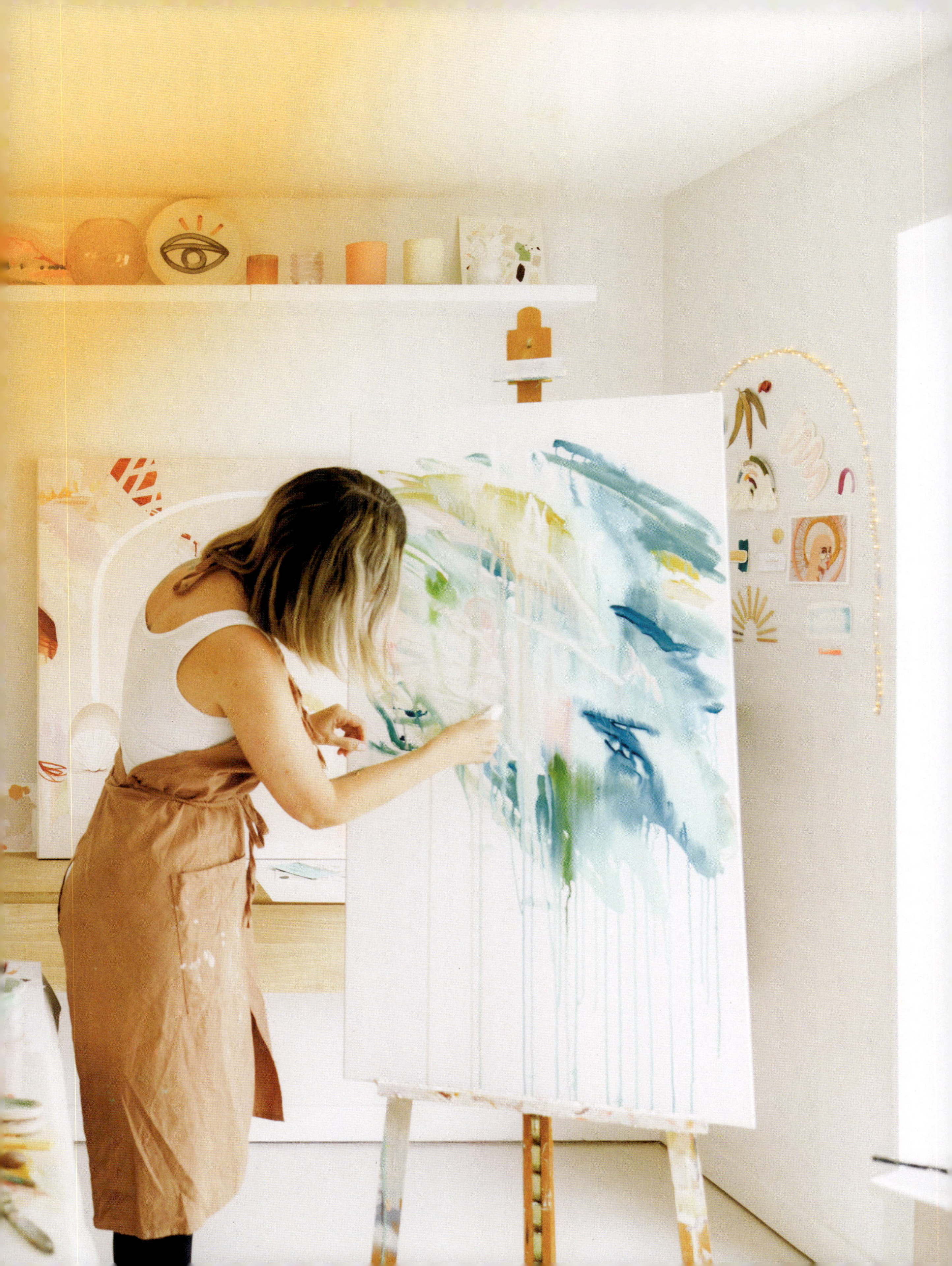

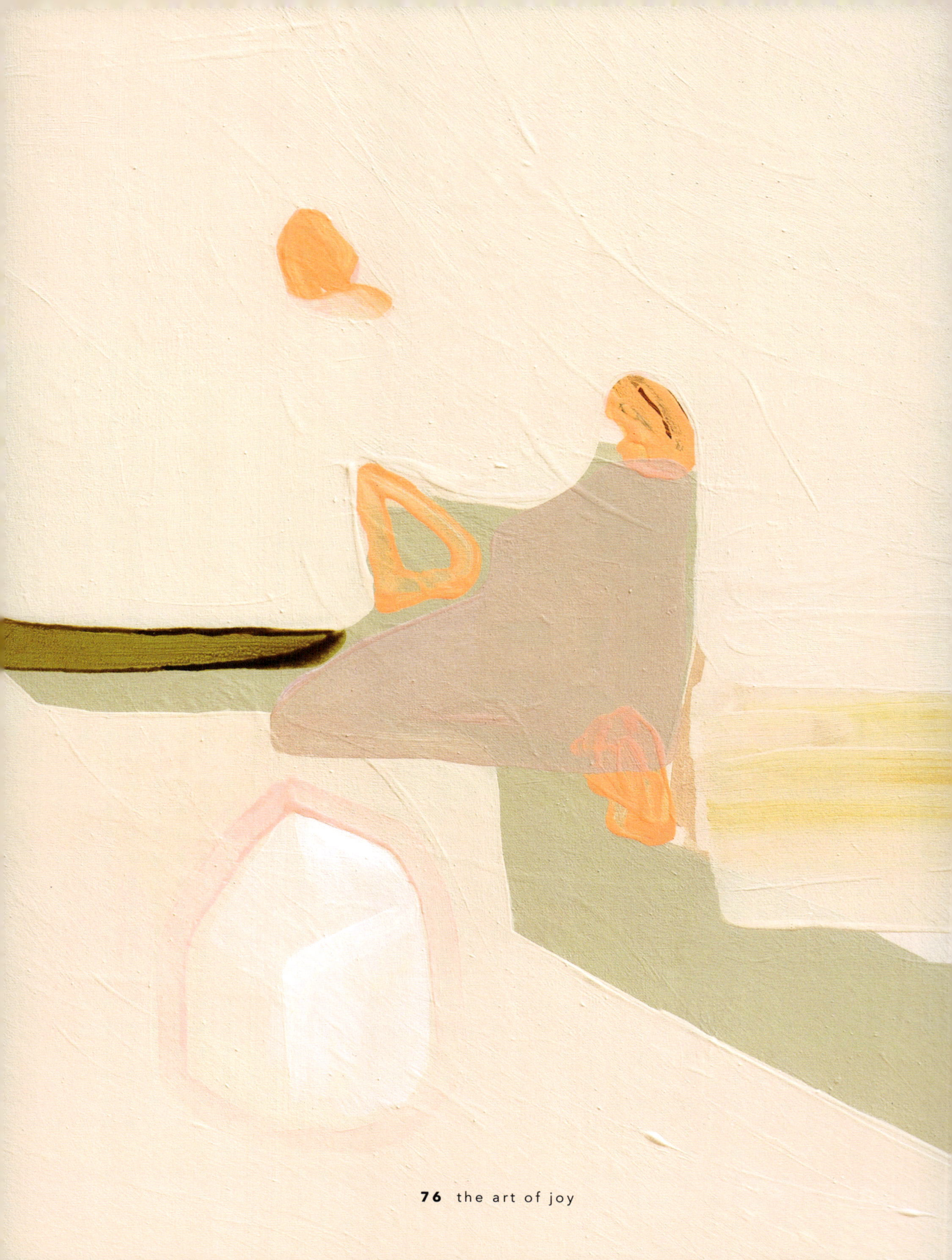

chapter six

JOY FOR DAYS

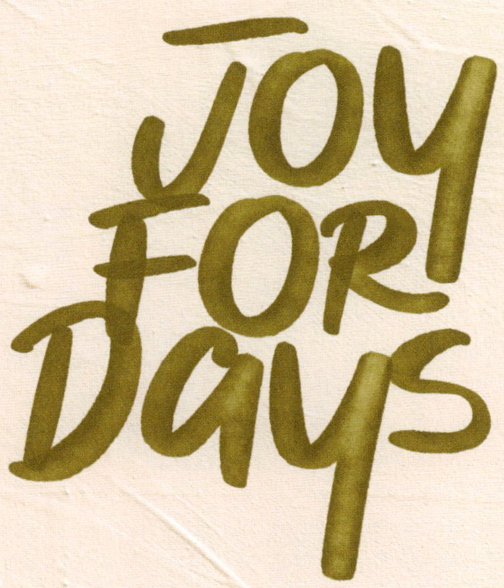

Foundational, daily practices to level up your happiness.

In the pursuit of identifying a recipe for what makes for a more happy and joyful life, some practices have been studied and tested more than others. One of my favourite happiness researchers and experts is Shawn Achor, who teaches Positive Psychology at Harvard (the most popular course in the university's history!). While traditional psychology focuses on how to treat people when things go wrong, Achor's classes, lectures and books are based on the scientific study of happiness.

Achor defines happiness as the joy we feel while striving toward our potential. He sees it not as a finish line, but rather a way of being. That's an important distinction because, as we've already explored, joy and happiness are not the same, though they are linked. Joy is internal, can be cultivated, and is lasting, while happiness tends to be external, more reactive, and momentary. They often show up together, but joy is the steady current running underneath, while happiness is the spark on the surface.

The good news is that happiness is largely a choice. While it's true that some of us are born happier than others due to our genetic make-up and environmental factors, our propensity to be happy or sad can be changed – and according to science, with minimal work. Studies have found that we all have the power to increase our baseline happiness.

I have said this already, but it's essential to come back to: this doesn't mean that we are aiming to be happy all the time. The ability to feel the full spectrum of emotions is necessary in order to live an authentic, balanced human life. Instead, this is about making a difference to how we feel when we're in 'neutral'.

Many of us have been raised to believe that if we work hard, we will become successful, and that success would make us happy. But this system is broken; what happens during all of the years we spend in the 'working-hard' phase? What happens if we never get to the level of success we crave? And if we do achieve our goals, we frequently discover that success is a moving goalpost. It brings us momentary happiness, and then we start dreaming up the next goal. I'm all for goals, I love challenging myself to see how far I can go, but this can't be the path to happiness.

Our dominant cultural belief about happiness is that it's mostly dependent on external factors (e.g. money, job title, good looks).

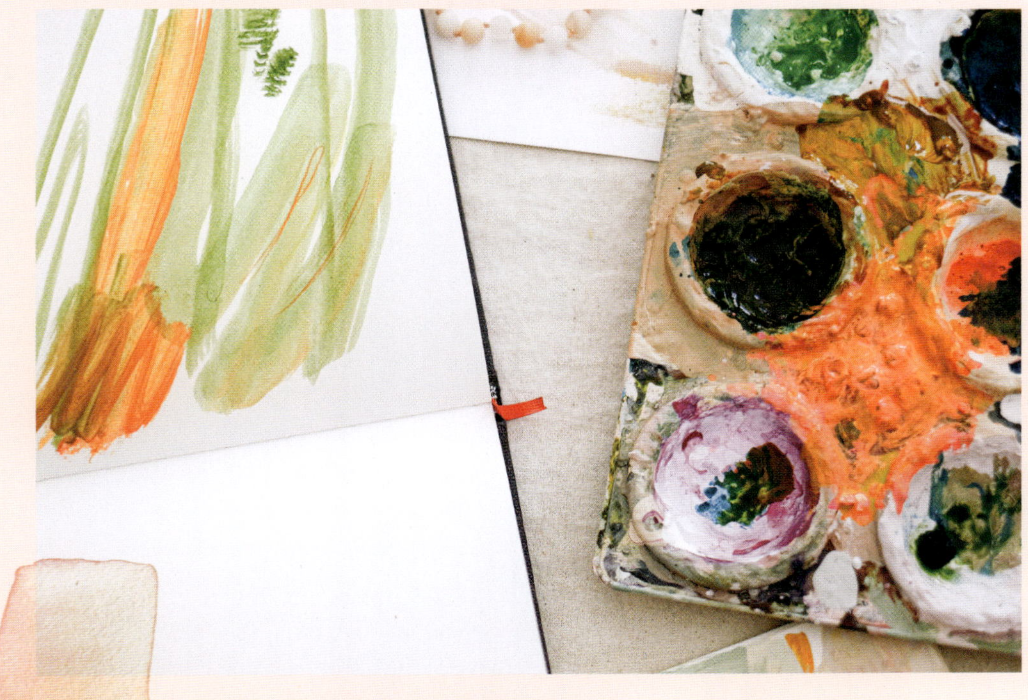

However, studies conducted by the top researchers in positive psychology, including Sonja Lyubomirsky, Kennon M. Sheldon, and David Schkade have flipped this belief on its head. Their research indicates that only 10 per cent of long-term happiness is based on life circumstances. Approximately 50 per cent of happiness is genetic, and the remaining 40 per cent is based on how we process the events in our lives and perceive the world around us. This is amazing because it means that WE have control over that 40 per cent, and therefore WE have the power to change how happy we are. If we focus on the negatives, our world feels negative; if we focus on the positives … well, we get happier!

Changing how we process and perceive the world might sound like a big ask, but according to Achor, it can be surprisingly straightforward and easy. He has developed six exercises to help people change their outlook, which we'll explore on the next couple of pages.

Participants in Achor's positive psychology studies were asked to spend two minutes a day on one of these exercises for 21 days, and the effects on their baseline happiness were profound. The study included people in their eighties who considered themselves low on the happiness scale. The results highlight these small tasks could override eight decades of negative programming and move their baseline happiness levels up.

TURN OVER FOR 6 EXERCISES FOR IMPROVING BASELINE HAPPINESS.

Shawn Achor's 6 exercises for improving baseline happiness

As most of these exercises can be done in two minutes a day, you can begin with one, building up to others as you feel so inclined. Start with the exercise that resonates the most with you.

1

Gratitude

Jot down three things you appreciated in the last day. These can include anything from a stellar cup of coffee to the warmth of sunshine. Try to find new things each day, rather than repeating yourself.

2

The doubler

Pick a positive moment from the past day and write about it in detail for two minutes. Reliving it is a form of savouring and re-experiencing the positive feelings, and this helps the good vibes to stick.

3

Meditation

Pause for two minutes daily to focus on your breath, or to do a quick guided meditation. There are oh-so-many of these on apps such as Headspace, Calm or Insight Timer, and also plenty on YouTube. It is a mini-break designed to bring calm and joy into your mind.

4

Conscious act of kindness

Begin each day by sending a kind message or compliment to someone. Achor suggests thinking of a person that you appreciate – maybe an old teacher or a current workmate – and writing them an email, or even better, calling them! Kindness is a powerful joy-maker.

5

The fun 15

Spend 15 minutes doing something active you enjoy, like dancing or walking. Regular light exercise works wonders for your mood.

6

Deepen social connections

Make time for loved ones. Strong relationships are key to happiness, success, and even longer life.

+

You'll notice that many of the exercises in this book fall into one of these six categories. This means every time you practise one of them, you're improving your baseline happiness!

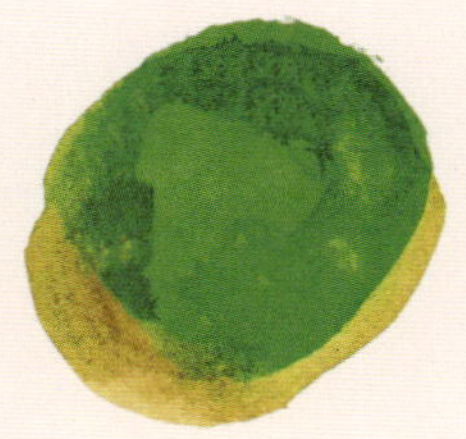

You are not your thoughts

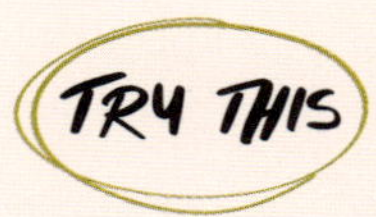

Next time you find yourself in a negative thought loop, stop for a few minutes and listen to your thoughts. Who is doing the listening and who is doing the talking? Which one of those is you? If you are the voice in your head, who is the *you* that is listening to that voice?

Have you ever noticed a voice in your head – almost like a narrator? The voice sounds so much like you that you may even think that it *is* you. It's there, giving a running commentary when you're annoyed, or berating you when you're messing up; at night, it runs through your increasing to-do list with a sense of urgency while you're trying to sleep. In fact, this voice babbles constantly – running over past situations and anticipating future possibilities, pointing out what might go wrong and trying to fix these fictitious situations before they happen.

This voice does an excellent job of pretending to be you, but it's most definitely *not* you. It is simply a stream of thoughts (repetitive ones, at that) formed from years of social conditioning and past experiences. The real YOU is the part observing those thoughts as they scroll past.

In some circles, this babbling voice is called the Ego (or small self), and the awareness that listens to that voice is called the Self (or true self). This division between the Self and the Ego underpins most mindfulness and meditation practices, but getting your head around this division of the Self can take a while, so don't worry if it's not making sense right now.

Here's another one of my favourite analogies: think of your thoughts as clouds. You are the clear, open awareness the thoughts are rolling through. You are not the storm or the rain, or the grey overcast days. Above and beyond those thought clouds is your true essence: calm, abundant, sky-like awareness.

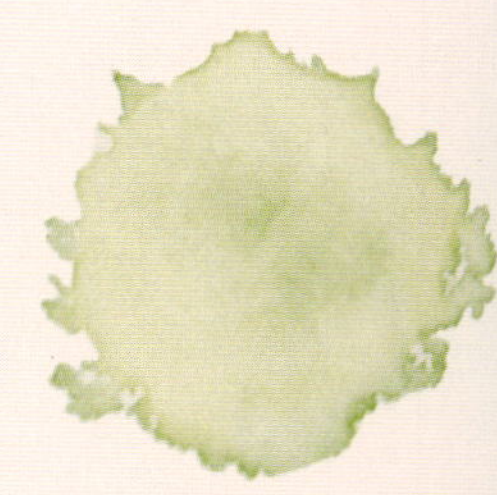

We can become so identified with our thoughts that if we have a series of storm clouds, we believe we are the storm. We might think, *I am an angry person* rather than *I feel angry*. There are ways to work with this – very well-researched and effective ways – that teach us to be more aware of our thoughts and to master them rather than them mastering *us*. One of the best ways to do this is by practising mindfulness, which we'll explore in more detail later in this chapter.

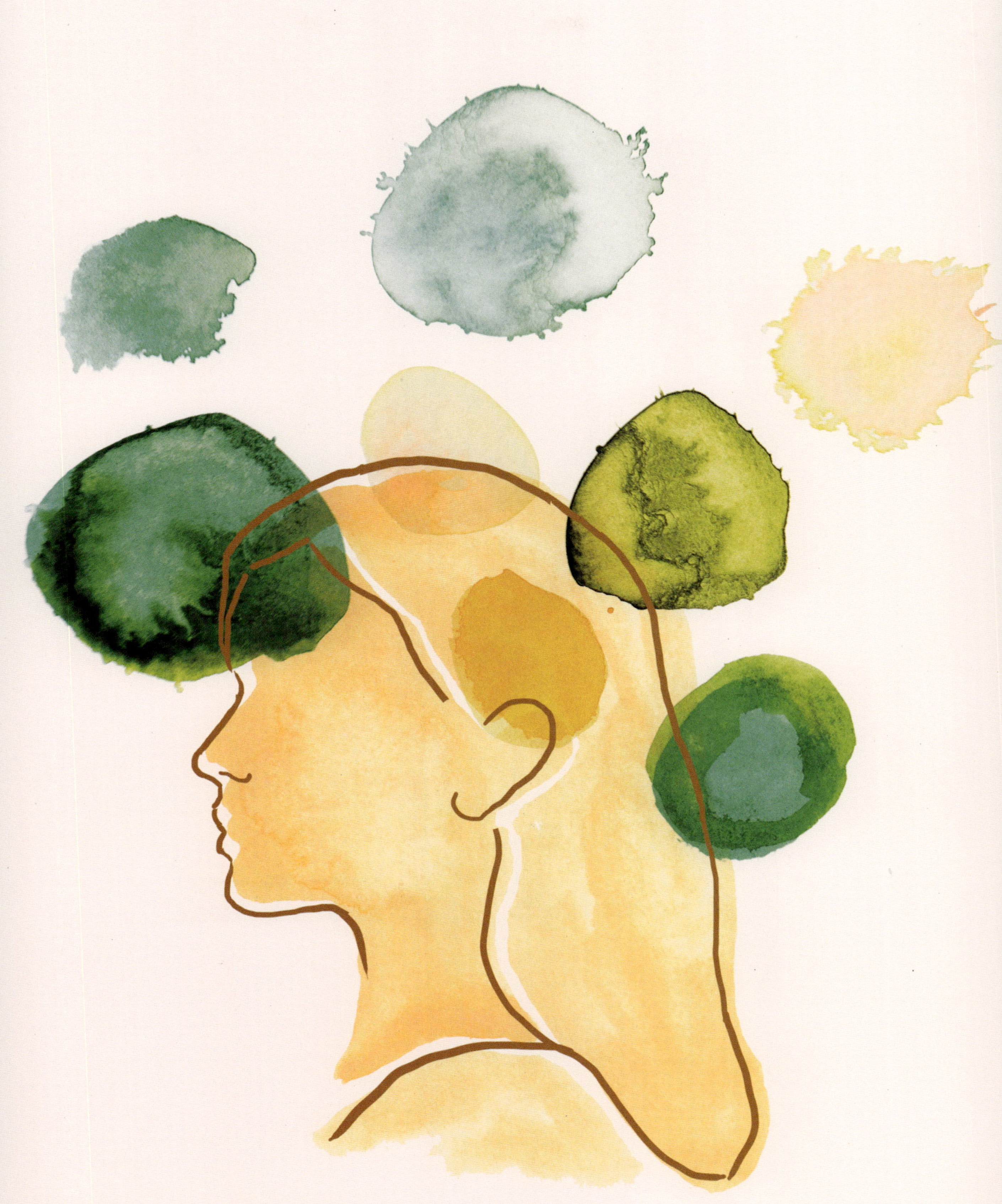

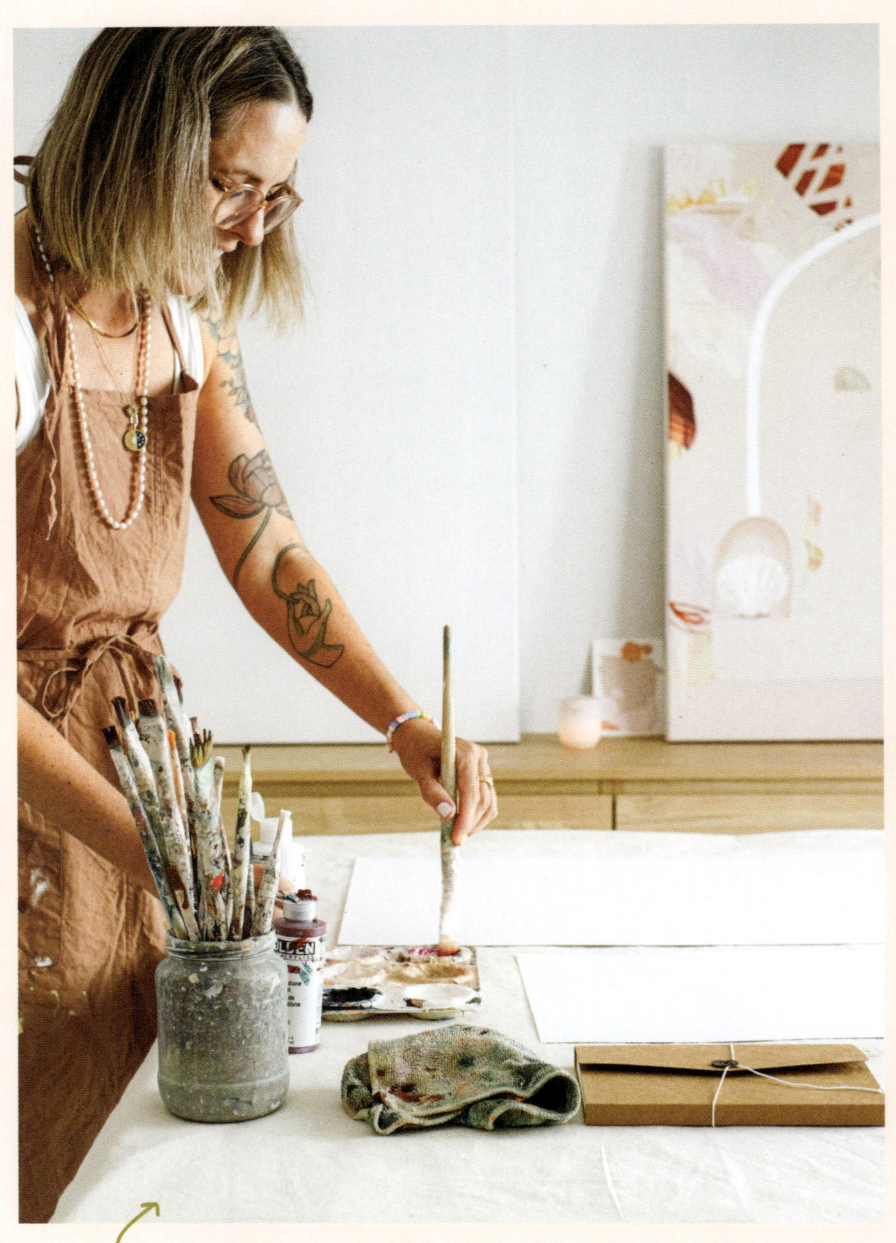

IN MY STUDIO, MY MIND CALMS DOWN AND I'M ABLE TO BE PRESENT AND CONNECT TO MY WORK.

The room-mate in our minds

Learning to distinguish between my inner voice and the thoughts in my head has been one of the most practical, transformative tools in my toolbox. In *The Untethered Soul* (this book will change your life btw!), author Michael A. Singer refers to this inner narrator as the 'know-it-all room-mate that you didn't choose, and who won't stop talking', and I've always found this analogy really helpful.

In an effort to protect you, your annoying room-mate will replay negative memories: e.g. *Remember how embarrassing it was when you got the wrong answer in class? Well, that could happen again today, so don't say anything. You'll sound like a fool.* Those negative memories are readily available thanks to your protective amygdala, and this is why it can be tough to stop the constant barrage of negative talk.

It can also be hard to separate truth from lies. After all, this voice has done such a good job of impersonating you over the years that you tend to believe it without question. But often, the story it's telling is totally unfounded in reality.

For example, say you text a friend to see if they want to meet up and they reply with a curt, *Sorry, can't*. Immediately, your noisy room-mate takes over. *Why is she being so rude?* it wonders. *Did I do something to offend her? Come to think of it, she was acting strangely last Friday, too. Well, if she wants to be like that, let's see how she likes it if I don't text for a few weeks. That will show her.*

In seconds, one rambling thought has taken over and escalated the situation. But if you stop for a moment to examine it more closely, you're likely to find there's no truth to it. Maybe your friend was in a rush and couldn't type more. Perhaps she pressed 'send' by mistake and plans to call you later. Any number of scenarios are possible, but your mind has jumped to the worst possible conclusion. Remember, don't believe everything you think. Your thoughts are not who you are.

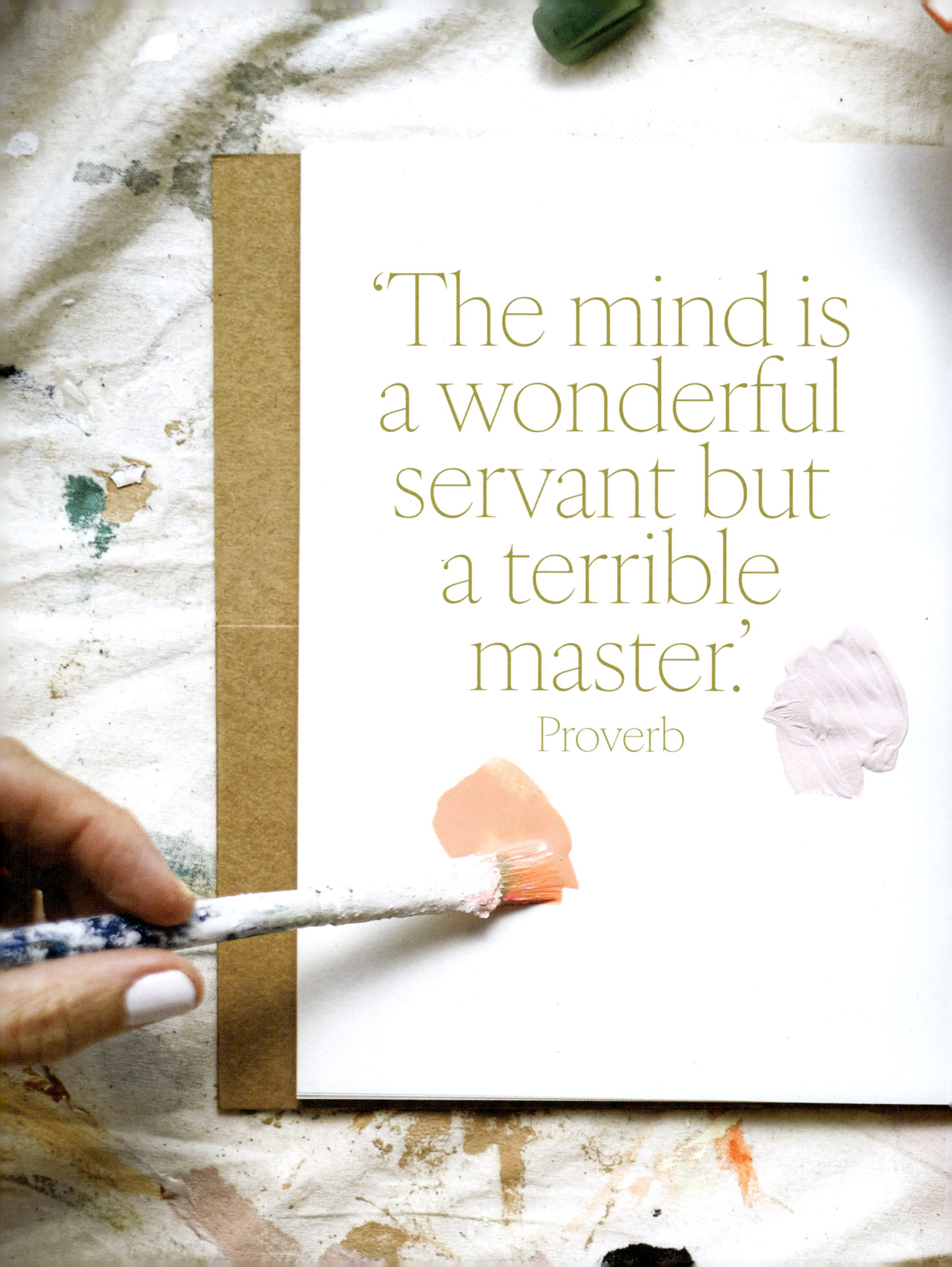

'The mind is a wonderful servant but a terrible master.'

Proverb

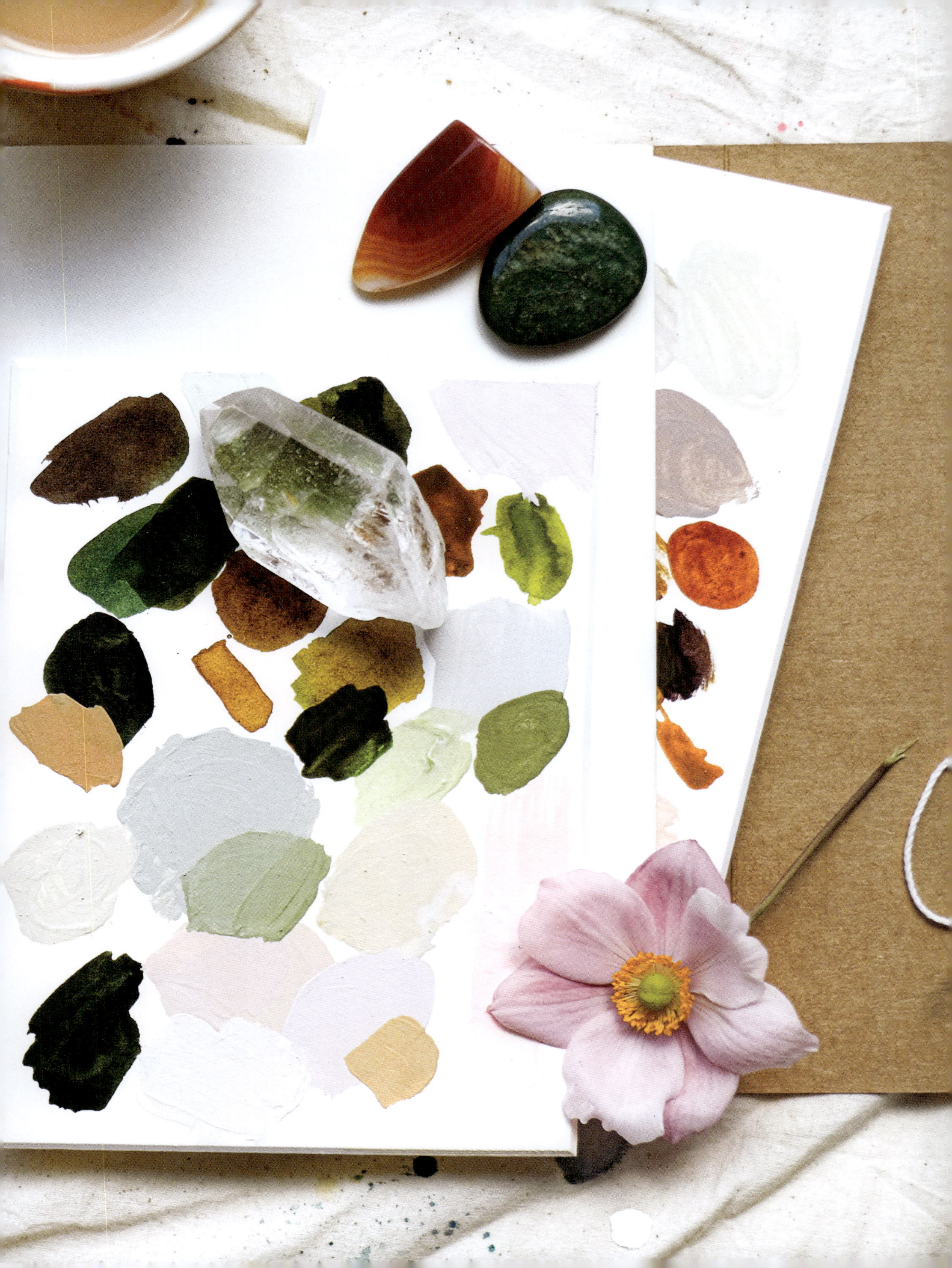

GRATITUDE IS THE QUICKEST, EASIEST PATH TO JOY. YOU CAN DO IT RIGHT NOW. SLOW DOWN, TAKE TIME TO APPRECIATE THE WONDERS AROUND YOU.

Gratitude

Gratitude is the quickest, easiest way to sculpt new neural pathways and enjoy a happier life. I am fascinated by the research on the dramatic effects gratitude practices can have on our state of mind, and I believe it's important to spread the word about it. Too often, we assume that something needs to be difficult in order to be transformative, but that's not the case here. There are so many ways to practise gratitude, and they couldn't be simpler.

Most studies on gratitude focus on subjects who are otherwise well, however the Greater Good Science Center at the University of California, Berkeley conducted research on people working through mental health issues such as anxiety and depression.

University students who had sought help from campus counselling services were randomly split into three groups. All three groups received the counselling they needed, but one group was also instructed to write one letter of gratitude to someone each week, for the first three weeks. The second group was asked to write about their thoughts and feelings about negative experiences, and the third group was given nothing extra to do beyond their counselling.

At four and twelve weeks, the letter-writing group felt better than both of the other groups after writing only three letters of gratitude! Minimal effort for great results.

The practice of gratitude has also been proven in studies to have lasting effects on the brain, making it one of the simplest pathways to a more joyful life. It almost seems too good to be true, and I urge you to try. What do you have to lose?

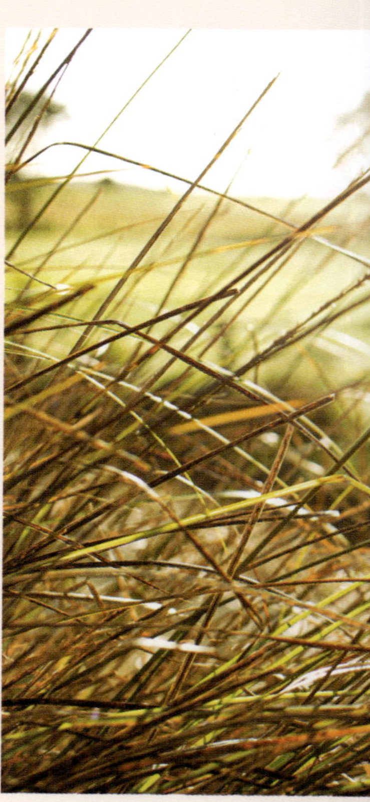

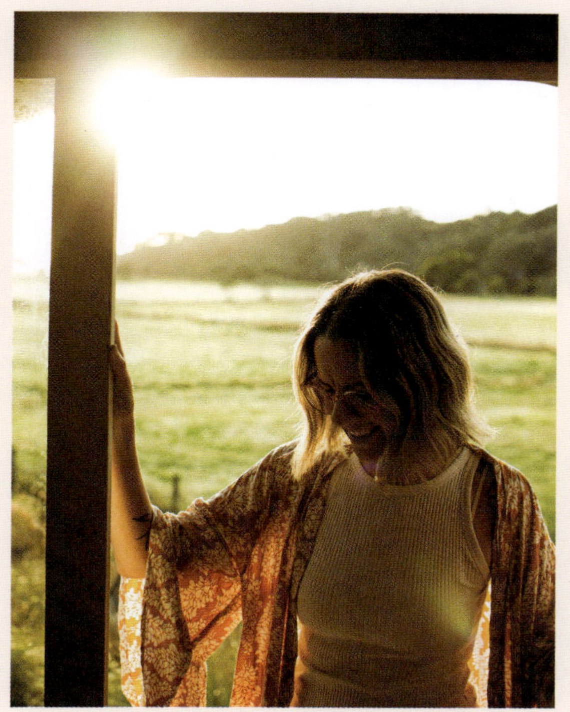

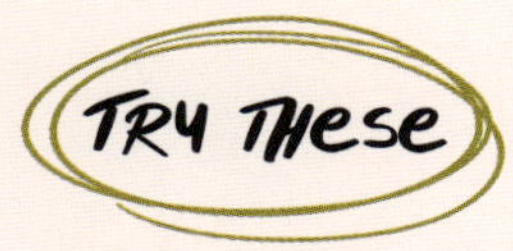

Pick one of these simple gratitude practices and stick to it for a few weeks to see how it helps.

1

Write and send a letter of gratitude once a week to someone you know. It could be a family member, an ex-teacher, a colleague, your partner or anyone you feel grateful for. It can be as simple as thanking them for their kindness, for inspiring you, or for a specific thing they have done for you.

2

Keep a journal next to your bed and each night, write down three things that you're grateful for. Try not to repeat the same things every time!

3

Start a gratitude chat group with some of your closest friends. Each day, send each other something you're grateful for. Sharing gratitude (or anything good!) with others always amplifies how good it feels.

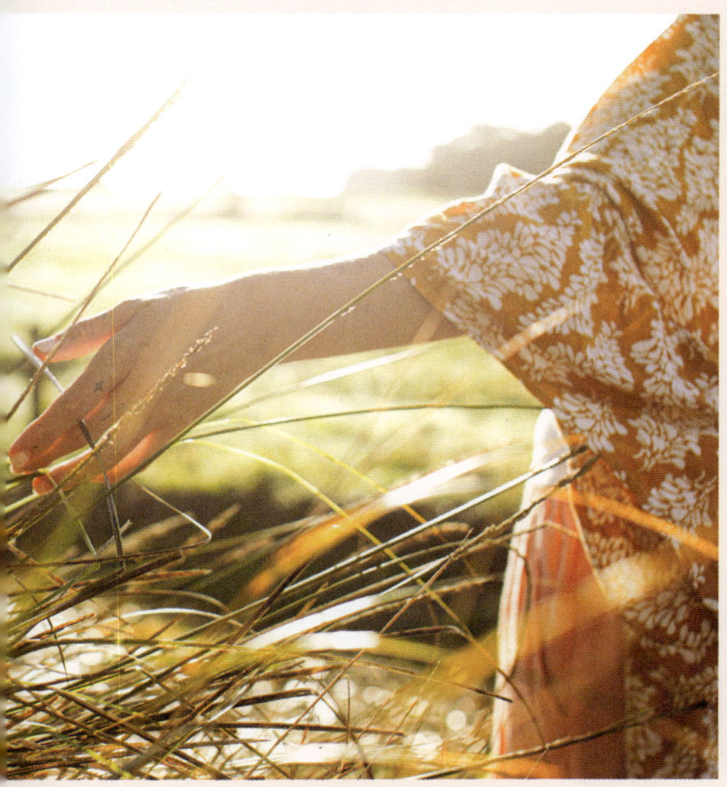

Mindfulness

Lots of us have dabbled in mindfulness, and a lot of us have probably become frustrated with it. Even if you've tried it, you might not have an answer to the question, *why practise mindfulness*? The answer is that it teaches us to observe situations and thoughts more objectively, and trains our brain to react appropriately to events.

With a consistent mindfulness practice, unimportant annoyances that once made us angry no longer trigger us. This doesn't mean we lose our passion or opinions; it just means that we're better able to identify what is worth being passionate or opinionated about. I'm here to tell you that you can pick your mindfulness mode. It doesn't have to be difficult or time-consuming; you don't have to do a 10-day silent Vipassana retreat (unless you want to). I have a few ways of looking at mindfulness that you might not have considered.

How does mindfulness work?

Buddhism teaches that when we are present in the moment, we cannot experience any suffering. The word 'suffering' might seem dramatic, but if you consider how much the voice in our head torments us on a daily basis – subjecting us to unnecessary stress and worry about scenarios that rarely materialise – that word suddenly seems a lot more accurate.

When we're being mindful of where we are and what we are doing in the present moment, that voice is temporarily silenced. Instead of ruminating about the past or the future, we are free to experience the reality of our sensations: what we feel, hear, smell, see and taste. And unless a real danger or issue interrupts us, those sensations bring us into a positive headspace where we are able to feel calm and at peace. Over time, we find that mindfulness helps us distinguish between real issues that need to be dealt with and things our brain is tricking us into worrying about.

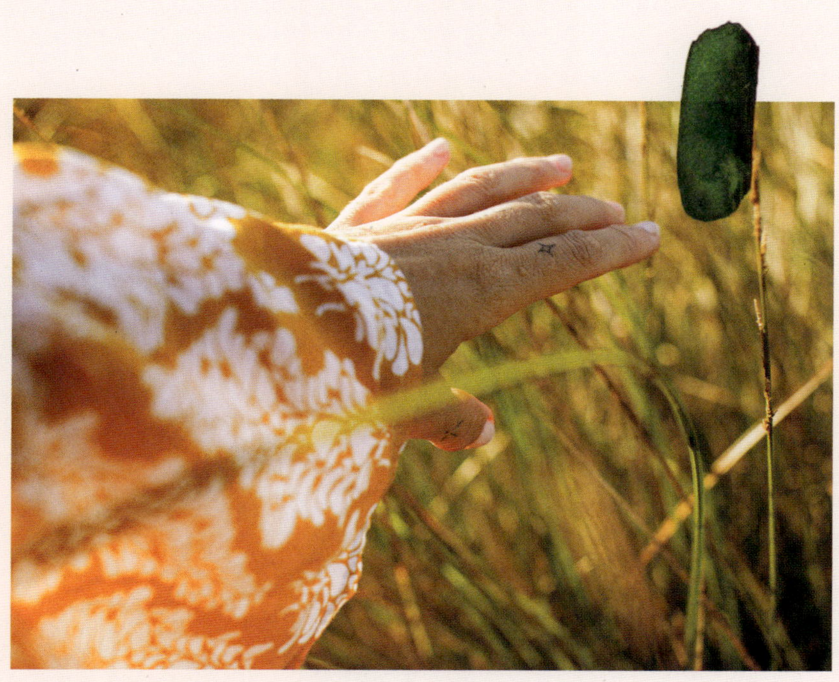

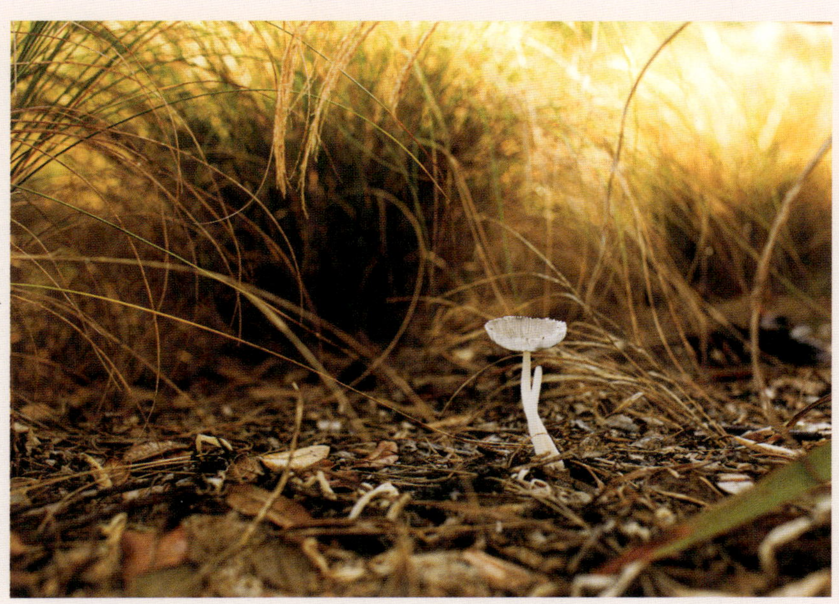

BE WHERE YOU ARE; THERE'S SO MUCH RICHNESS IN THE PRESENT. I SPOTTED THIS DELICATE LITTLE MUSHROOM ON AN EARLY MORNING ADVENTURE.

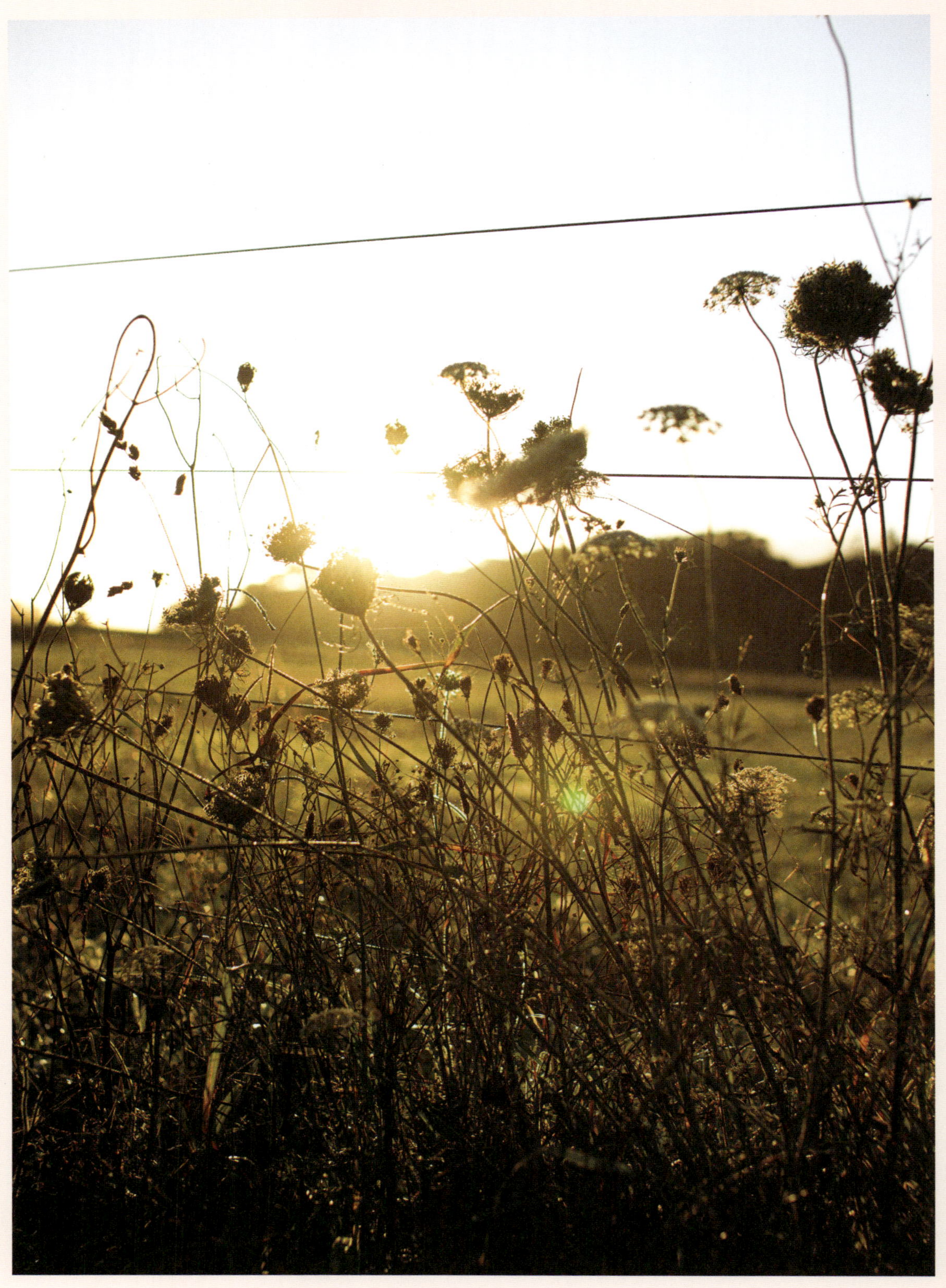

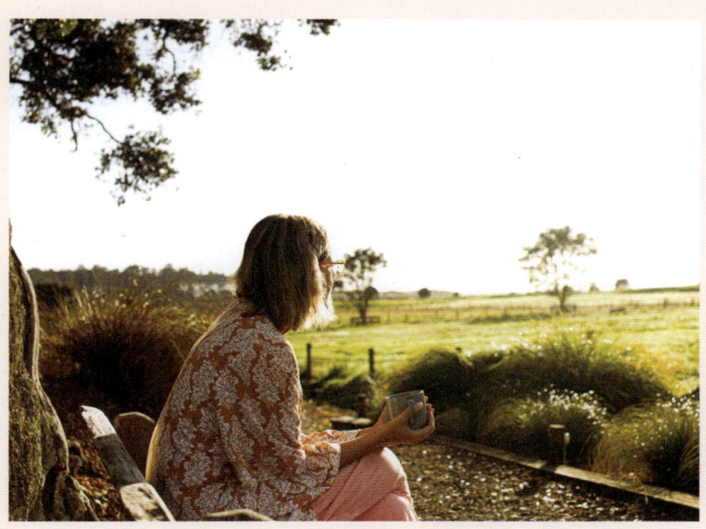

It's *being* without the baggage

The aim of practising mindfulness is to help us enjoy our lived experiences as they really are, rather than seen through the lens of whatever stories our brain tells about them. Take standing in a long queue, for example: we're conditioned to dislike queues, so we're likely to feel agitated or even angry when stuck in one.

But, if we pause for a few seconds and direct our attention to the sensations we're feeling rather than the story our brain is telling, our perception of this event can change. We might start to notice the aromas of freshly brewed coffee and warm pastries, we might tune into the music playing over the speakers, or notice the flowers on the table. From this vantage point, the actual sensation of being in a queue starts to be far less tedious.

You don't have to be a Zen master to reap the rewards of mindfulness, either. Even after many years of practising meditation, I still don't enter a transcendent state of nothingness. My brain ticks over at a rate of knots, yet now and then I experience a few moments of peace. I keep returning to this practice because I see how it benefits my life. Cultivating small pauses of mindful observation between an event and your reaction to it can completely change how you live your life.

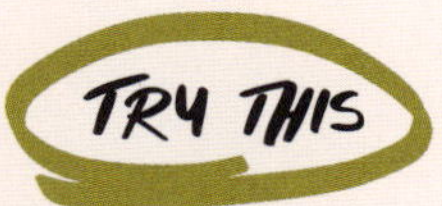

Mindfulness can be quick and easy. This first approach is an espresso shot of mindfulness that can be done anywhere, at any time.

1

Right now, put down this book.

2

Squeeze your hands into tight fists for the count of 20.

3

Close your eyes. Notice your attention shift from the world around you to your internal world and the sensations of the body.

Four different ways to practise mindfulness

1

Mindfulness vs mindlessness

Professor Ellen Langer, a social psychologist and researcher at Harvard University offers a new way of looking at mindfulness. She sees it as 'actively noticing'. It's simple really, no meditation is necessary, and you reap the same benefits. Most of us are constantly in a state of mindlessness where we are doing one thing and thinking of another.

When we actively notice things around us, we are in the present moment. Langer suggests making a point of noticing five new things in each situation (particularly situations that you partake in every day). Her research shows that this simple act enlivens us, bringing context to our situation, and improving our mental state.

2

Mindful moments

This is a practice I love because it fits in with my lifestyle, and the benefits are real. Pick a few daily rituals, for example, brushing your teeth, getting into the car, getting a drink of water, or having a cup of tea. Make these habits reminders to take a mindful moment. If you're brushing your teeth, take a deep breath first, then focus intently on your brushing, rather than checking your phone or tidying your bathroom while you do it. Be in the moment.

When I'm driving, I like to notice the feeling of my hands on the steering wheel – it's a simple, powerful way of coming out of my mind, and into my body. If you tend to forget to do this, jog your memory by placing a few dot stickers wherever your habits take place.

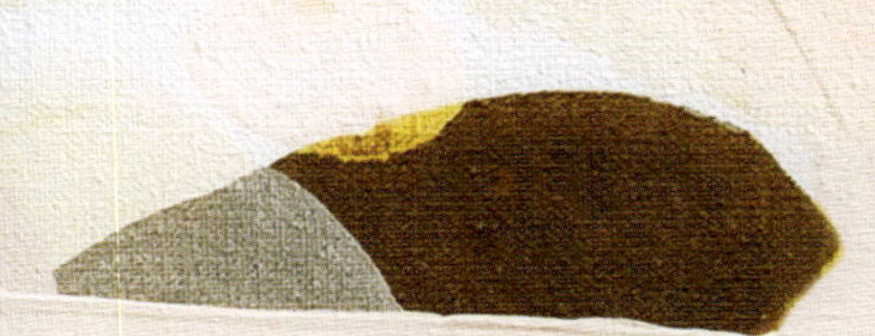

3

Mindful activity

Engaging in a consuming physical activity can be very mindful. For me, it's yoga. I recommend *Yoga with Adriene* on YouTube because her classes are free and she is incredible.

✦

Focusing on every movement and sensation in my body leaves me with a complete joy buzz, even after just a 15-minute practice. If the idea of yoga has you yawning, never fear. Rock climbing and surfing are two unbelievably mindful endeavours. You are so focused on your next move and the environment around you that you are present.

✦

Not into physical exertion? Art can also be a powerful mindfulness tool, which is why I've included some wonderful mindful art exercises in chapter eight.

4

Mindfulness meditation

Mindfulness meditation has been highly researched, and shown to be hugely valuable with countless benefits. If you're new to meditating, don't fear, there are many easy ways of starting that don't include becoming a Buddhist monk or chanting with your crystals under moonlight (although both options could be enticing).

✦

Mindfulness meditation can be as simple as paying attention to your breath and noticing your thoughts. There are some fabulous apps such as Headspace and Insight Timer to help you get started. You can also find guided meditations on YouTube. Try one out, and if you enjoy it, do it again tomorrow. If you don't, try another one. There are so many options, you're bound to find one that you enjoy.

✦

If you would like to take your meditation further, there are many ways to do this. I started my journey with a 10-day Vipassana retreat. This was quite an extreme way in, but very beneficial. Research meditation courses in your area or any online options that feel like they are at a level you are comfortable with.

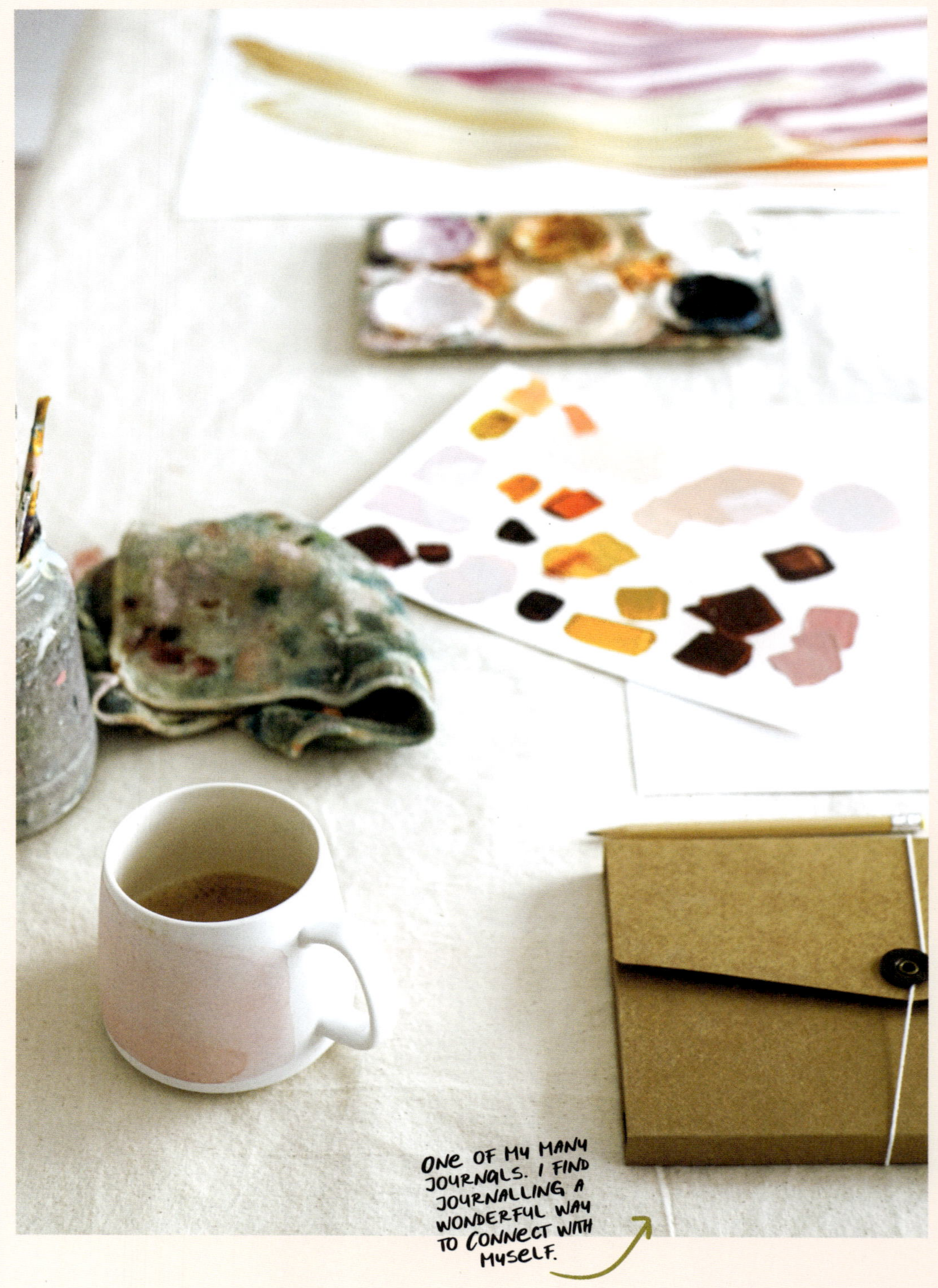

ONE OF MY MANY JOURNALS. I FIND JOURNALLING A WONDERFUL WAY TO CONNECT WITH MYSELF.

Journalling

One of my favourite practices is journalling. Though I try to be consistent with it, there are many days I don't open my journal. But that's okay, I know that I get a lot of benefits from the practice, even though it isn't 'perfect'. Journalling happens to be one of the most effective ways to explore what's going on inside of us, and it can help us reconnect with our true self. Writing things down has been shown to have many benefits.

- It helps us to process emotions and release stress.
- Improves mood and emotional regulation.
- Increases clarity and self-awareness.
- Increases the likelihood of following through on goals.

Putting thoughts down on paper not only gives shape to them, it also helps us better understand our inner landscape and find clarity. You don't need to be a 'writer' to journal because this practice is for you, not anyone else.

There are many approaches to this daily practice, so if traditional journalling isn't your thing, try another style until you find one that works for you. A good old-fashioned brain dump or daily gratitude list works for some people, while others find that a soulful, emotional style feels natural. Jotting down song lyrics that reflect your mood might do the trick some days.

Alternatively, you might lean into visual journalling, either by sketching, or by pressing leaves, scraps and other little treasures from daily life into the pages. This can be a great way of noticing what you love, what you long for, or just what's on your mind. This is your space, so make it yours.

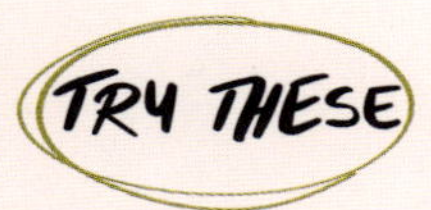

Start a love list

Grab a pretty book. At the top of the page write the words 'I Love', then list everything that you love – big, small, beautiful, insignificant, silly or strange. You can do this once, or start an ongoing list that you add to every now and then.

Morning pages

One of the most well-known journalling practices comes from Julia Cameron's book, *The Artist's Way*. The goal is simply to write three pages, by hand, first thing in the morning. No editing, no overthinking – just a stream of whatever's on your mind. This practice clears mental clutter, helps you hear your own voice, and often leads to unexpected insights. Think of it as a brain dump meets a gentle self-check-in.

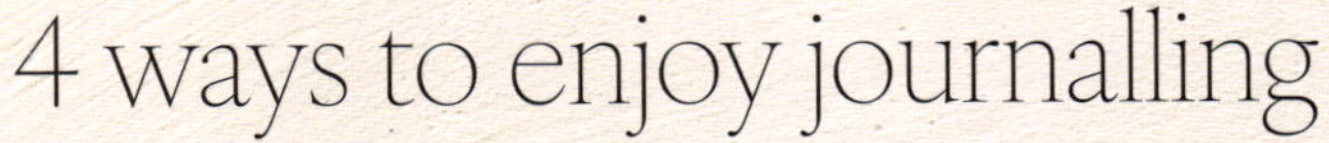

4 ways to enjoy journalling

There's no one 'right' way to journal. Here are a few playful and creative twists to get you started. Which ones resonate with you?

1
Scrapbook

Glue in ticket stubs, receipts, photos, dried flowers, or mementos from the week. Let your journal become a time capsule – messy, tactile, and completely yours.

2
Doodles

Draw your coffee cup. Sketch your dog's ears. Fill a page with swirls or nonsense shapes. Visual journalling is a brilliant outlet if words aren't flowing.

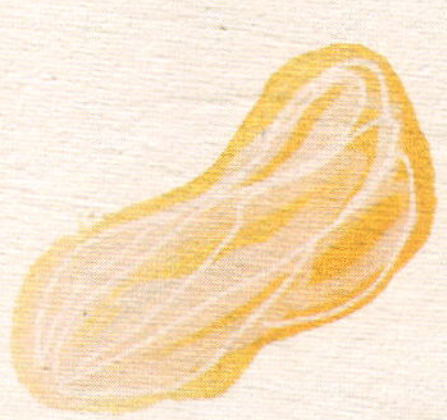

3
Colour your mood

Pick a colour that matches how you're feeling, and use it to fill a page. Scribble, draw blocks or loose shapes, anything goes. Let colour do the talking when words don't quite fit.

4
One-line reflections

At the end of each day (or week), jot down one sentence that captures something real: a moment, a mood, a thought, or a win. No pressure to explain – just one line to mark that day as lived.

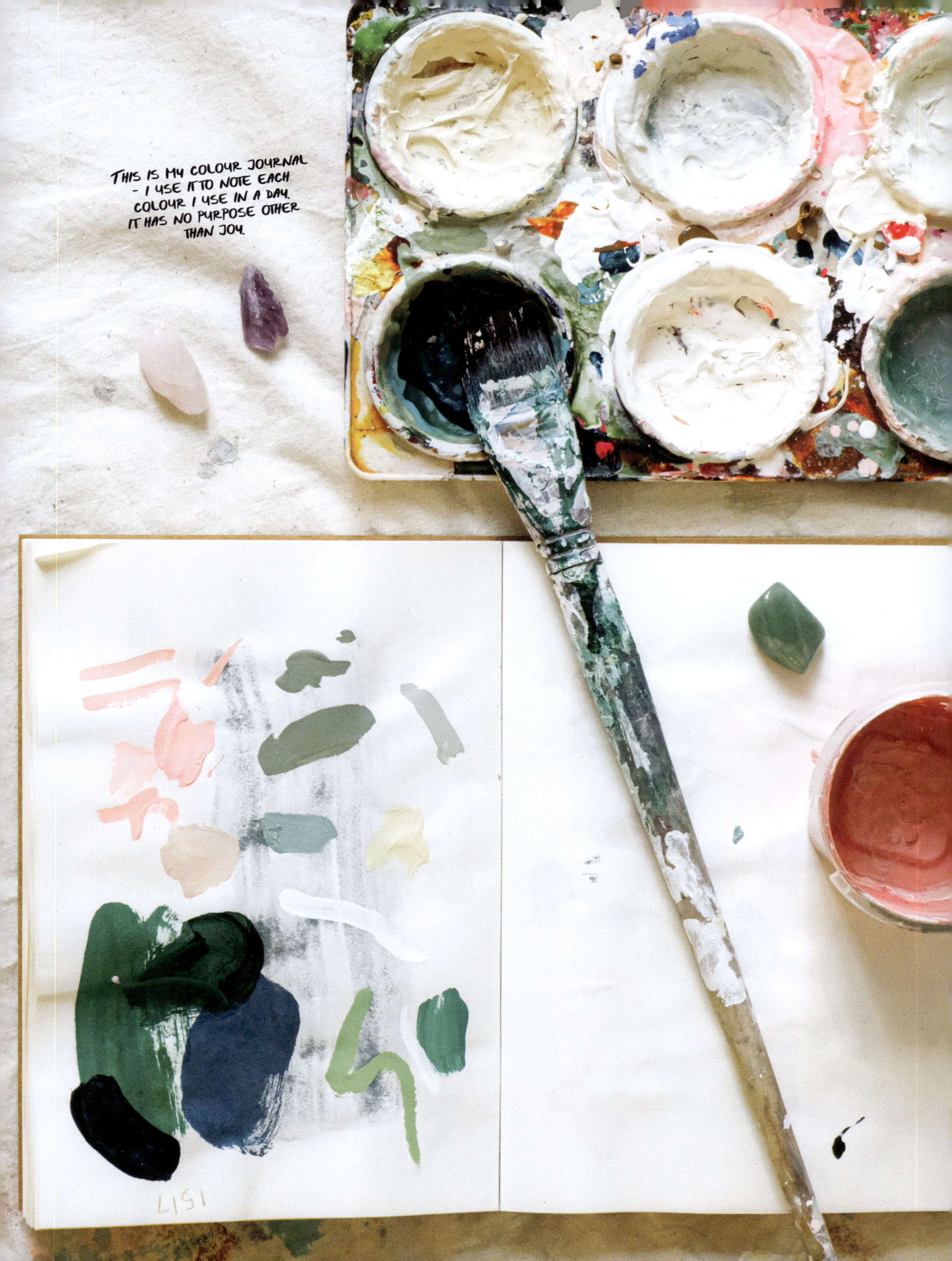

THIS IS MY COLOUR JOURNAL - I USE IT TO NOTE EACH COLOUR I USE IN A DAY. IT HAS NO PURPOSE OTHER THAN JOY.

Elizabeth Gilbert's 'Letters From Love'

In 2023 I came across a new journalling practice thanks to writer Liz Gilbert. I'm a massive 'Liz fan girl' (yes, I like to refer to her as Liz) because her enthusiasm for life is contagious, and it's impossible not to fall a tiny bit in love with her presence. When it comes to the hard things in life, it feels like she really 'gets it'. Liz's daily journalling practice is called 'Letters from Love', and the intention behind the practice is to ask 'Love' a question and then channel Love's response to you in the form of a written letter. It feels very mystical, and I believe it is, but even if you don't have a mystical bone in your body – this practice still works!

Liz thinks of 'Love' as being a higher power: God, Spirit, the Universe, Source, or whatever you call it. Personally, I love the idea of calling God 'Love' because it removes the image of an old bearded white man on a cloud throwing lightning bolts down at those who don't obey his rules. I grew up Catholic, so that image was quite heavily etched into my mind.

I think of 'Love' as the energetic field that holds us all together and creates all things, but if you don't believe in a higher power, think of 'Love' as being the wisest, most loving part of yourself. Interestingly, when 'Love' replies to me, it comes through as a collective energy, referring to themselves as 'we'. Connecting to Love – whether it's an internal or external force – always results in beautiful advice that can hold you through challenging times and celebrate with you when things are going well.

All you need is paper, a pen and a quiet place. As you start writing, the reply will naturally form itself. It doesn't take long, and you might be amazed at how easily the words flow. Write without thinking, and keep going until the letter feels done. This practice is part journalling, part channelling, and part connecting to a soothing, loving energy that makes you feel safe and adored.

On her Substack, Liz shares letters written by her, as well as by some of her wonderful friends, such as Glennon Doyle, Martha Beck, Abby Wambach and Pico Iyer; members of the public can share their letters too. Through this sharing of letters online, I began to understand the magic of the practice, and I fell in love instantly after trying it for myself. It's now something I do on a near-daily basis. If you try ONE thing in this book, I think it should be this.

I think of 'Love'
as the energetic
field that holds us all
together and creates
all things, but if you
don't believe in a higher
power, think of 'Love'
as being the wisest,
most loving part
of yourself.

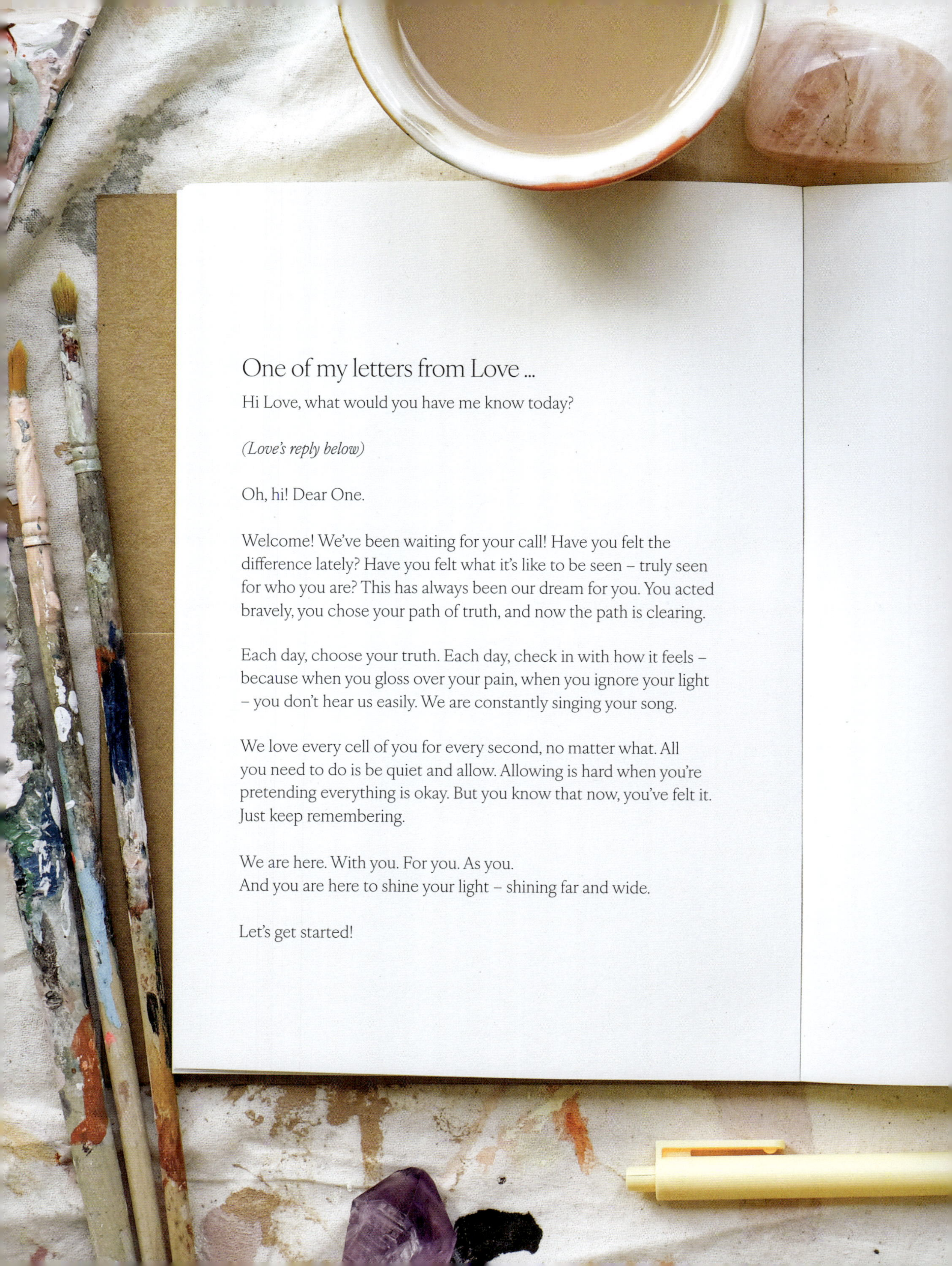

One of my letters from Love ...

Hi Love, what would you have me know today?

(Love's reply below)

Oh, hi! Dear One.

Welcome! We've been waiting for your call! Have you felt the difference lately? Have you felt what it's like to be seen – truly seen for who you are? This has always been our dream for you. You acted bravely, you chose your path of truth, and now the path is clearing.

Each day, choose your truth. Each day, check in with how it feels – because when you gloss over your pain, when you ignore your light – you don't hear us easily. We are constantly singing your song.

We love every cell of you for every second, no matter what. All you need to do is be quiet and allow. Allowing is hard when you're pretending everything is okay. But you know that now, you've felt it. Just keep remembering.

We are here. With you. For you. As you.
And you are here to shine your light – shining far and wide.

Let's get started!

JOURNALLING IS MY DAILY INTUITIVE PRACTICE.

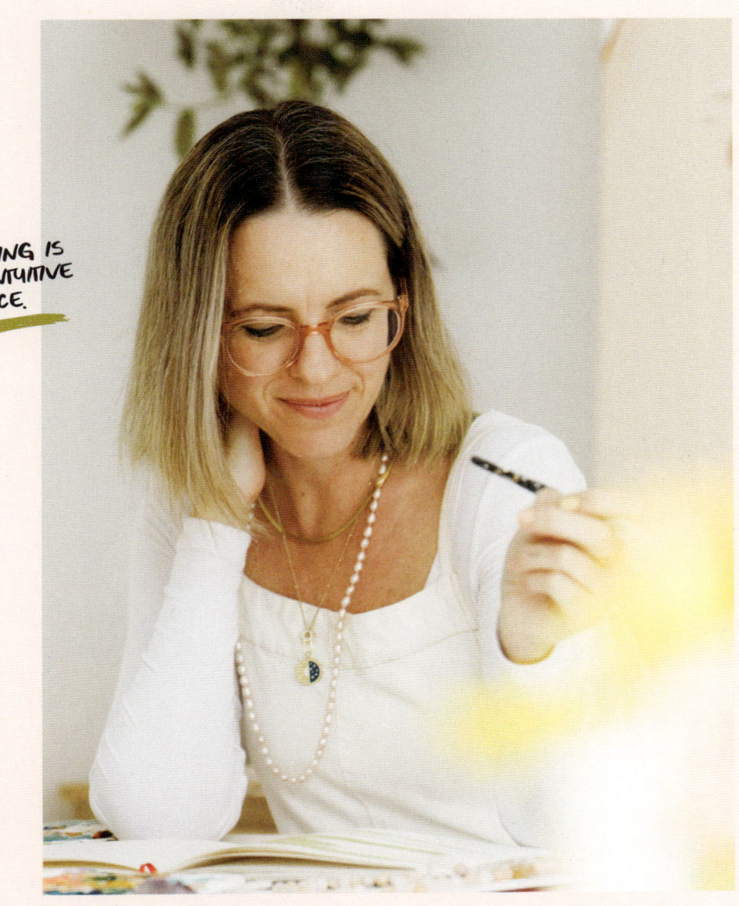

For the first few years Liz wrote these daily letters, the responses from Love were the same: it told her that she was incredibly loved and that it was there for her whenever she needed it. It was only when Liz started believing that message at her core that Love started giving her specific life advice.

The beauty of writing these letters, for me, has been discovering that Love thinks I'm special. And the thing is, it thinks that of all of us – that's the incredible thing about connecting with this energy. It's here to remind us of how magical we all are. We spend so much time listening to the angry, inner critic that it often rules our lives. We make choices based on what it says and live in fear and worry. The voice of Love is a powerful replacement that will guide us in ways that open beautiful doors and create a joy-filled life.

Try it. Just once. Even a single letter might have a huge benefit – but I have a feeling you will want to do it again and again – and maybe even turn it into a daily practice.

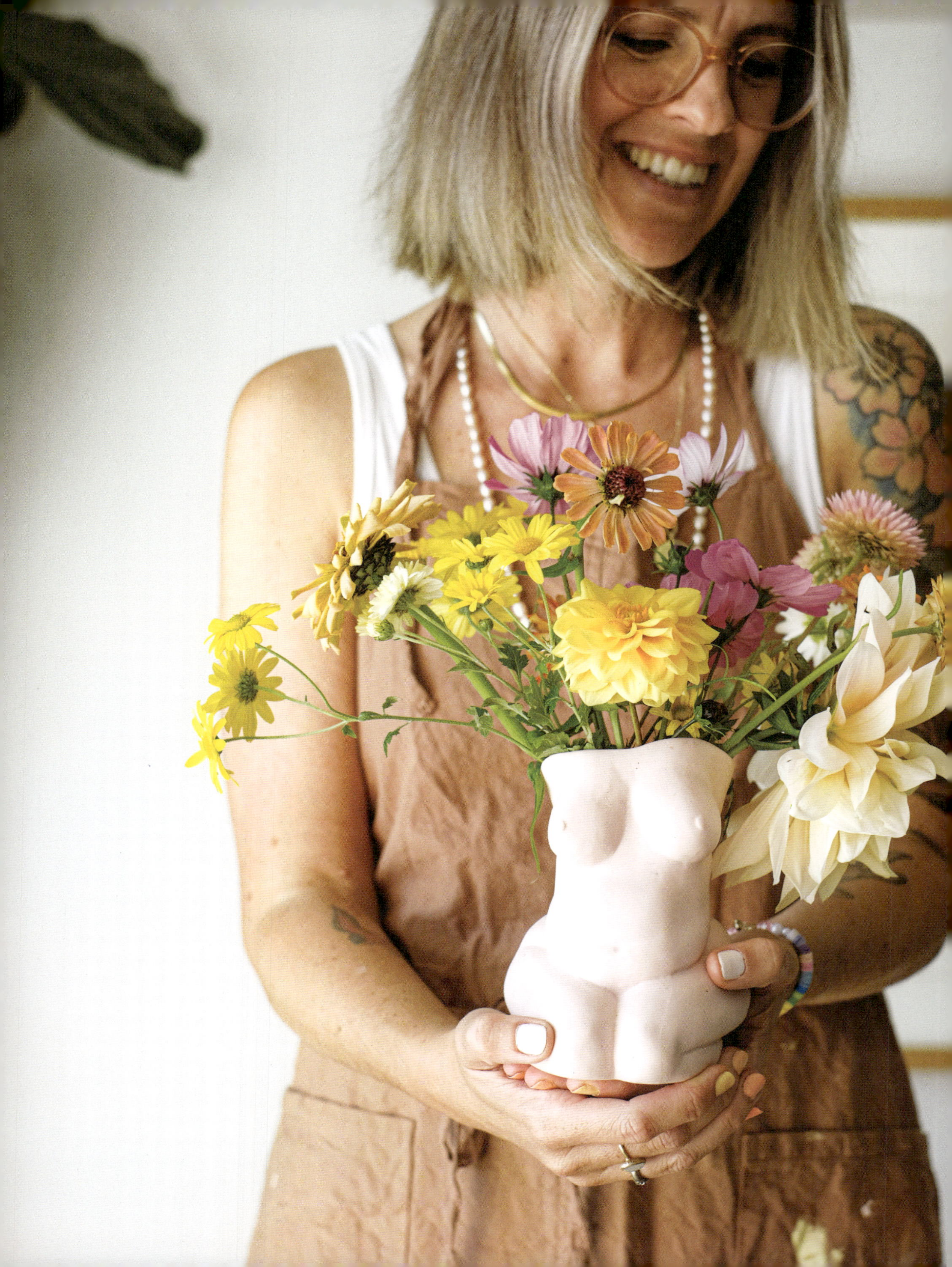

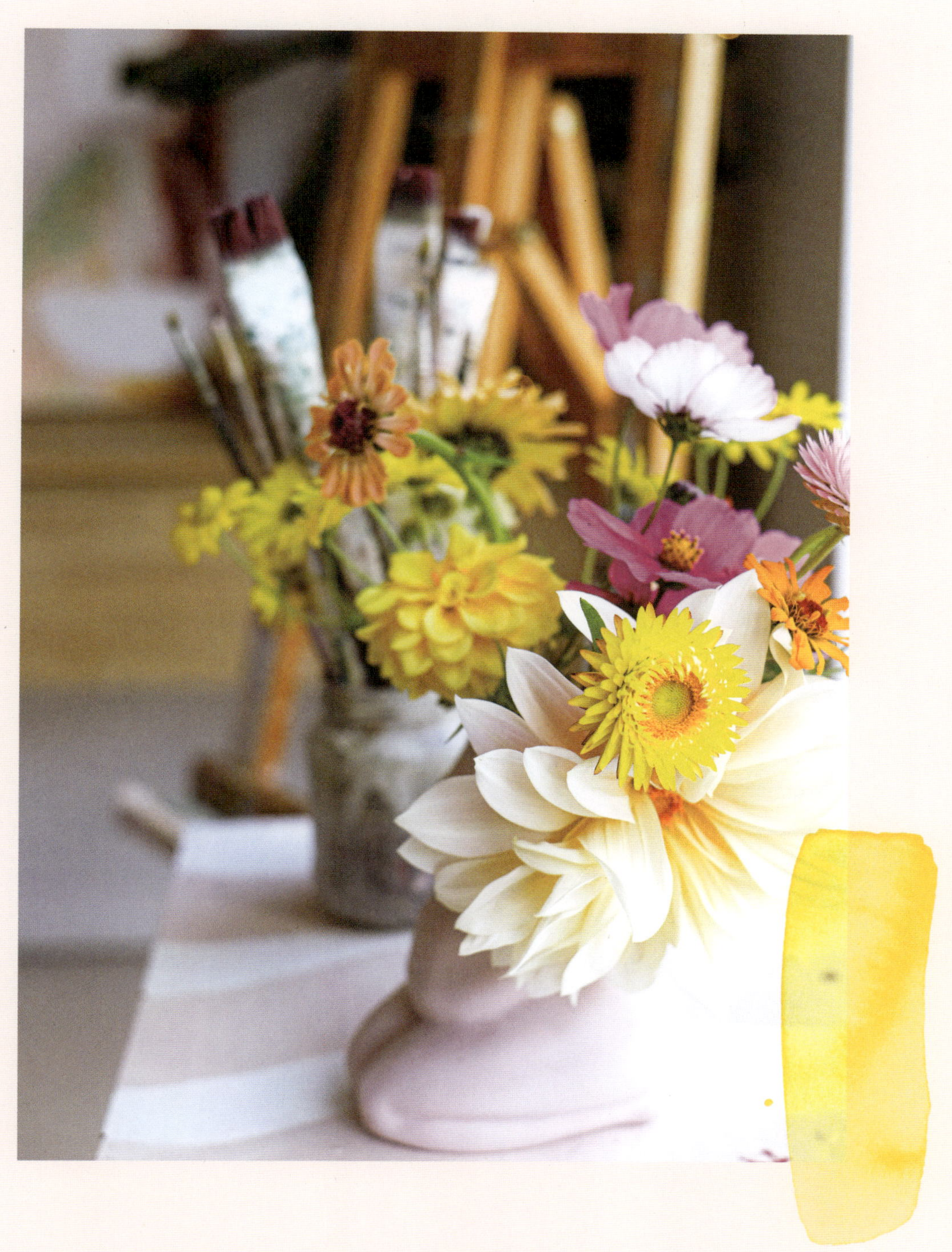

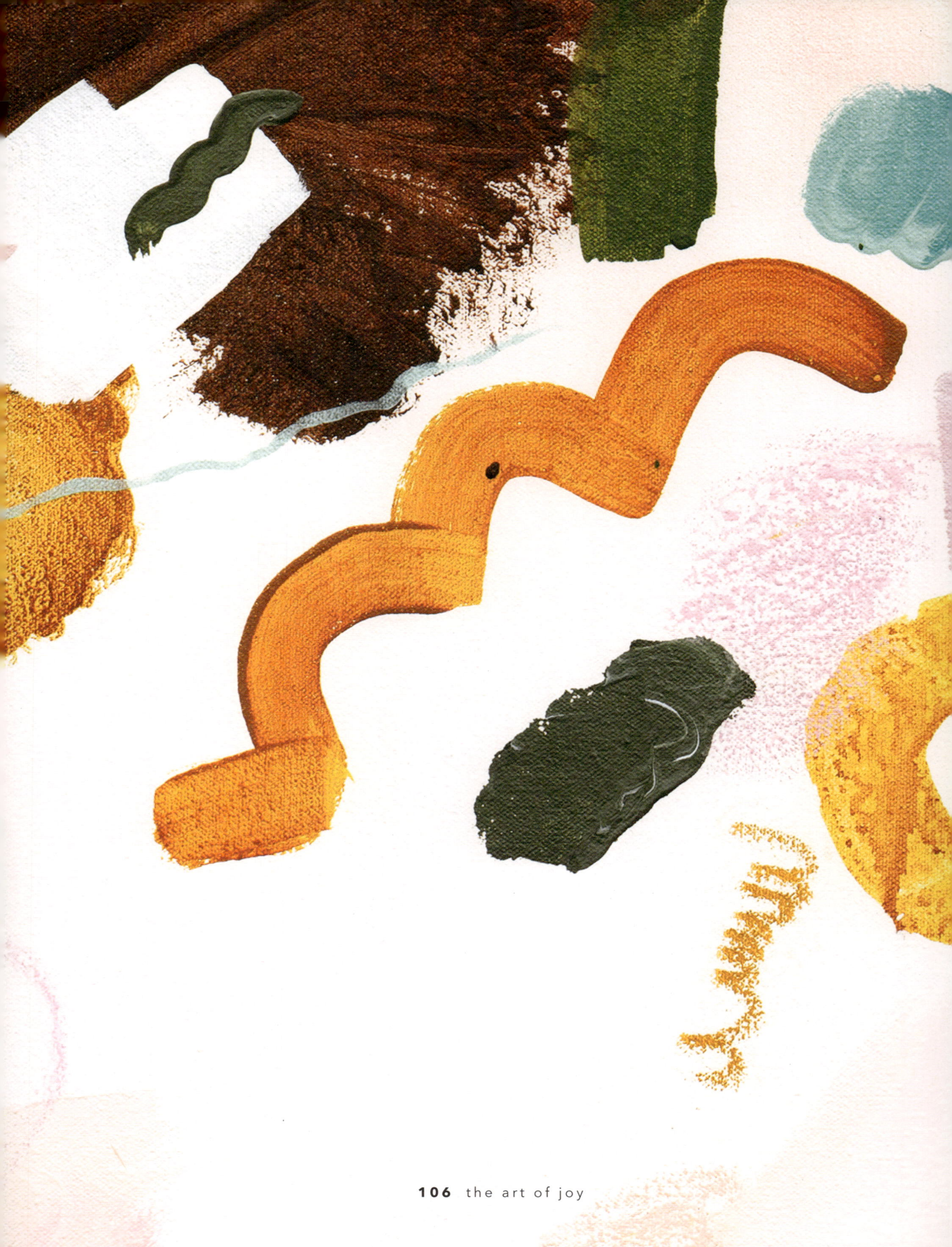

chapter seven

You're never too old to play

The art and power of play for grown-ups.

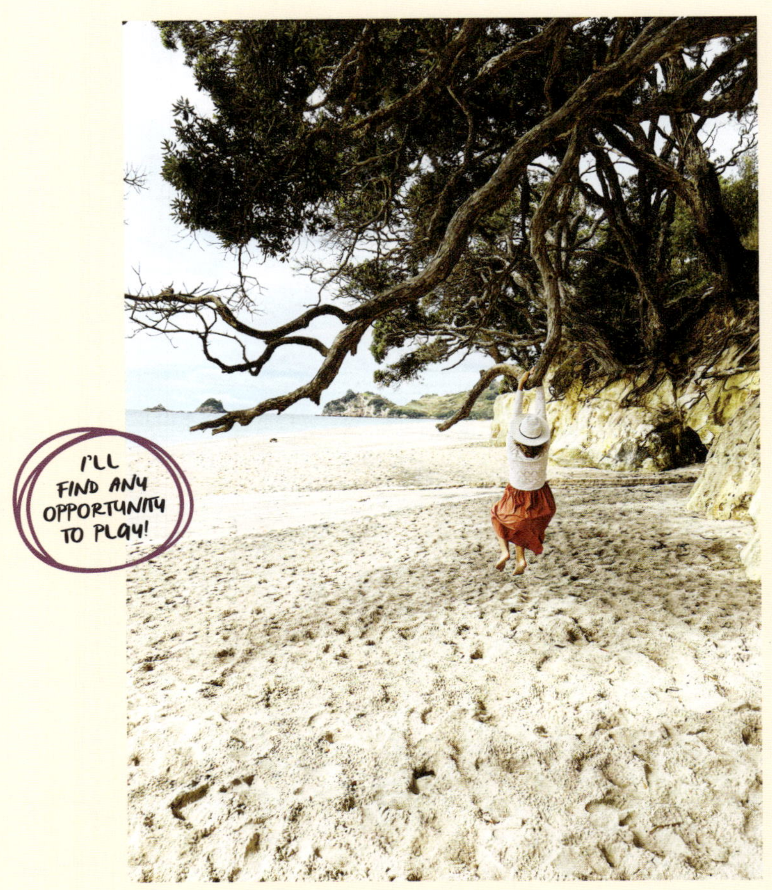

Play is synonymous with childhood, and often viewed as a frivolous pursuit to be swapped for paying taxes and doing the dishes. As we grow up, we're conditioned by society and circumstances to make every minute of the day as productive as possible – what use are we without productivity? The reality, though, is that if we lose our capacity to play, those parts of ourselves calcify. We get sucked into the mundane and lose our ability to do something for the sheer joy of it.

Play isn't just fun; it has some quite wonderful neurological benefits (not that I'm trying to justify it as productive, but it's fascinating to know and might get a few more of you over the line!). It stimulates the prefrontal cortex, that part of the brain that helps regulate emotions, makes decisions and connects the other parts of our brain to each other. As we explored earlier, the prefrontal cortex is the calm, measured cousin of our guard dog, the amygdala. Play has been known to improve cognitive function, decrease stress and improve creativity. Without play we can become irritable and overwhelmed.

Reclaim the magic of play

When I started painting again, the freedom and playfulness it provided were exquisite. The sheer delight of mixing colour, creating things that weren't there before, and watching what would unfold was absolutely an act of play. While I slowly turned it into something productive, an art business, the play part of my work slowly diminished. I was still enjoying it, and it definitely beat sitting at a desk in an advertising agency, but the freedom of play was no longer there. To counter this, I occasionally take a break from painting things to sell and let myself have a few days (or sometimes only a few hours) to create without an outcome – to play with paint. It invigorates my creative mind (ha, there I go, trying to turn it into something productive!), and it feels good. I think the main difference in this case is not having a plan – letting my own joy and little surprises along the way guide the process.

I can hear the mums reading this saying, 'Oh gosh, play is *not* fun for me. My child is constantly asking me to play a game with them and spending that entire time bossing me around. It's equal parts dull and frustrating!' I hear you, and I have something controversial to say … playing with your child is often not playing. It's work. It is parenting. The way particularly smaller children play is not enjoyable for adults. We do it (lovingly) to connect with them and make them feel loved and seen, but that doesn't necessarily mean that it's fun for us.

We each need to find our own ways of playing, and uncovering yours might not be as simple as it was for me. What if you're not arty? What if you don't want to go surfing or play a game of tennis? (For me, sport is terrifying.) It's okay if finding your way of playing is a process. It's okay if you don't know what you like to do for fun. Remember, as adults, we have been heavily conditioned to leave play behind.

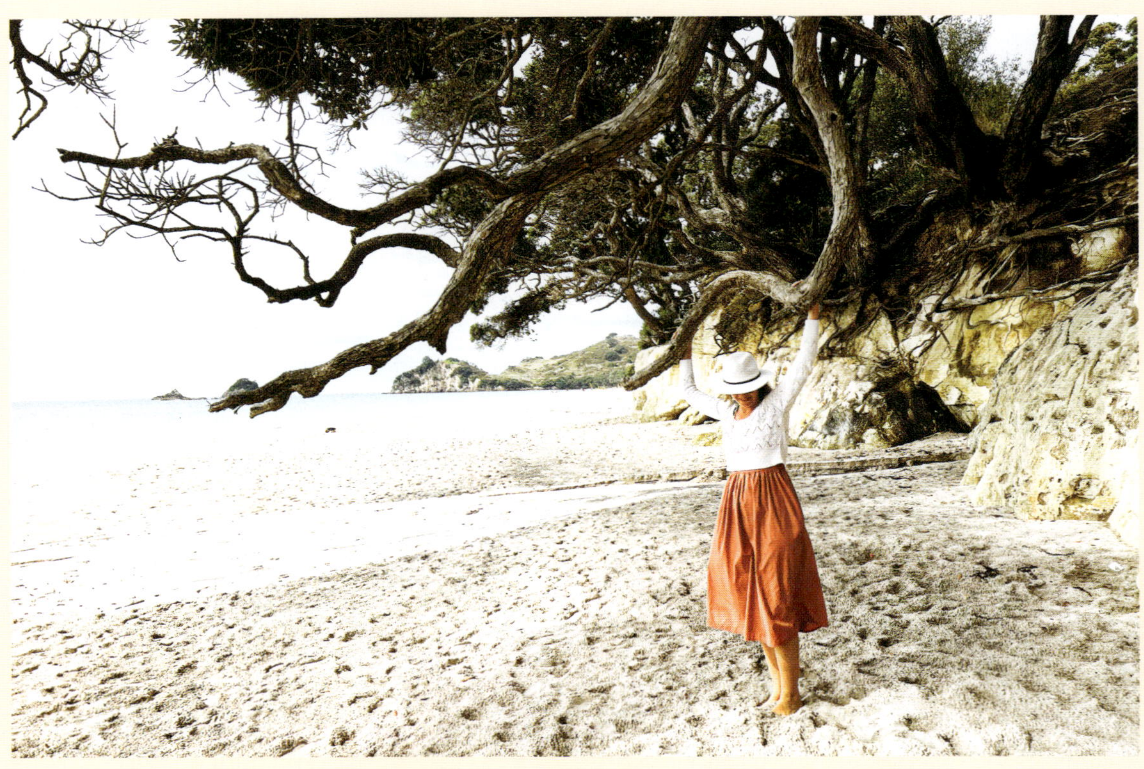

Three tips to bring play into your life

1. The first step is to carve out time for yourself with no productive goal. You'll most likely have to schedule this so that you take it seriously. Start with just 15 minutes a week (if you can find more time or do this more often, even better!). Whatever you do, don't let yourself stare at your phone during this 'play' time. Phones are the thieves of so many excellent opportunities.
2. If you aren't sure what you want to do with this time, try writing in a journal. Start by writing *Right now, I feel like* ... and list any ideas that come to you. If nothing comes up, next time, have some crafting materials nearby, or plan to follow a vague curiosity you had a few years ago but never pursued (like pressing wildflowers, or going roller skating).
3. Another way to explore how you'd like to play is to look to your childhood for clues. If you loved collecting shells, head to a beach and find some. You might be happy with that, or you might want to try arranging them in patterns or towers (see Transient Art on page 66).

In time, you will find something that brings you absolute joy. Something you can do for the sake of it – wholly unproductive and filled with delight.

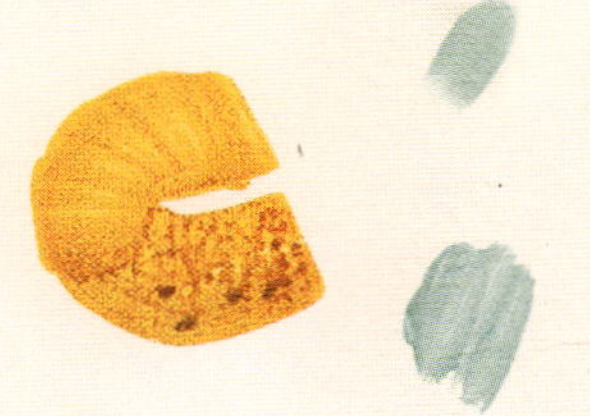

Dr Brown's 8 play personalities

Dr Stuart Brown MD, founder of the National Institute for Play (yes, that exists!), has identified the following eight play personalities in adults. Which ones resonate with you?

1 The Joker

Delights in making people laugh – the class clown.

2 The Kinesthete

Finds joy in moving their bodies.

3 The Explorer

Loves discovering new things and going to new places – physically or mentally.

4 The Competitor

Loves to win – whether it's against others or competing against their own previous records.

5 The Director

Finds joy in planning and organising – planning an event could be play for them.

6 The Collector

Plays by creating collections of things that interest them.

7 The Artist/Creator

Adores creating – whether it's art, crafts, music, gardening or any other creative pursuits.

8 The Storyteller

Loves to spend time in their imagination – they love writing, imagining or telling stories.

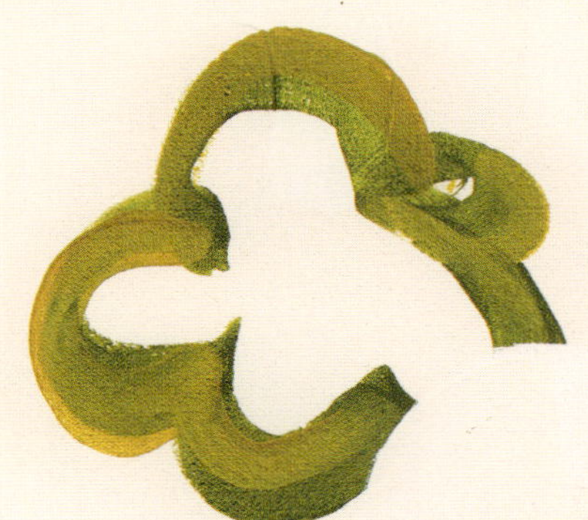

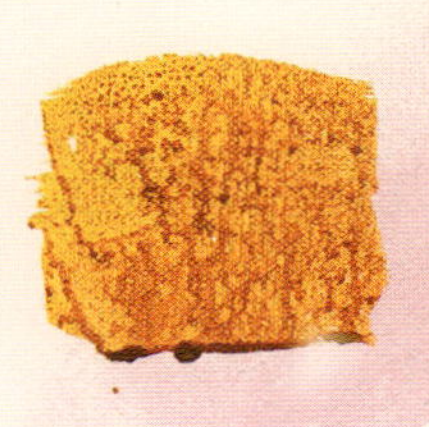

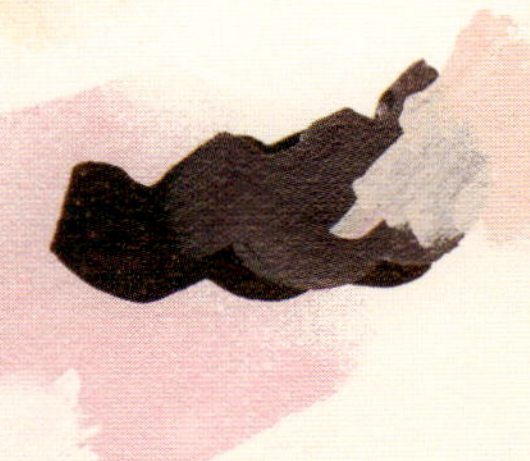

How do I play?

Play is our soul's way of reminding us that we're here to live, not just function. When we start to express this part of ourselves, even in small, quiet ways, we turn the volume up on our intuition, joy, and sense of self.

The play personality I most align with is Artist/Creator, though I also have aspects of a Storyteller and a Collector. Obviously, painting is one of the ways I play – though for it to truly count as 'play', I separate that creating from the painting I do for work.

I've also developed a few other modes of play over the years that enrich me and help me express my me-est me. As a child, I loved playing dress-up. My mum had the most glorious old suitcase full of costumes from her days in a ballet company. Whenever friends came to visit, we'd pull that suitcase down from the cupboard and mix and match the colourful, silky treasures, then swan around like princesses.

That passion for dressing up crept into my adult life, and today, I take dress-up parties very seriously (or playfully). I plan my outfits ages in advance, especially for music festivals, which give me a great excuse to spend months creating custom outfits and hats. The child in me delights in these moments, and I truly feel like myself wearing a home-made multi-tiered cake hat, or a sparkly crown with colourful ribbons.

Another way I inject moments of play into daily life is by being silly or creative with my daughter. Sometimes, this is as simple as tickling her, dancing, pulling faces or saying ridiculous things. (I think she's a Kinesthete/Joker/Creator.) It's important to play with her in ways that excite her and meet her interests. She loves making beaded bracelets, so sitting on her bed and making those together is such a special way to play.

MILA AND I WILL TAKE ANY OPPORTUNITY TO DRESS UP AND PLAY!

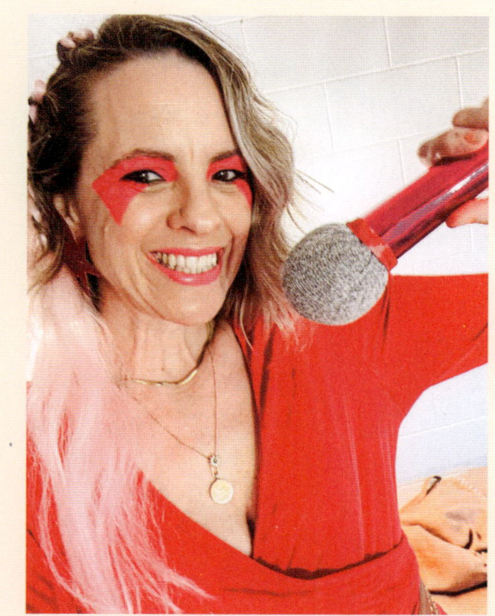

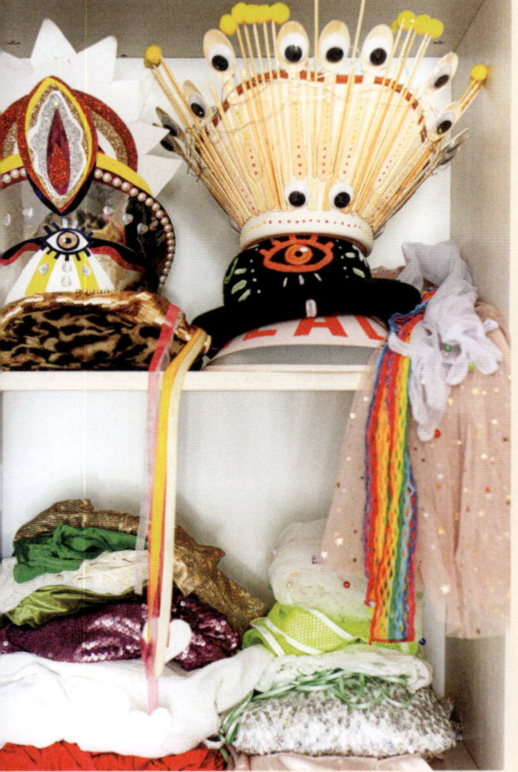

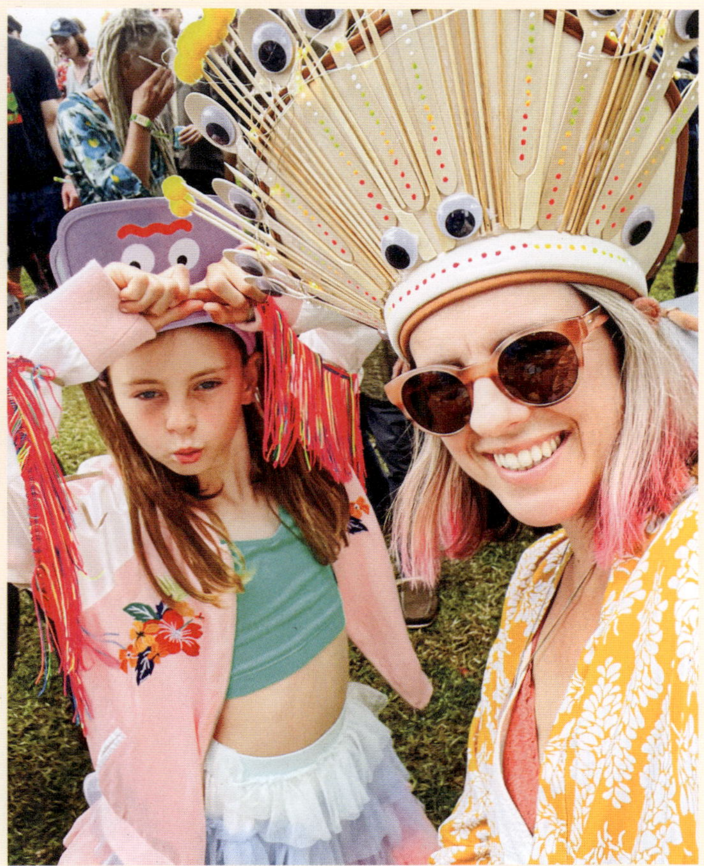

WHEN I'M FEELING STUCK, I LOVE TAKING A FEW MINUTES OUT TO PLAY AND CREATE SOMETHING JUST FOR THE JOY OF IT, EXPRESSING MYSELF THROUGH COLOUR AND MARK-MAKING.

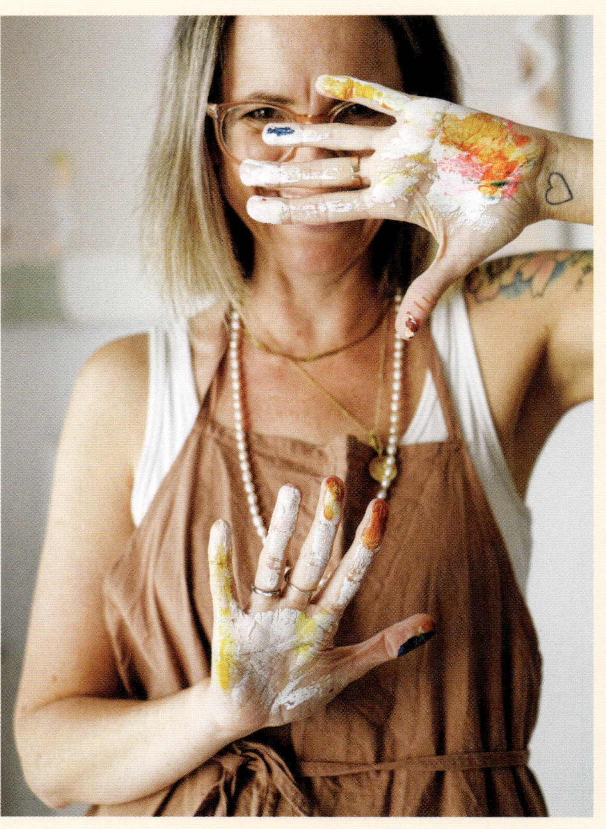

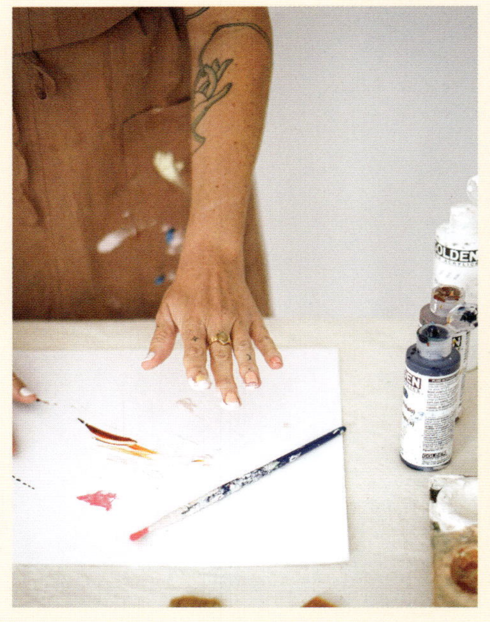

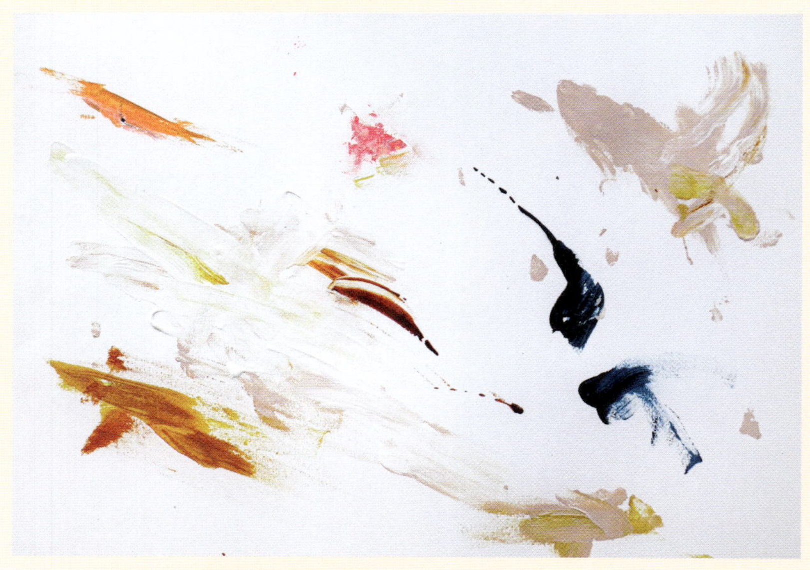

Play has been known to improve cognitive function, decrease stress and improve creativity. Without play we can become irritable and overwhelmed.

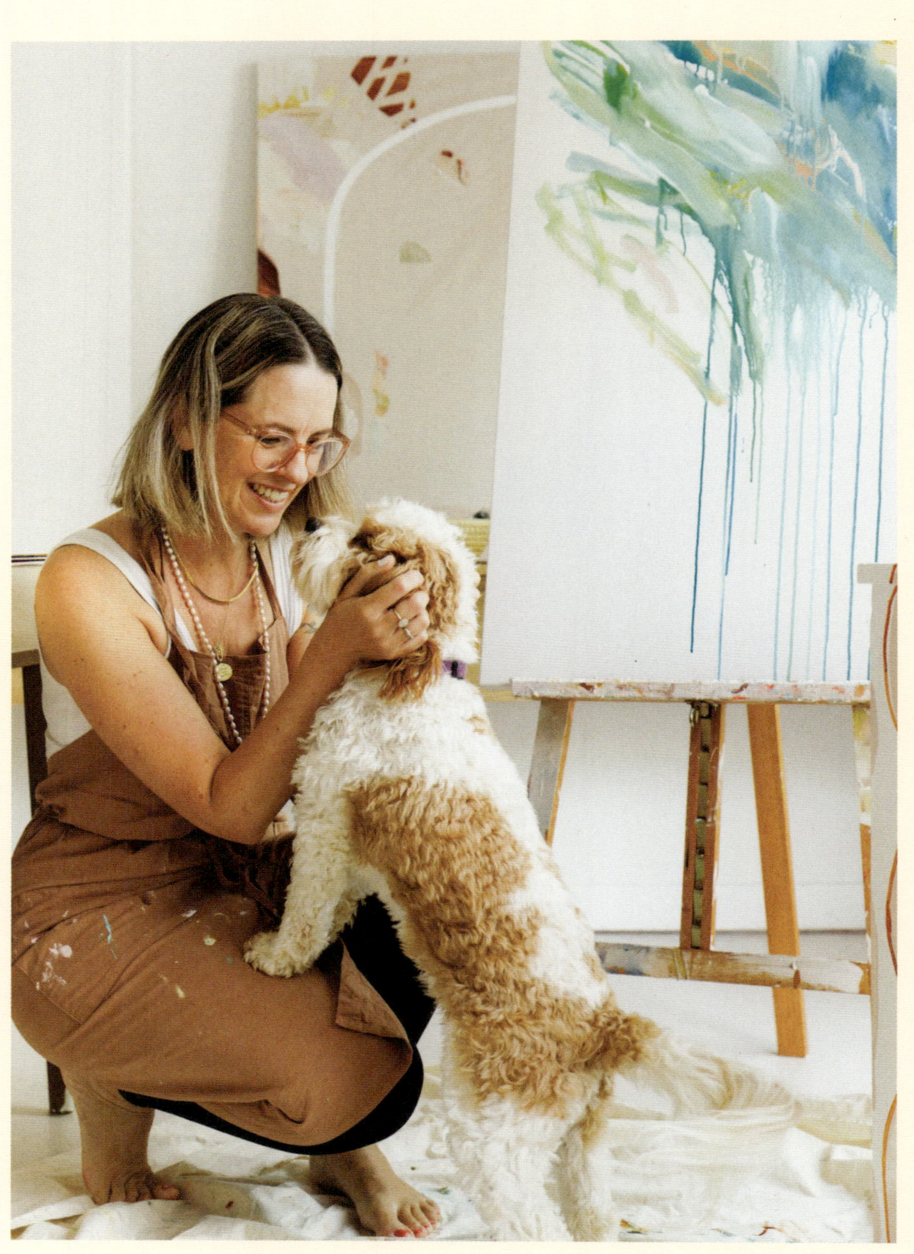

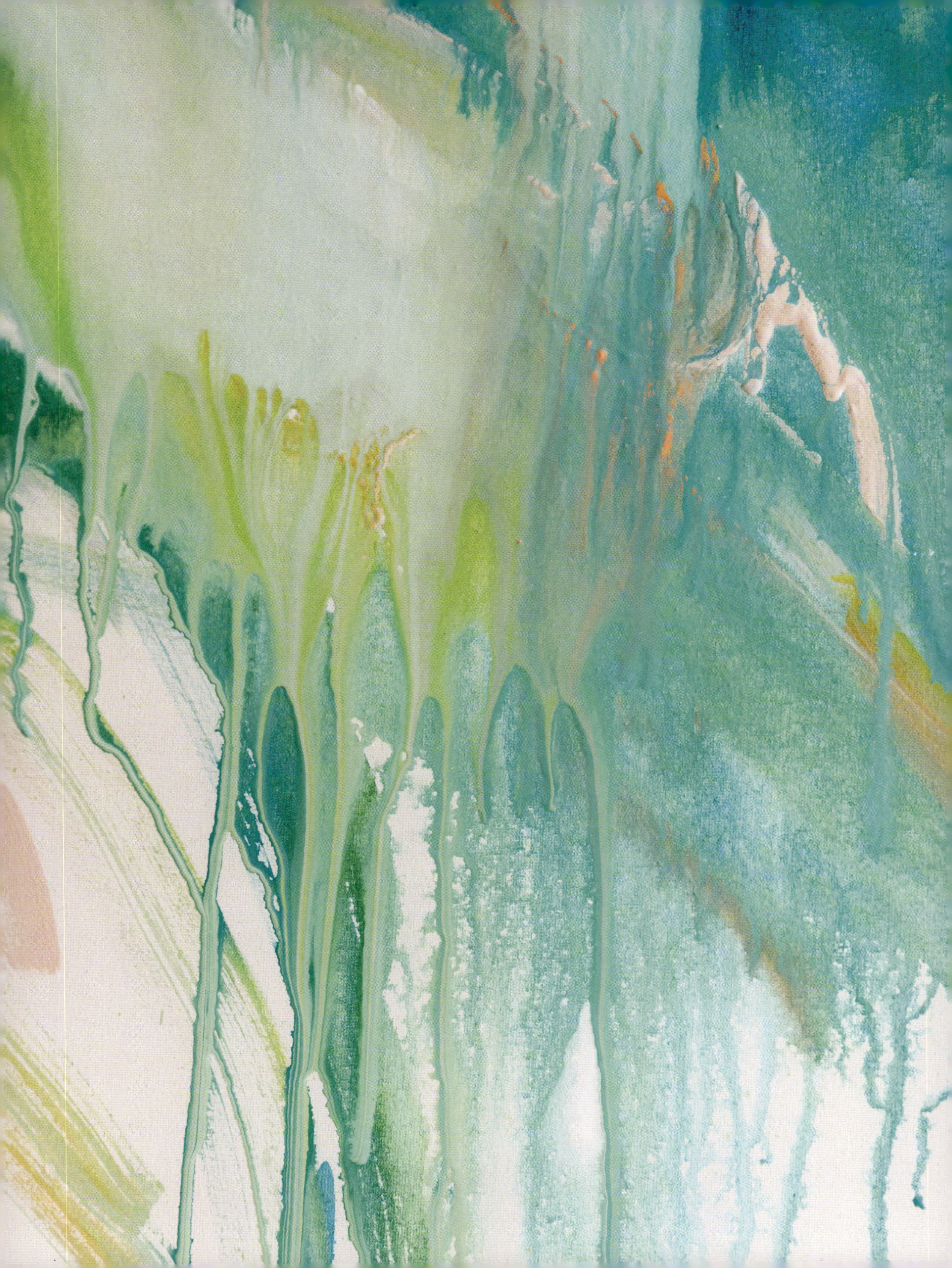

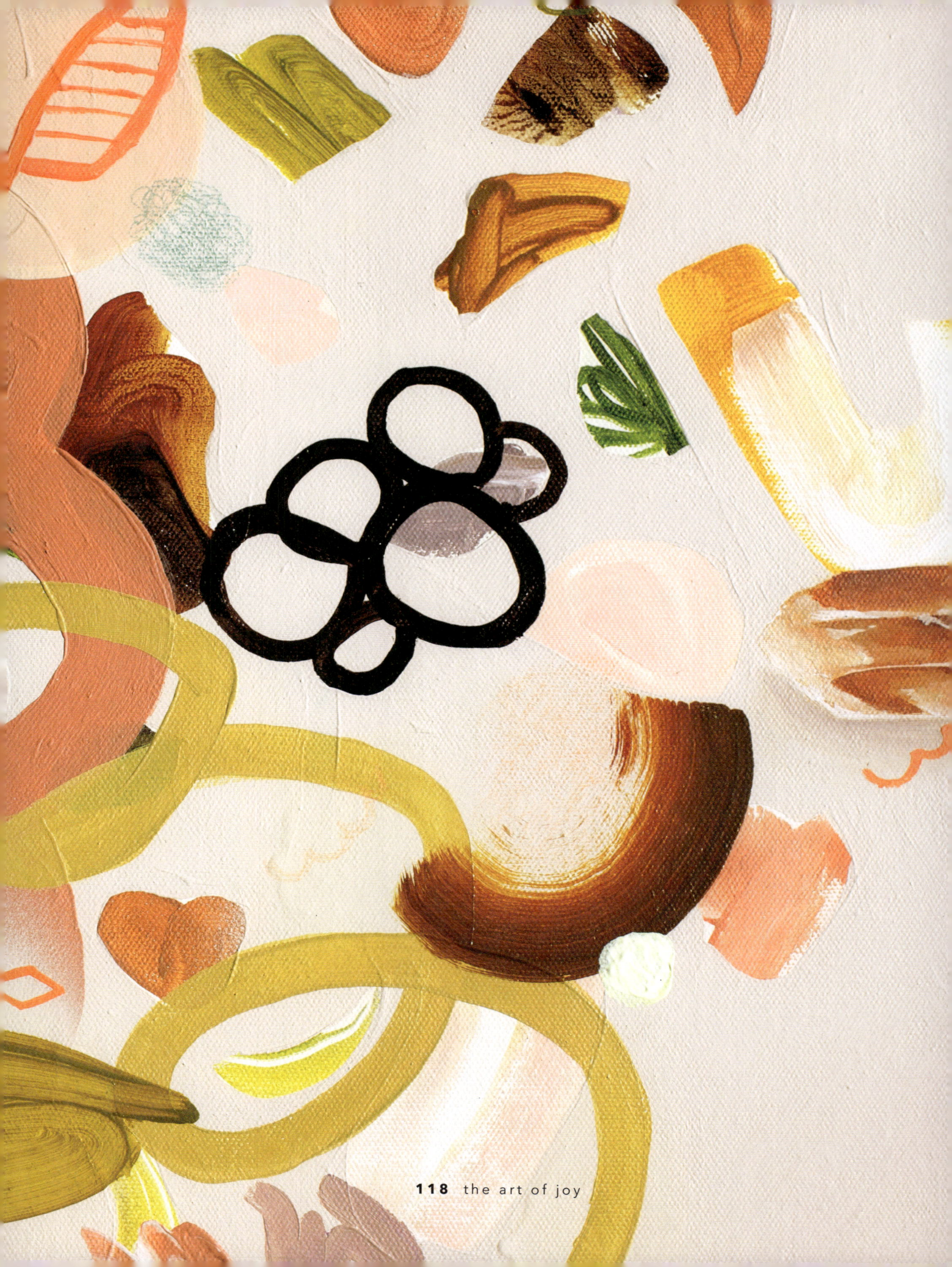

chapter eight

We Are All Creative

You don't need to be an artist to make something for fun.

So many people are brought up believing that because they don't write, create art, sing or dance they're not 'creative'. Society often has a limited view of what creativity is. It's been sold to us as a rare and unusual talent; something bestowed on the lucky few, rather than a quality inherent in every human.

However, you only have to think of everything we humans have created (some good, some not so good), and it's clear that we are an incredibly creative species, capable of conceptualising and innovating in all facets of life. The way we build, cook, garden, code, decorate and even organise our lives are all creative acts. Broadening our view of creativity not only helps us embrace our unique strengths, it can create an immense amount of joy in our lives.

It's no accident that this chapter comes directly after play because creativity and play are intrinsically linked. The purest moments of creativity feel like play, and can open us up to beautiful flow states.

A flow state, particularly in the context of creativity, is a deeply immersive mental state where you are fully absorbed and engaged in the activity at hand. When we experience flow, we feel a profound sense of focus and enjoyment. Time seems to blur, and self-consciousness fades.

Creativity, at its essence, is problem-solving in many different forms. It's how we find novel solutions and come up with new ways of doing things – whether that's sculpting a masterpiece, fixing an issue at work, or finding a new way to relate to our children.

If the idea of being creative feels intimidating, or out of your comfort zone, try implementing 'micro moments' of creativity. You don't need to take up watercolour painting or grow a show garden; you can start simple. Doodle, journal, or go rogue with your usual dinner recipes. Perhaps your creative heart yearns to rearrange the furniture or colour-code your bookshelf. All of these small creative actions are opportunities for you to tap into joy and express yourself.

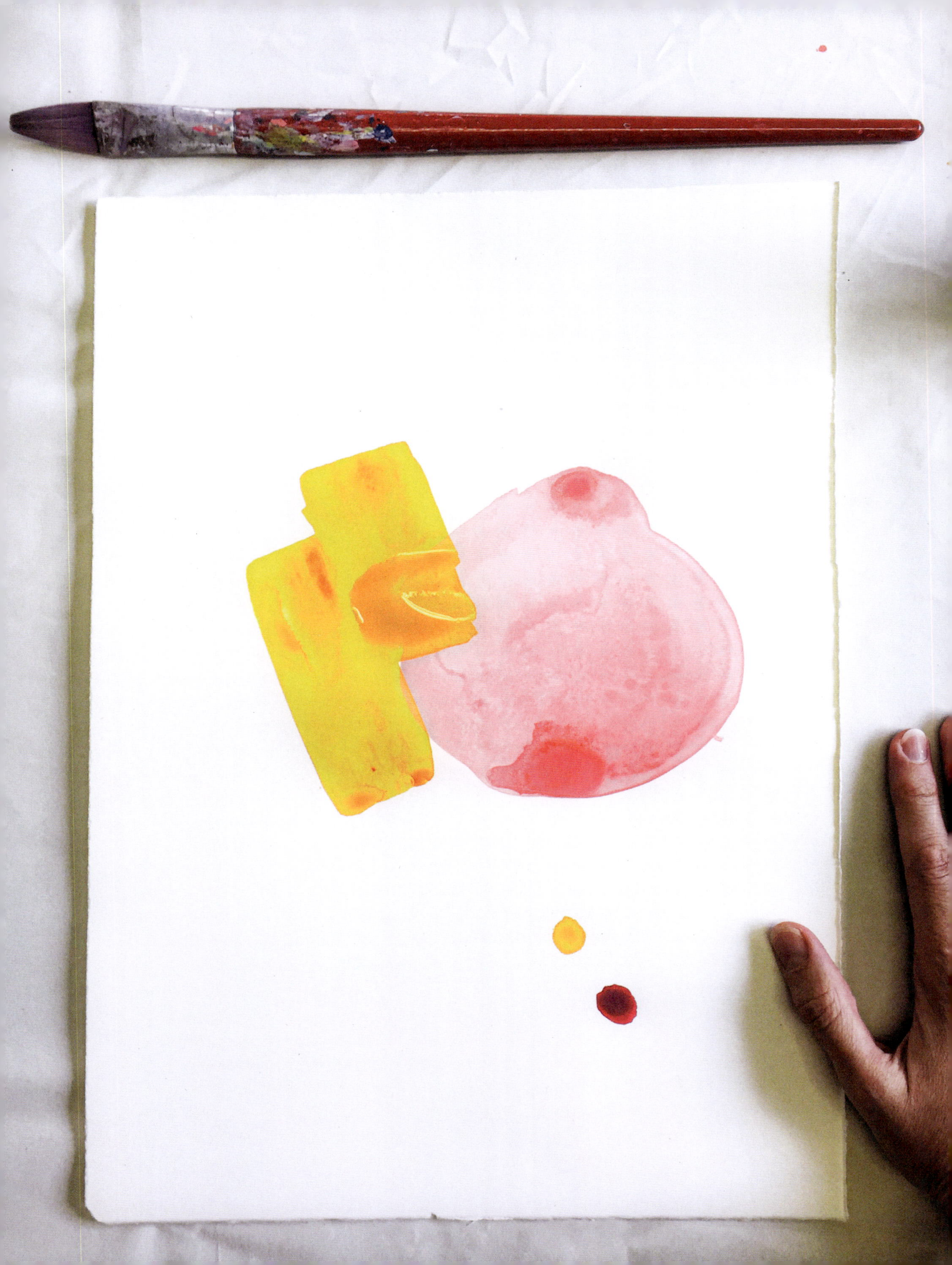

The link between creativity and joy

Creativity enhances joy in several ways. Being absorbed in a creative task takes us out of a state of mental clutter, so it can act as a form of mindfulness. Some of my most beautiful creative moments have led to a flow state where the ever-present chatter in my mind is replaced with a quiet witnessing of how my work is unfolding. Time passes without me realising when I reach that state of flow.

Creative activities also provide a powerful outlet for self-expression, allowing us to explore and articulate our thoughts, feelings and experiences. This process of expression can lead to a greater understanding of ourselves and a feeling of personal growth. When we see our inner thoughts and feelings reflected in our creations, it validates our experiences and helps us to understand the world and our place in it.

Novelty, whether it's in thinking, making, or perceiving, stimulates the brain, and creative activities provide an endless supply of these. The joy of discovery, learning new skills and seeing the world in new ways can awaken our sense of wonder and keep us engaged with the world around us.

Engaging in creative activities can be a powerful coping mechanism for dealing with stress, anxiety and depression. The act of creating can serve as a distraction, helping to break cycles of negative thoughts, and a means of processing emotions and experiences. Many people find joy in the tranquillity and mindfulness that come from creative expression.

The pursuit of creative activities often leads to the development of new skills and the mastery of new techniques. This process of learning and improving is inherently rewarding and can lead to feelings of achievement and pride. The joy of mastering a new craft or solving a creative problem is a significant source of happiness and fulfilment. It can also create a feeling of purpose and meaning in a life that might otherwise get lost in the day-to-day.

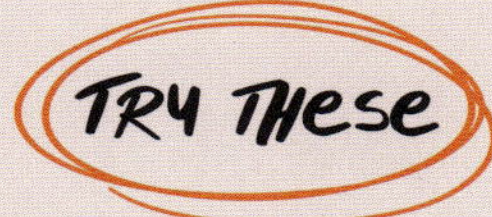

Four simple ideas to help you get creative.

1 Writing with a twist

Start a one-sentence story journal. Each day, write down a single sentence that tells a story or captures a moment, thought, or feeling. This activity nurtures narrative thinking and can be surprisingly expressive, encouraging you to think about how much meaning can be packed into one well-chosen sentence.

2 Digital storytelling

Using your smartphone, create a short, one-minute video about a day or a moment in your life. Focus on capturing small details, like the way light enters your room, or the sound of the city or nature around you. Edit the video using a free app such as CapCut and try adding music or text to enhance the storytelling. This activity blends creativity with technology, encouraging you to tell stories through visual means.

3 Culinary creations

Challenge yourself to invent a new dish using only the ingredients you already have at home. This encourages improvisation and creative problem solving. Document the process and the recipe. If you like, you can compile a cookbook of unique recipes that tell the story of your culinary experiments.

4 DIY décor

Choose an object in your home that you'd like to give a new life to – this could be a piece of furniture, a lampshade, or a plain notebook. Use whatever materials you have (fabric scraps, washi tape, markers, etcetera) to decorate or upcycle the item. This project taps into your design creativity and can transform the way you see and use everyday objects.

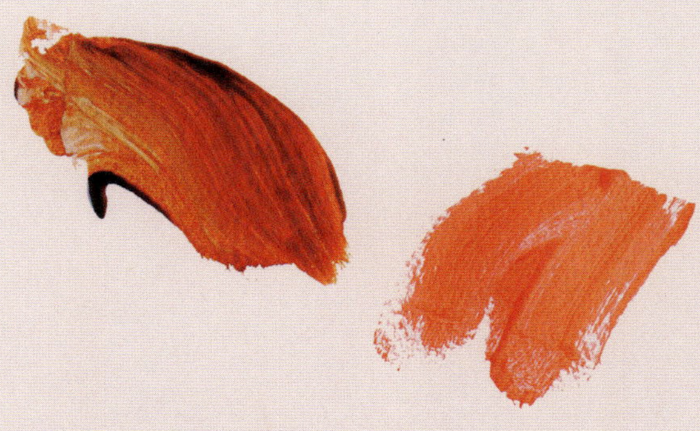

WANT TO PLAY WITH PAINT? TRY THE IDEAS ON THE NEXT FEW PAGES

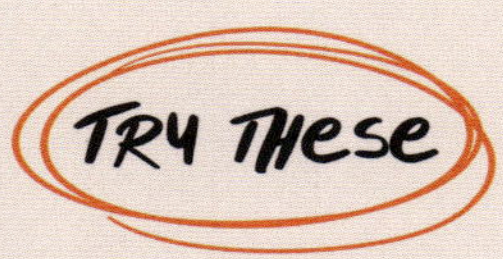

I have created three artistic tasks that are fun, simple and zero pressure. If you're not inclined to try one of these, check in with yourself and ask whether you're holding back because you're afraid the end result won't be beautiful or perfect. If that's the case, don't let that stop you. The intention here is to focus on the *doing* – the play of it – rather than the final product. This way, you're much more likely to find joy in the process.

Creative play #1: Brush stroke collage

Due to dry time, this exercise is best done over two sessions.

You will need:

- Some relatively thick paper that will hold paint without breaking or dissolving, like watercolour paper
- Paints – if you don't have some already, even a small watercolour set would work well. My absolute favourite paints are Golden Fluid Acrylics – but if you're not an artist, you might have a heart attack at how much they cost
- Brushes of a few sizes
- Scissors or a craft knife
- Glue

1 Put on some music to set the mood. Choose or mix a handful of colours you love. Mindfully fill your page with brush strokes of different sizes, colours and textures. Keep each stroke separate. You are going to cut them out later. Use this time to focus on the joy of paint on paper. Try some brush strokes with a lot of water and some dry, scratchy strokes. Consider which colours are catching your eye and use them again. Notice how some colours hold more depth between light and dark and play with that. Fill in as many pages as you want to. If you get sidetracked from single strokes and feel the need to connect them and create something completely different, follow that curiosity!

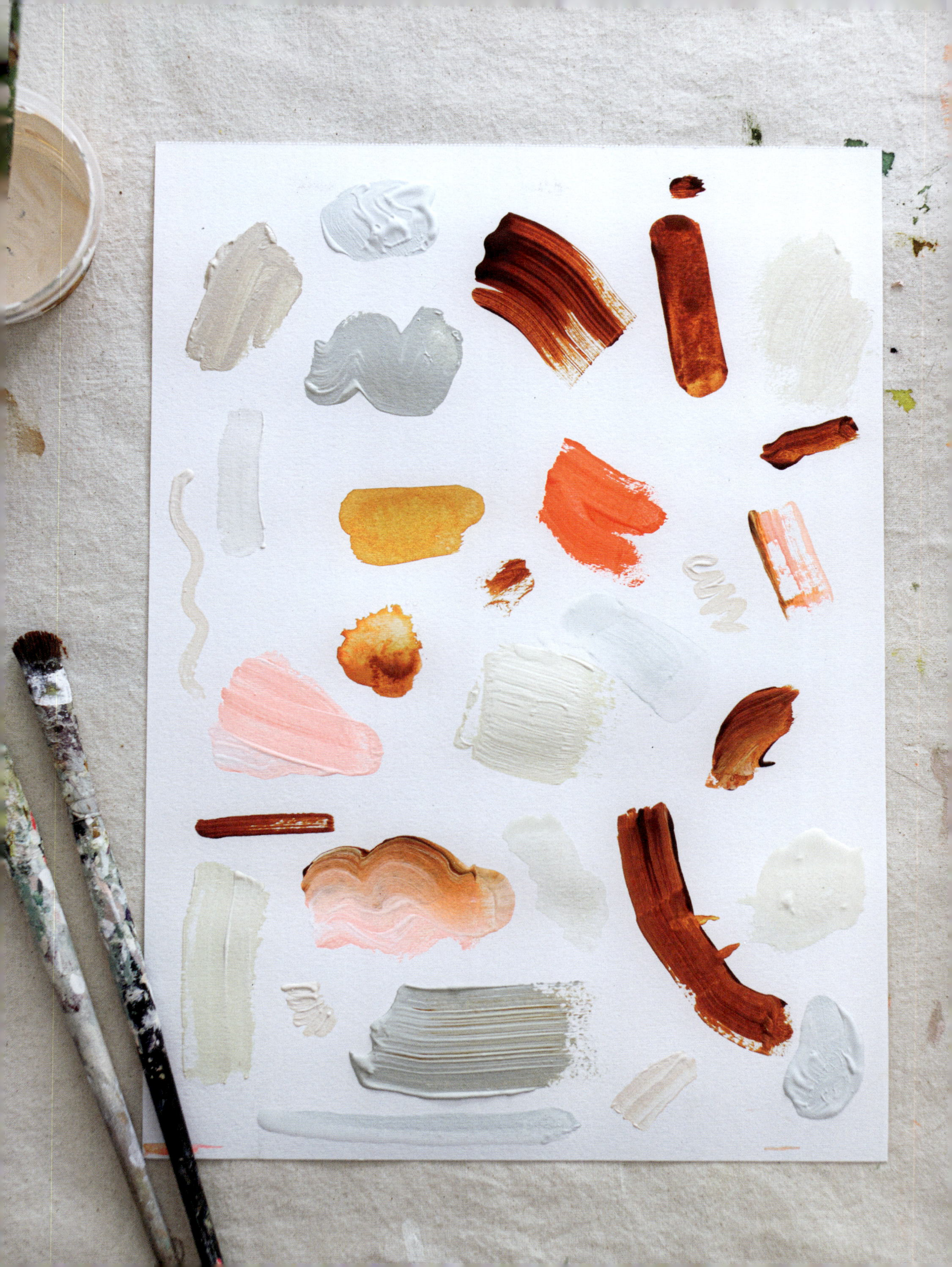

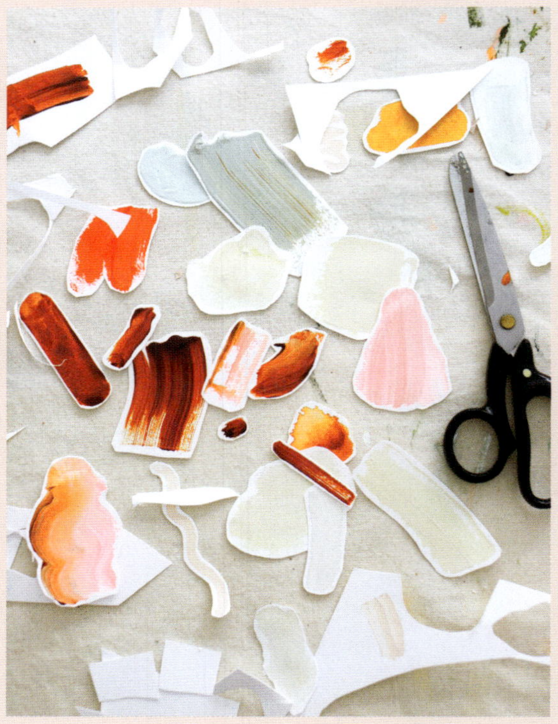

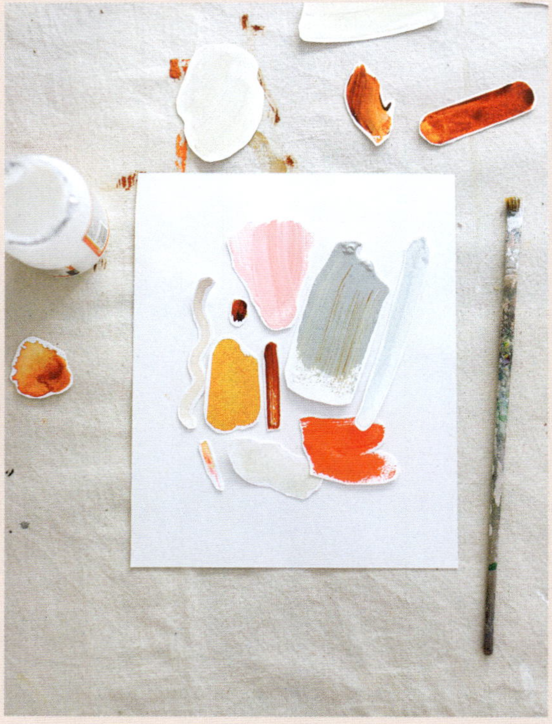

2 Leave the paint for an hour or two to dry completely. Once dry, cut out your favourite brush strokes. Admire the beauty of each one of them as you cut. Remember, this is an abstract creation, so it doesn't need to look like anything specific. The joy is in how the paint has been applied to the paper. If you notice that the paint has caused the paper to warp and curl up, you can place some heavy books on top of them for a while to flatten them.

3 Next, take a fresh piece of plain or coloured paper and either drop the brush strokes on the page randomly to see how they land, or arrange them into an intentional composition. Once you have an arrangement that feels good, glue the brush strokes to the paper. You might need to get your heavy books out again so that they stick down flat. If so, place a sheet of baking paper between the composition and your book to prevent them sticking together.

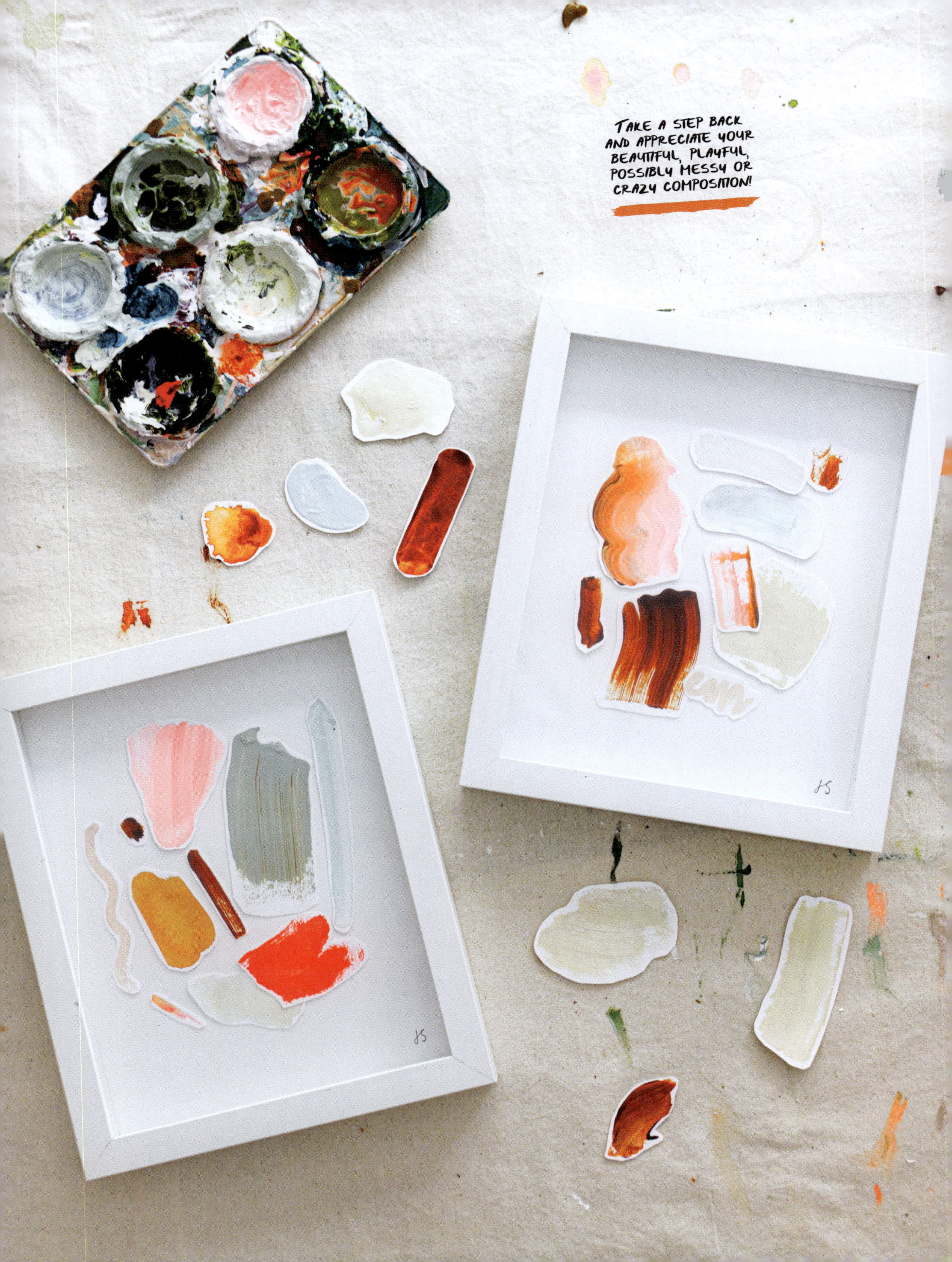

TAKE A STEP BACK AND APPRECIATE YOUR BEAUTIFUL, PLAYFUL, POSSIBLY MESSY OR CRAZY COMPOSITION!

Creative play #2: Brush stroke blends

This is a simple mindful exercise that celebrates the unpredictability of paint and water. It can be done in one sitting.

You will need:

- Some relatively thick paper that will hold paint without breaking or dissolving, like watercolour paper
- Paints that can be diluted with water – acrylics, watercolours, etcetera
- A medium to large brush and a smaller one
- A jar of clean water

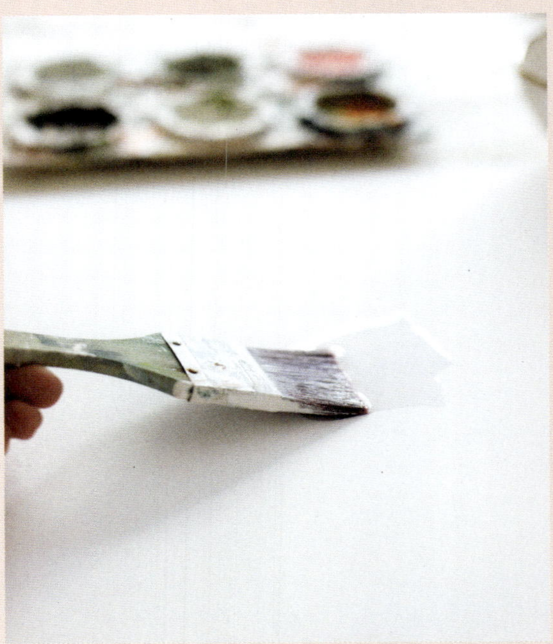

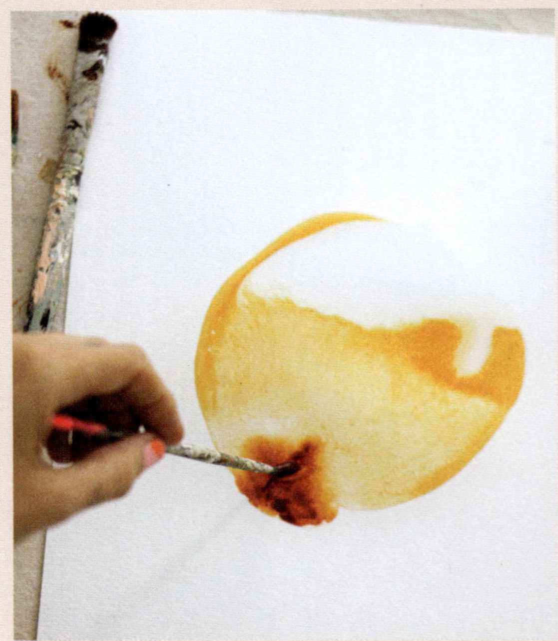

1 Use your medium to large brush and water to paint a shape onto your paper. Use enough water so that it doesn't dry instantly. You want it to stay wet for a few minutes so that you can apply paint to the wet shape.

2 Use any brush with some paint on it to gently touch one side of your water shape. Watch how the paint blends beautifully into the water. Add more of the same colour if you'd like to, or watch it move through the water until it stops. Add more colours next to your current colour or on the other side of the shape.

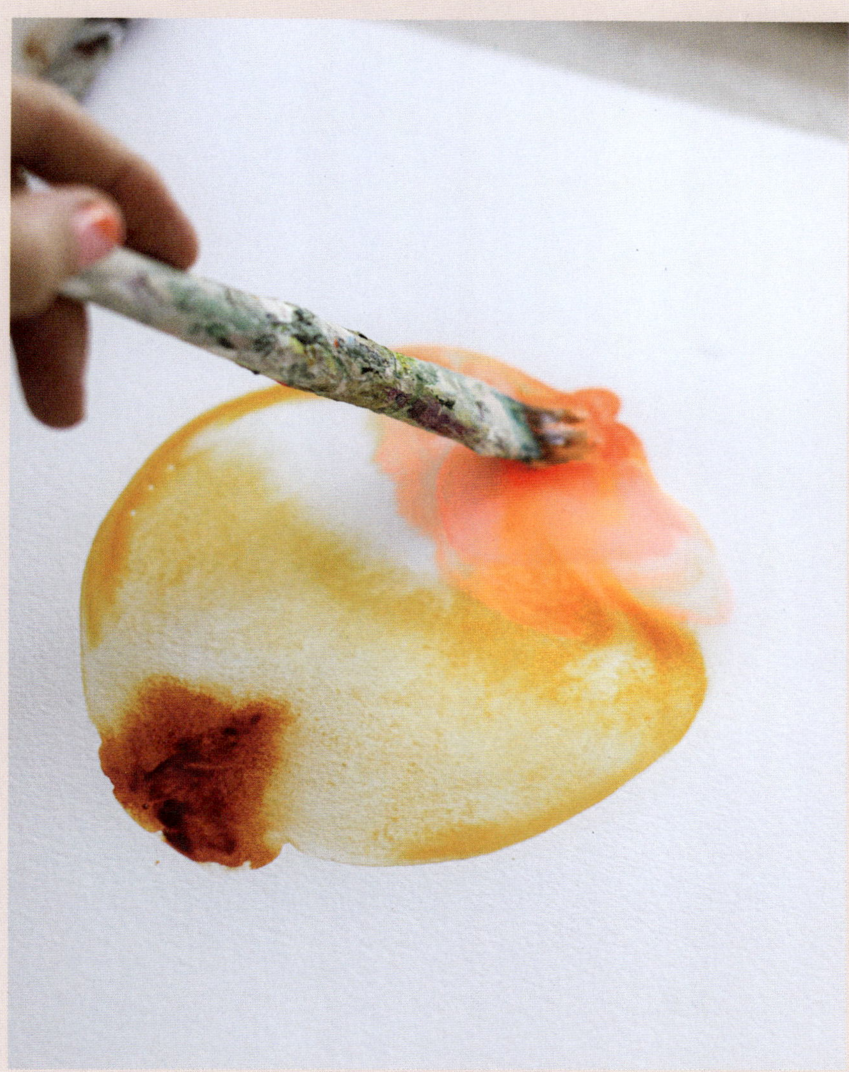

3 Play with the water shapes and paint to your heart's content. You can try adding more to the water shape, or seeing what happens if you use white paint over the others. Just play. It's likely to be a messy outcome, but remember, it's the process, not the result that matters.

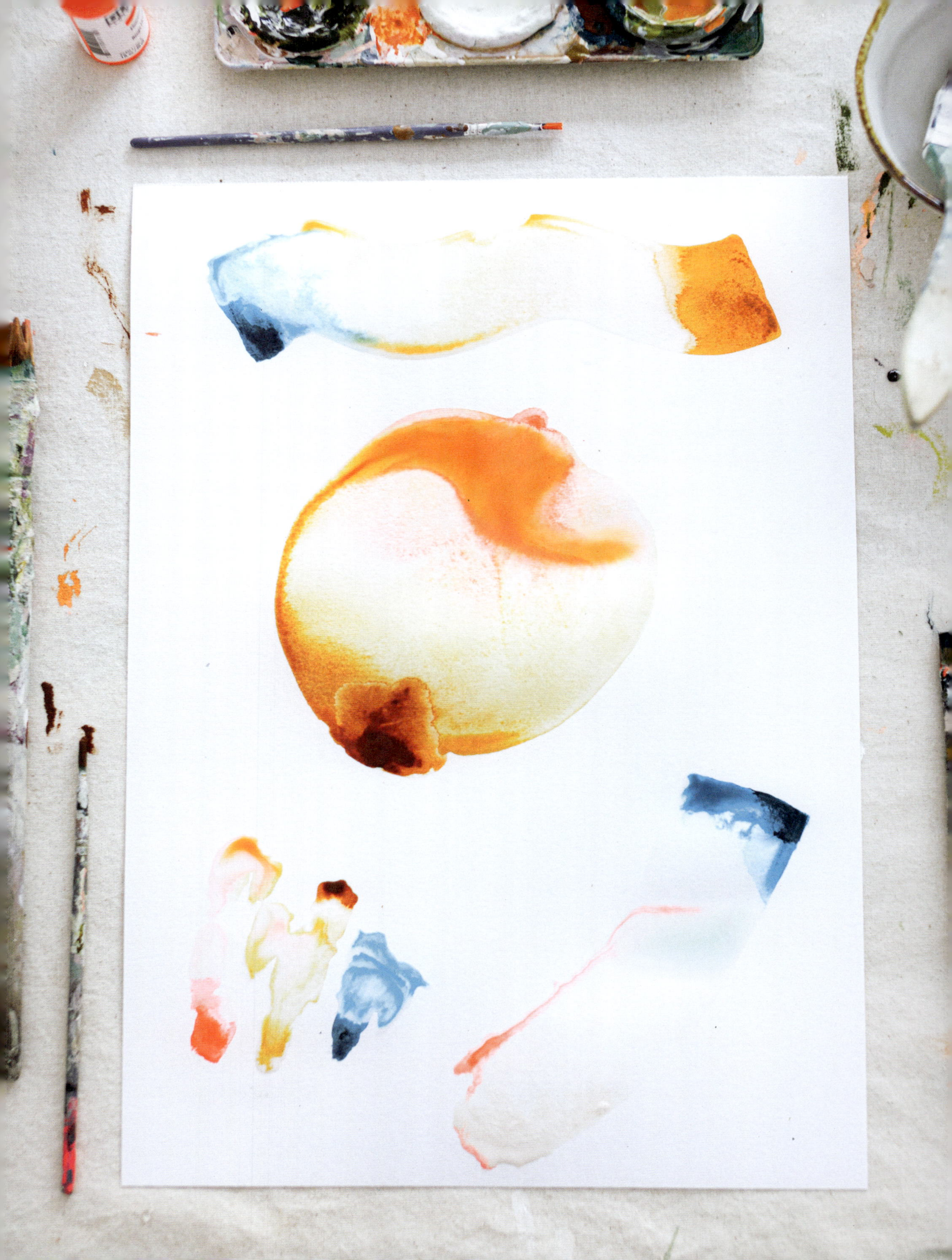

Focus
on the *doing*
– the creative
play – rather
than the final
product.

Creative play #3:
Flower vase collage

Due to dry time, this exercise is best done over two sessions. I love how this exercise plays with chaos and order. We start with something completely wild and free, then give it form.

You will need:

- Some relatively thick paper that will hold paint without breaking or dissolving, like watercolour paper
- Paints (any type), other art materials such as pencils and pastels are optional
- Brushes of a few sizes
- Scissors or a craft knife
- Glue

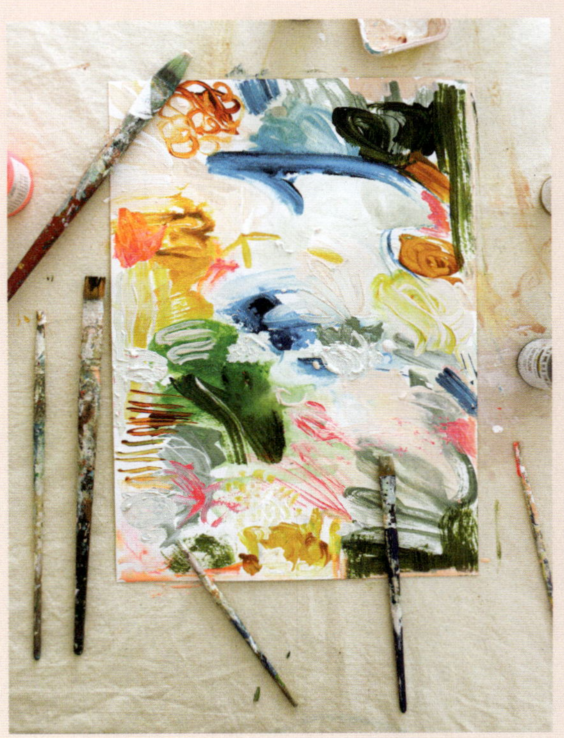

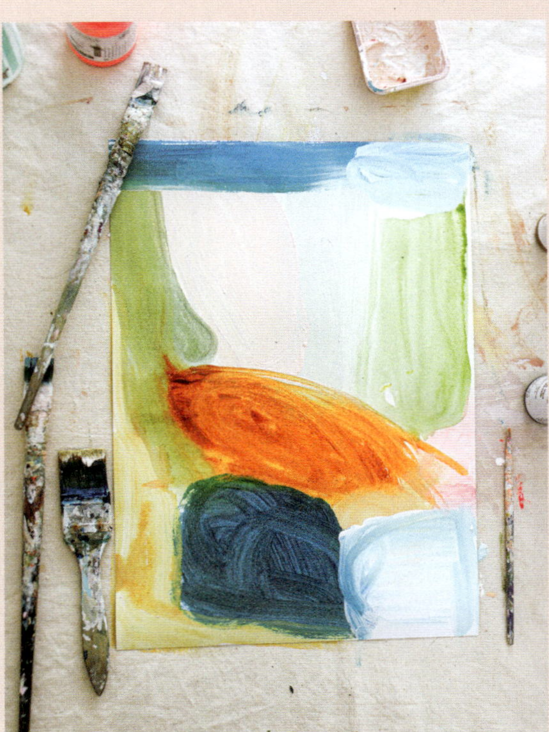

1 Fill an entire page, edge to edge with fun, crazy, messy paint. Use as many colours, shapes, textures and brush strokes as you can. Use your fingers if you feel like getting messy. Add in textures and marks with pencils and pastels if you want to. The goal is to fill the page with lots of variety in colour, texture and marks.

2 Start a new page. This time fill it with larger areas of colour, less texture and less variety. Again, the goal is to fill the entire page. Try to use different, smoother textures and shapes in comparison to the messy shapes on the previous page.

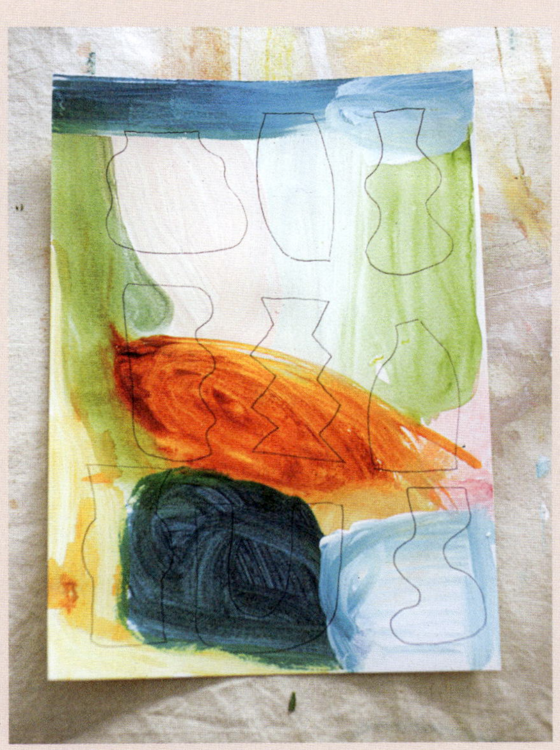

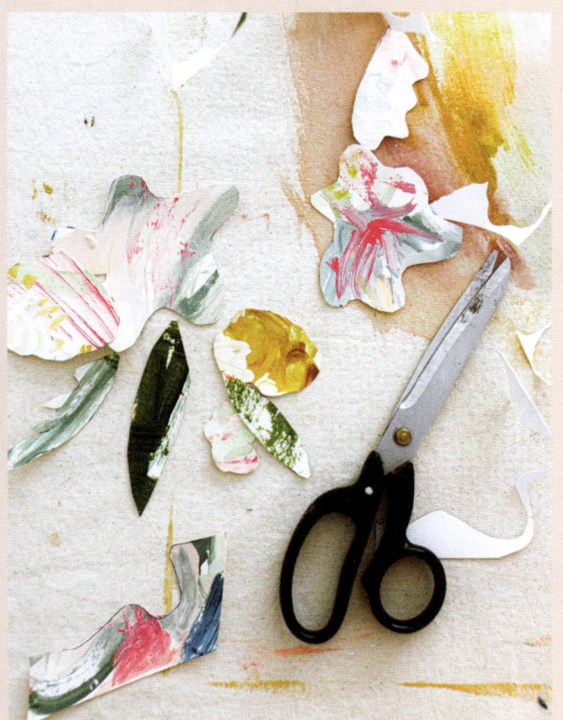

3 Once the pages are dry you are going to draw shapes over the paint. For the first, messier page, draw outlines of flower shapes. These can be messy and random – like squiggly circles – but you could make them pretty and perfect too. I opt for messy! On the second page, draw a few vase outlines.

4 Cut out the flower shapes and vases. Don't worry about being too precise – the charm is in the looseness. Let the shapes be a little wild or wobbly. You can always trim them more neatly later, or layer smaller pieces on top. Enjoy the process and let the colours and shapes surprise you.

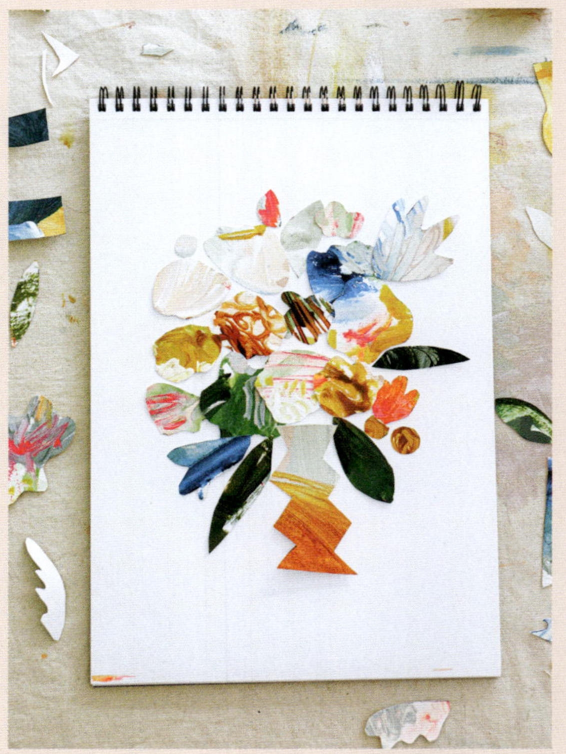

5 Grab a piece of thick white or coloured paper, and arrange your flowers in the vase shapes on the page. If you like what you see, glue it down! If not, keep playing around with combinations. If you want to turn these into little artworks for your home, you could do a set of three or four and frame them, then hang them together.

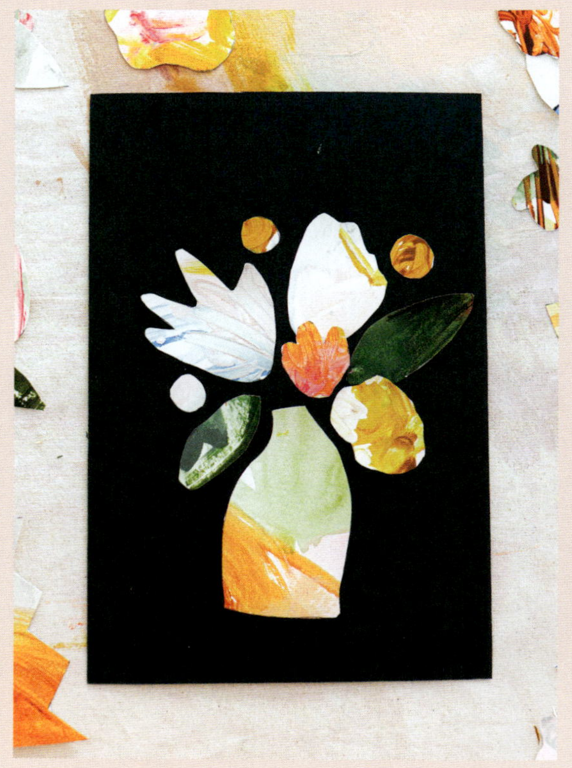

DON'T FORGET, EVERYONE IS CREATIVE, EVEN IF YOU HAVE CONVINCED YOURSELF OTHERWISE!

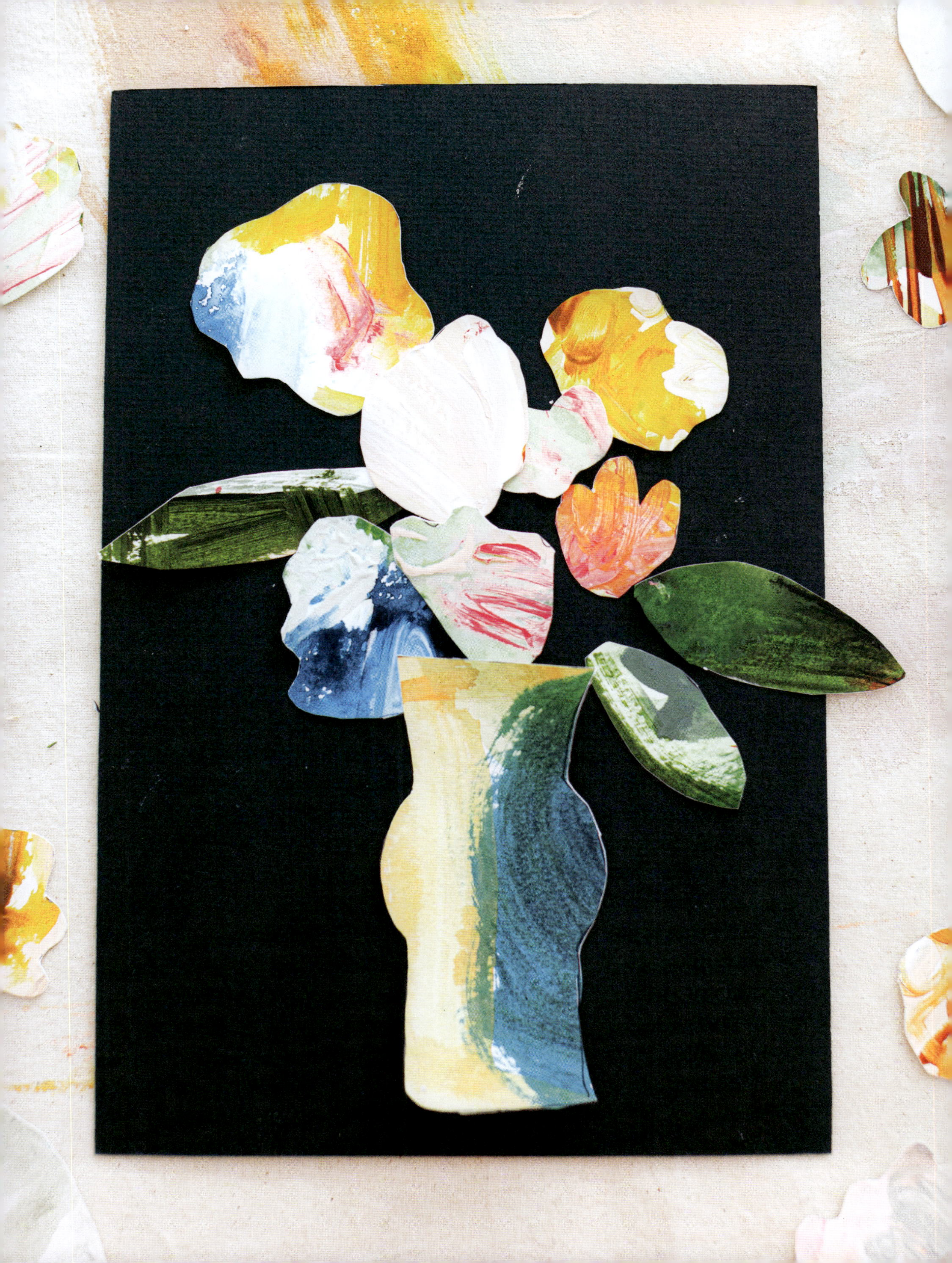

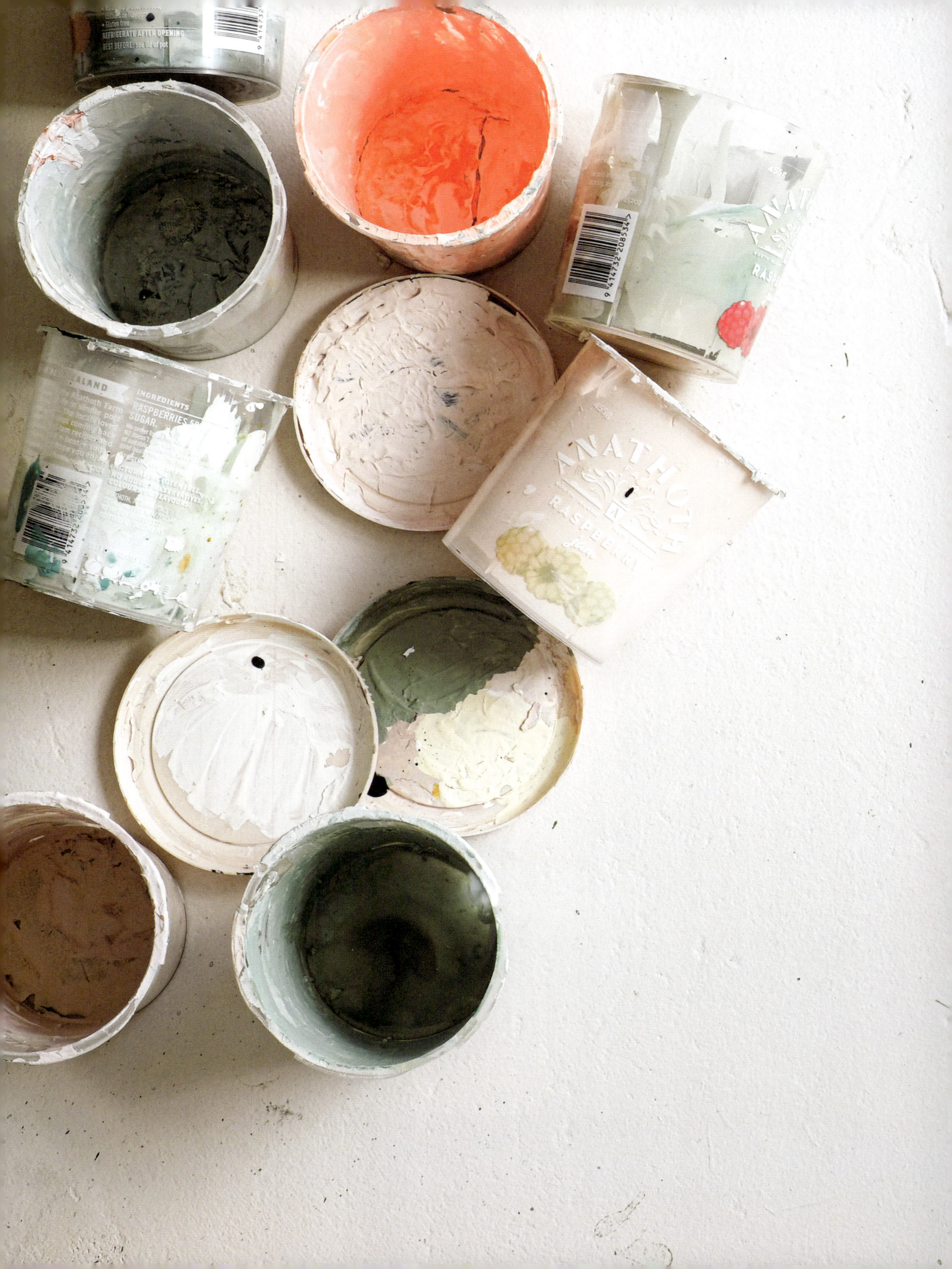
Gluten free
REFRIGERATE AFTER OPENING
BEST BEFORE: see lid of pot
INGREDIENTS
RASPBERRIES
SUGAR
ANATHOTH
RASPBERRY

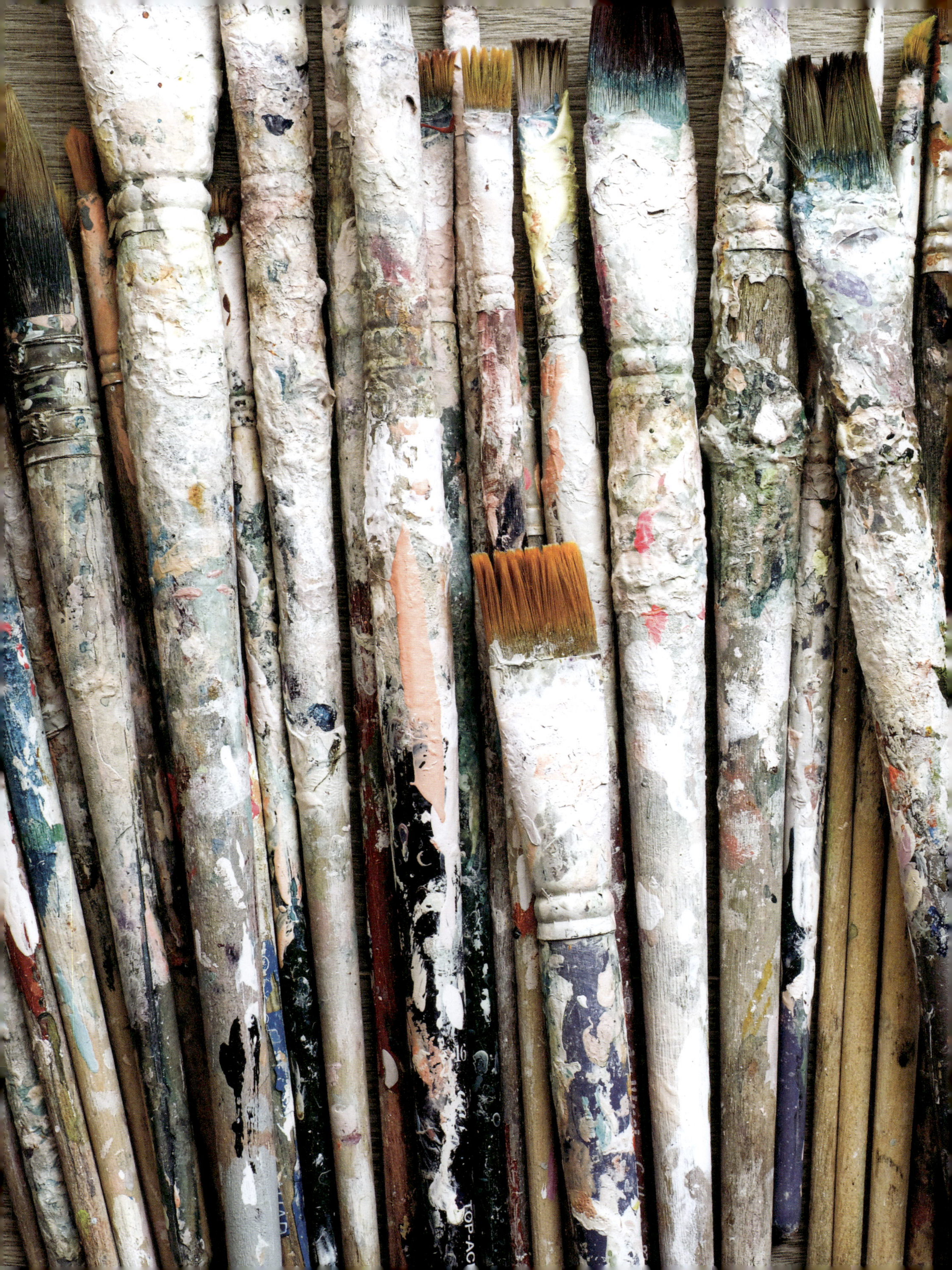
16
TOP-AC

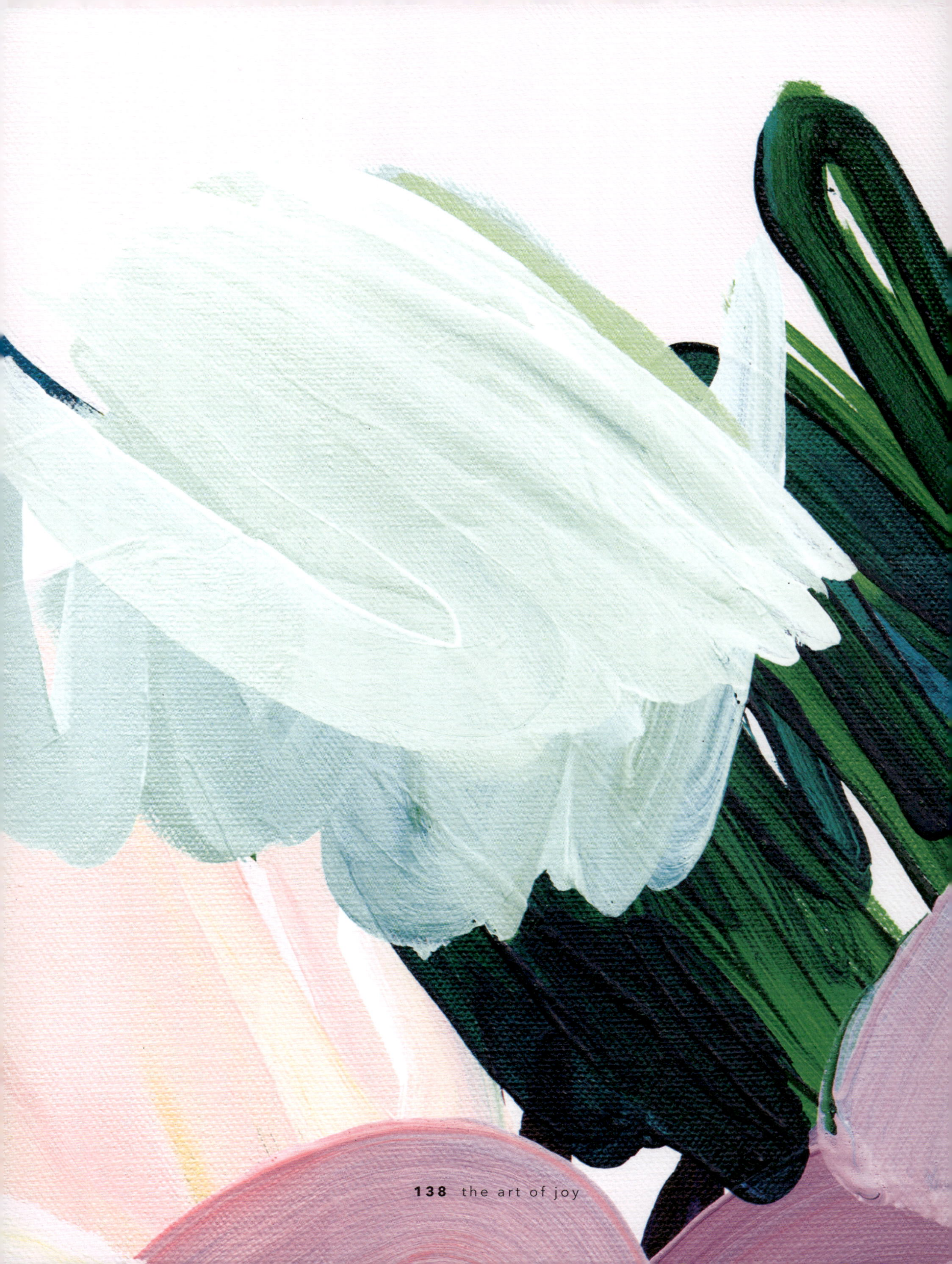

chapter nine

Find the Buried Treasure

The art of uncovering gold when life hits hard times.

Experience has taught me that there's joy to be found in every situation, even earth-shattering, awful ones. I believe we're here to learn and grow, and that more often than not, growth and learning come through hardship.

We have the capacity to hold pain and joy simultaneously. I know that might sound glib, particularly if you're currently going through one of life's doozies, but hear me out.

In December 2010, I was on holiday with my then-partner near Hot Water Beach, a small, coastal town on the North Island of New Zealand. It was the start of my first-ever road trip, and I was excited for this new experience. We had just finished an evening of delicious food and wine and gone to bed in the old bus we'd converted into a campervan when my phone rang.

Phone calls at 10.30 pm are rarely good, and this one was the worst I've ever received. I crept out of the van so as not to wake my partner. My brother-in-law was on the other end of my phone while I stood in the dark outside the bus. 'I'm sorry, Jen, I have bad news – your sister, Kerry, was in a car accident. Jen, she's dead.'

The ground fell away beneath me. Everything that was solid or had made sense in my life was suddenly vaporous and flimsy, lurching me around a now very unsafe world. I remember feeling that I was completely unprepared for this moment – no one ever gives you the tools you'll need when your big sister suddenly no longer exists. What are you supposed to do, think, or, worst of all, feel?

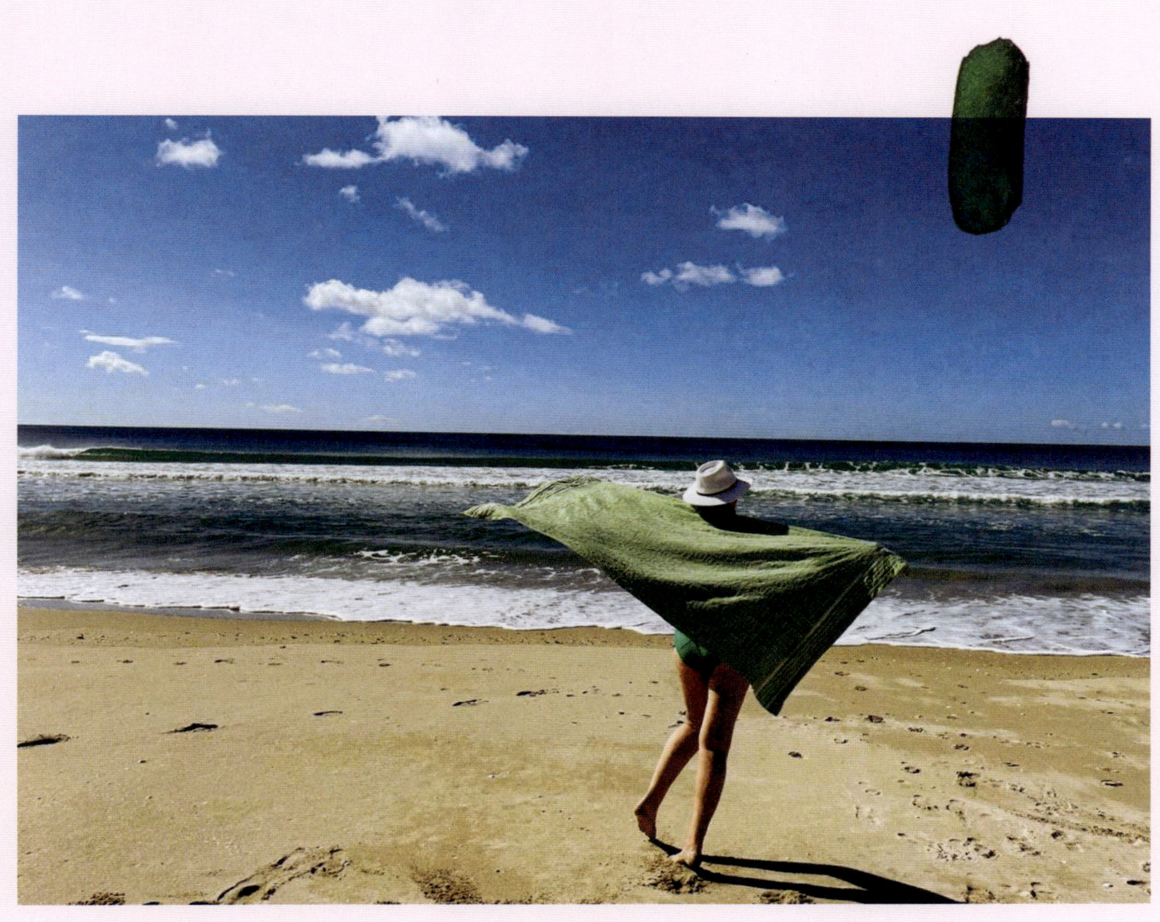

RETURNING TO THE COROMANDEL WAS HEALING. A CELEBRATION OF LIFE, RATHER THAN A SAD JOURNEY INTO MY MEMORY OF THAT NIGHT.

I believe we're here to learn and grow, and more often than not, growth and learning come through hardship.

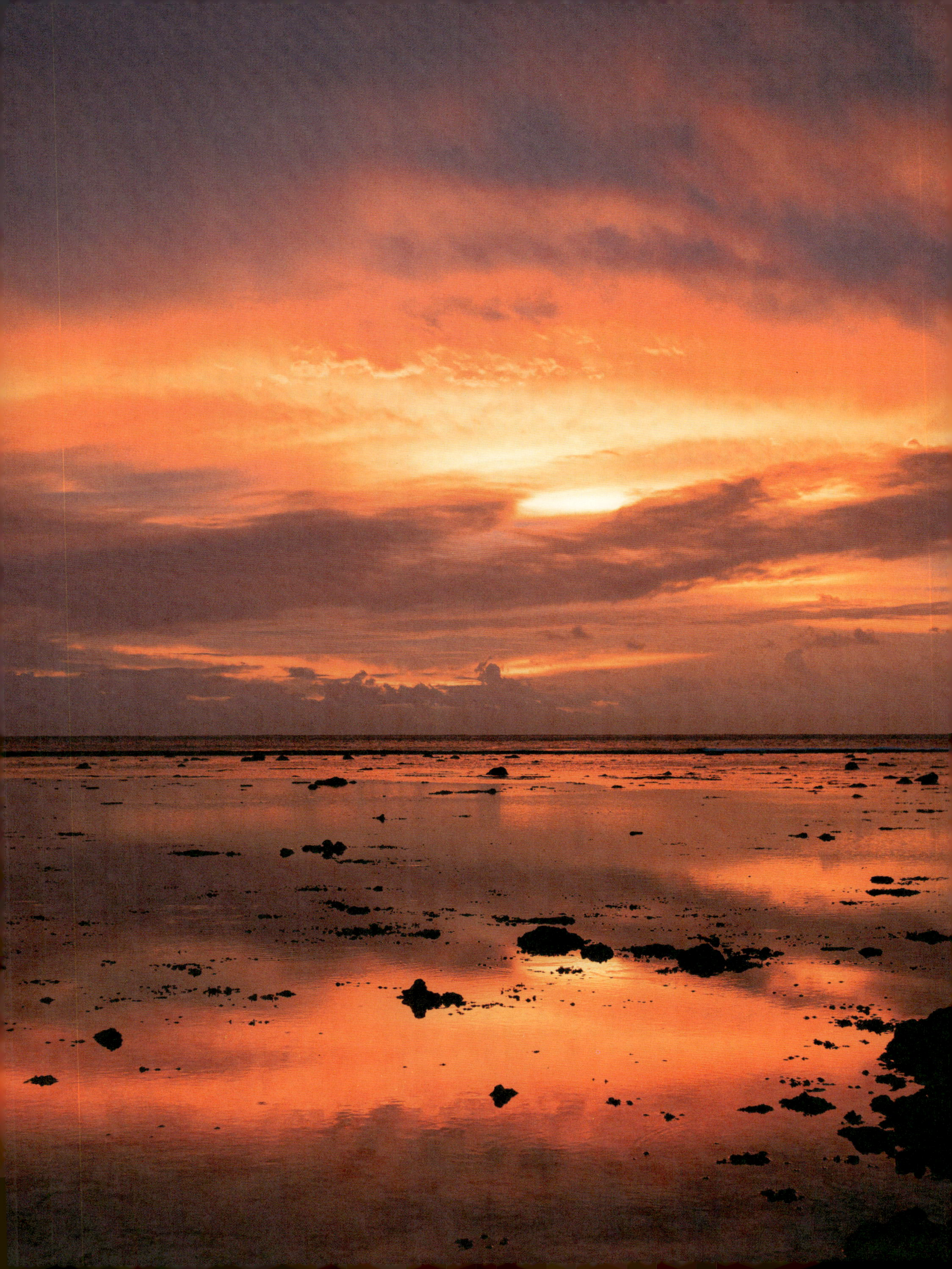

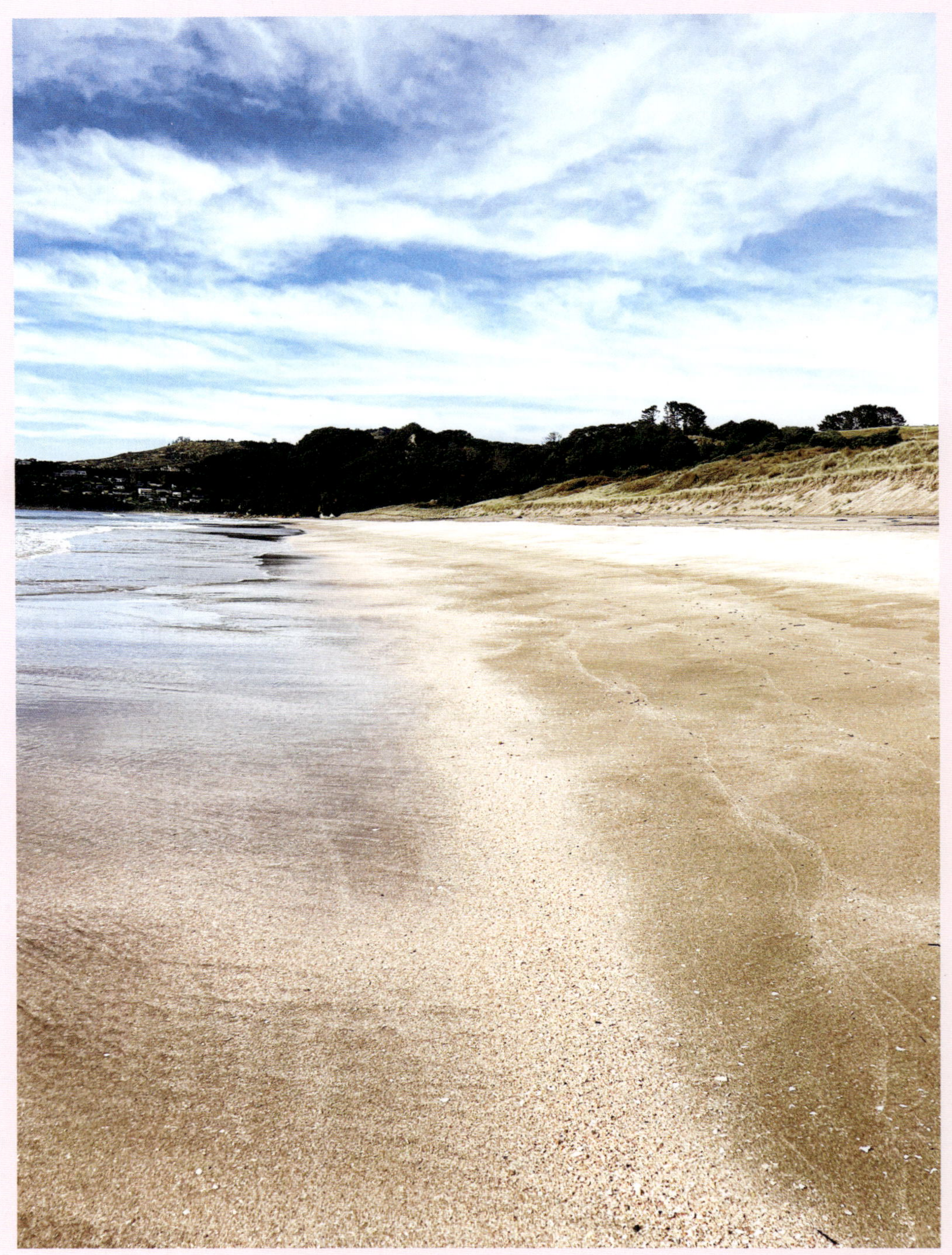

The next 24 hours were spent driving to Auckland and then flying to Wellington, where my mum and my other sister are based so we could fly together to Cape Town, South Africa, where Kerry had been living.

In the midst of this nightmare, moments of love and connection started to appear. On each step of our journey, friends, family, flight attendants, and so many other kind people held us up. There was an outpouring of love from around the globe. In South Africa, an old friend and his wonderful mum drove an hour just to stand with us in the transit lounge of the airport for half an hour while we waited for a connecting flight; to be close to us, hug us, and wrap us in their love. There was joy, even in our pain. It didn't make the hurt go away, but it was there; it was huge, and it made the ache in our hearts much more bearable.

We held two memorials for my sister – one in Cape Town and one in our hometown of Johannesburg. At both of these, we met friends of Kerry's that we hadn't known – people from the parts of her life that we hadn't been involved in, such as work. We heard stories of how she had mentored people, inspired those around her and changed lives. It was beautiful. We would never have known all of this without her passing. Joy was present in those stories. And this is where it starts to sound strange because *of course*, I would rather that Kerry was alive – spending time with us and watching her son grow into the wonderful young man he is now. But that doesn't negate that her death also brought beauty and connection to our lives.

We tend to think that when something is bad, it can't include anything good – but even devastating times can hold moments of tenderness and love, and opening to those is what reconnects us with joy. Finding both good and bad in a situation can be referred to as 'both/and' thinking, in contrast to 'either/or' (aka binary) thinking. 'Both/and' thinking encourages us to see all parts and nuances of a situation.

Learning how to hold negative and positive feelings within one situation can enhance your life dramatically. There is still joy underneath the pain and stopping to access it (usually through connection with other people) doesn't mean denying the pain or being okay with it – it's simply a way of experiencing the full spectrum of what life has to offer.

Use life's daily dramas to train for hard times

Annoying traffic, missed appointments and awkward moments are the perfect training ground to build resilience. Practising 'both/and' thinking whenever you encounter one of life's small challenges strengthens your ability to stay open to the good, even during tough times. Train yourself to find small moments of perspective, even beauty, during everyday setbacks, and you'll be better equipped to do the same when life gets really hard.

Recently I was in a fantastic mood, it was the start of the year, and I'd had a few really great realisations and let go of many things that were no longer serving me. I felt unstoppable – in a fresh new energy. I popped into the supermarket and all of the fruit and vegetables seemed brighter than usual; I felt like I was connecting with the people around me (mostly shop assistants) on a soul level.

The sun was out, I had just sold a painting, and I thought, 'Wow, this is a wonderful day,' as I walked to my car. The car park was bustling, and somehow, in the chaos, I reversed into a car. I had never crashed into anyone in all my years of driving, and I immediately went into a shaky state of shock.

I got out of my car and the other driver shouted, 'Look where you're driving!' Heart racing, I took a deep breath and smiled at him, apologising and making sure he could see me as a human being who'd made a silly mistake. Immediately, he calmed down, and after exchanging details, I got back into my car and burst into tears – my body needed to release all that emotion and energy. But after that quick cry, I checked in with myself and made a conscious decision to put the idea of radical joy to the test. Was I still feeling happy? I was! Five minutes of drama in an otherwise perfect day meant this was still a good day!

A previous version of me might have become caught up in the story of it all, and slipped into self-loathing mode for being so careless. I might have veered towards victim consciousness and asked, 'Why me? Why on such a good day?' Instead, I was able to extend myself some kindness, access my sense of perspective, drop the story and return to my awesome day.

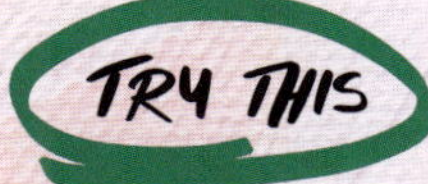

During a difficult time, open yourself up to moments of beauty, and allow yourself to accept the 'both/and' idea. Good things can happen in bad moments. Small resets like the ones below help us to build emotional resilience and keep the bigger picture in view.

+ After the 'day-ruining' event is over, do your best to let it go. Don't re-hash the moment in your mind or go into a mental cycle about it. That only causes more suffering than necessary. Don't let it darken your whole day.

+ Acknowledge your humanity. Mistakes and awkward moments happen to everyone.

+ Pause and breathe deeply to interrupt the rush of emotion.

+ Redirect your thinking. Don't let one small event dominate your perspective.

+ Shift your body language – smile, stand tall, loosen your posture.

+ Give yourself a reality check by asking, 'Will this still matter tomorrow?'

+ Stay open to the good. Believe that the rest of the day can still be great.

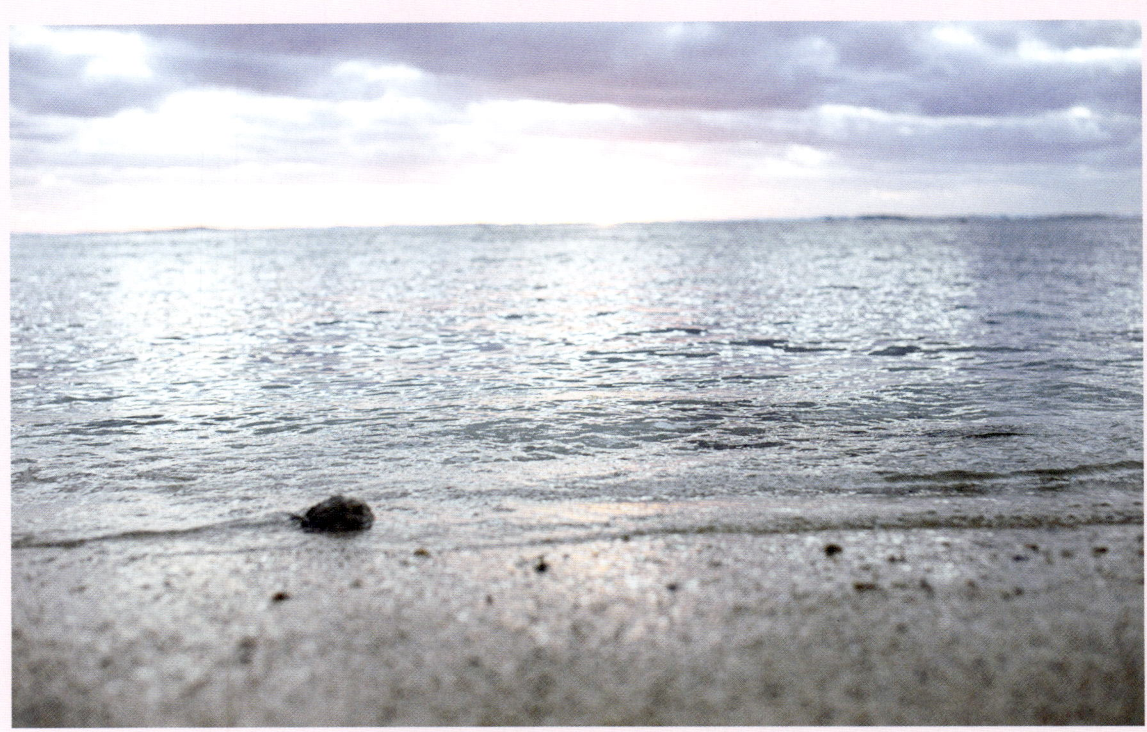

A gift in dark places

One of the biggest pitfalls of hardship, especially when a tough situation occurs over a long period of time, is falling into a victim mentality. Our brains are wired to look for the bad things and worst-case scenarios (as early cavemen, this kept us safe), so it's naturally much easier to hunt for the bad during a challenging time than it is to mine a tough situation for hidden treasure. But, with practice, we can train our brains to look for the good.

In April 2019, I was lucky enough to be on holiday in Thailand with some of my favourite family members and friends. My twin brother lives in Phuket (I know, not fair), and we were celebrating our 40th birthday together.

After a gorgeous day at the beach, I had a shower and noticed a hard lump on my ribs, just to the side of my right breast. It felt strange – like a spiky stone about the size of a pea – and unlike any other bump I'd ever noticed. I made a mental note to check in with my general practitioner when I returned to New Zealand.

A few months passed before I did anything about it – life felt completely crazy and busy, and going to the doctor seemed like a waste of time. It wasn't until I got a cough I couldn't shake that I finally asked my doctor to check the lump. She was concerned

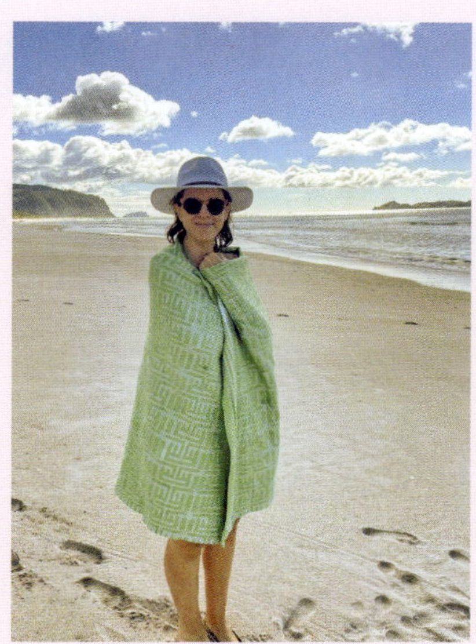

and sent me for a fine-needle aspiration – a type of biopsy. When she called a few weeks later and asked me to come in for a chat, and suggested that I might want a support person with me, I knew that it wasn't good news.

The test showed a 'suspicion of malignancy', but they needed more tests to be sure – mammograms, ultrasounds and biopsies were all necessary for an accurate diagnosis. It took ages to get an appointment in the public health system, and each step dragged on – made even less bearable with the worried, sleepless nights of not knowing.

I was diagnosed with stage one breast cancer in early October 2019 – at the age of 40, and just as I was about to start my solo exhibition of works depicting goddesses painted on Perspex (I still believe that the goddesses had chosen me to paint them so that they could give me the strength I needed over that period of my life). I was fortunate with my diagnosis, and I know so many people aren't. As the breast cancer specialist said to me, 'You got the good breast cancer, the kind we can cure.'

WHO KNEW THAT CANCER WOULD END UP BEING ONE OF THE BIGGEST BLESSINGS OF MY LIFE SO FAR.

The next two months were a blur of appointments, decisions, worry, surgery, results, more surgery and a cloud of upcoming radiotherapy hanging over me. I realised how lucky I was that I didn't need chemo on top of that, and I got to keep my breasts.

At the time, I was also making some big decisions in my career. I had built my art business to the point that it might be safe to quit my day job – a goal I'd been working towards for five years and a thought that was constantly in my head shouting at me loudly. I was desperate to go full-time with my art, but it was a scary financial decision, and my then-husband was (understandably) not keen for us to take the risk.

One thing that a cancer diagnosis gives you in spades, is perspective. Being faced with your own mortality reframes what is important to you – a lot like if someone close to you passes away. Suddenly, financial security didn't seem as important as following my most joyful path. I was convinced, but my husband wasn't – the risk seemed too great. That's where radiotherapy became my greatest gift of all.

Radiotherapy is a painless treatment; while it doesn't make you sick like chemotherapy does, it does make you exhausted and depleted for quite a while afterwards. One of the worst parts of radiotherapy is the schedule. I had to go to the hospital every weekday (five times a week) for three weeks. The treatment takes only about 15 minutes – add half an hour for waiting around and getting in and out of those gorgeous hospital robes. The hospital was about a 40-minute drive from my home. As much as my wonderful day job was incredibly understanding of what I was going through, I couldn't deny that I had a big scheduling problem. Every hour of my day was already filled with the morning school run, rushing to work, finishing early to do the afternoon school run, then working a few hours at home on my day job before doing my art business at night and on the weekends … oh, and being a parent. How would I fit a return trip to the hospital into that time and get any work done at all? I'd used up all of my sick leave and taken some extra from all the appointments and surgery before that. Something had to go. It was time to quit my job.

So, in January 2020, I became a full-time artist, and I haven't looked back. It turns out that I wasn't forgoing a good wage to follow my dreams, in fact, the opposite happened: I very quickly started making more money from art than ever before. Strangely, the timing turned out to be perfect. Covid hit not long after I took the leap, and my last few sessions of radiotherapy were undertaken during New Zealand's national Level 4 Lockdown, which was scary and strange.

Although lockdowns were crippling for so many businesses, mine was not one of them. I, along with a lot of artists, benefited from the fact that our clientele was not able to spend their money on overseas trips or restaurants. Instead, they were stuck at home, staring at their walls and making their homes beautiful with online shopping.

My cancer, and the treatments that cured it, were like a beautiful, fated gift from the universe. Yes, it was a hard time, and I still live in the shadow of knowing that the cancer could come back, but had it not happened, I don't know if I would ever have had the courage to quit my day job. My art journey would never have flourished like it has, and I probably would not be writing this book.

TRY THIS

When things go wrong, look for lessons, skills learned, or opening doors. Life gives us hardships so we can grow and learn. Sometimes, it's hard to see them while they're happening, but when you get to the other side, write in your journal and ask yourself, 'What were the gifts of this difficult time?'

+

I recently did a delightful exercise to identify the treasure from a tough 2023; you could try it, too. I drew a page of fictional Girl Scout badges I'd earned last year, acknowledging what I had learned from the tough times. I created badges such as self-compassion, resilience, boundaries, valuing heart over money and one that I called the 'creative explorer' badge. Seeing them drawn on my page gives me so much joy and makes me feel like I really accomplished a lot in a tough year!

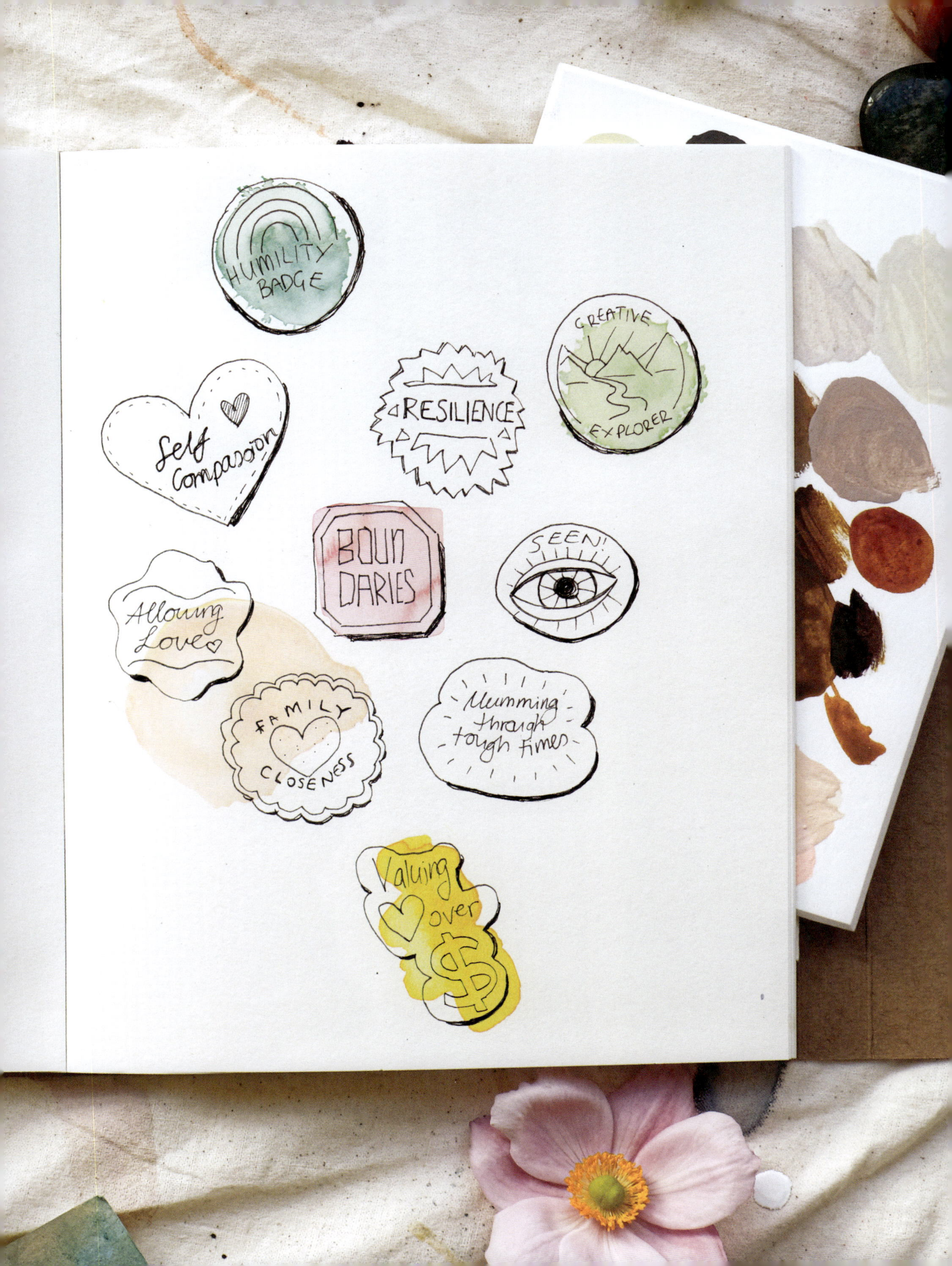
HUMILITY BADGE
CREATIVE EXPLORER
RESILIENCE
Self Compassion
BOUN DARIES
SEEN!
Allowing Love
FAMILY CLOSENESS
Humming through tough times
Valuing over $

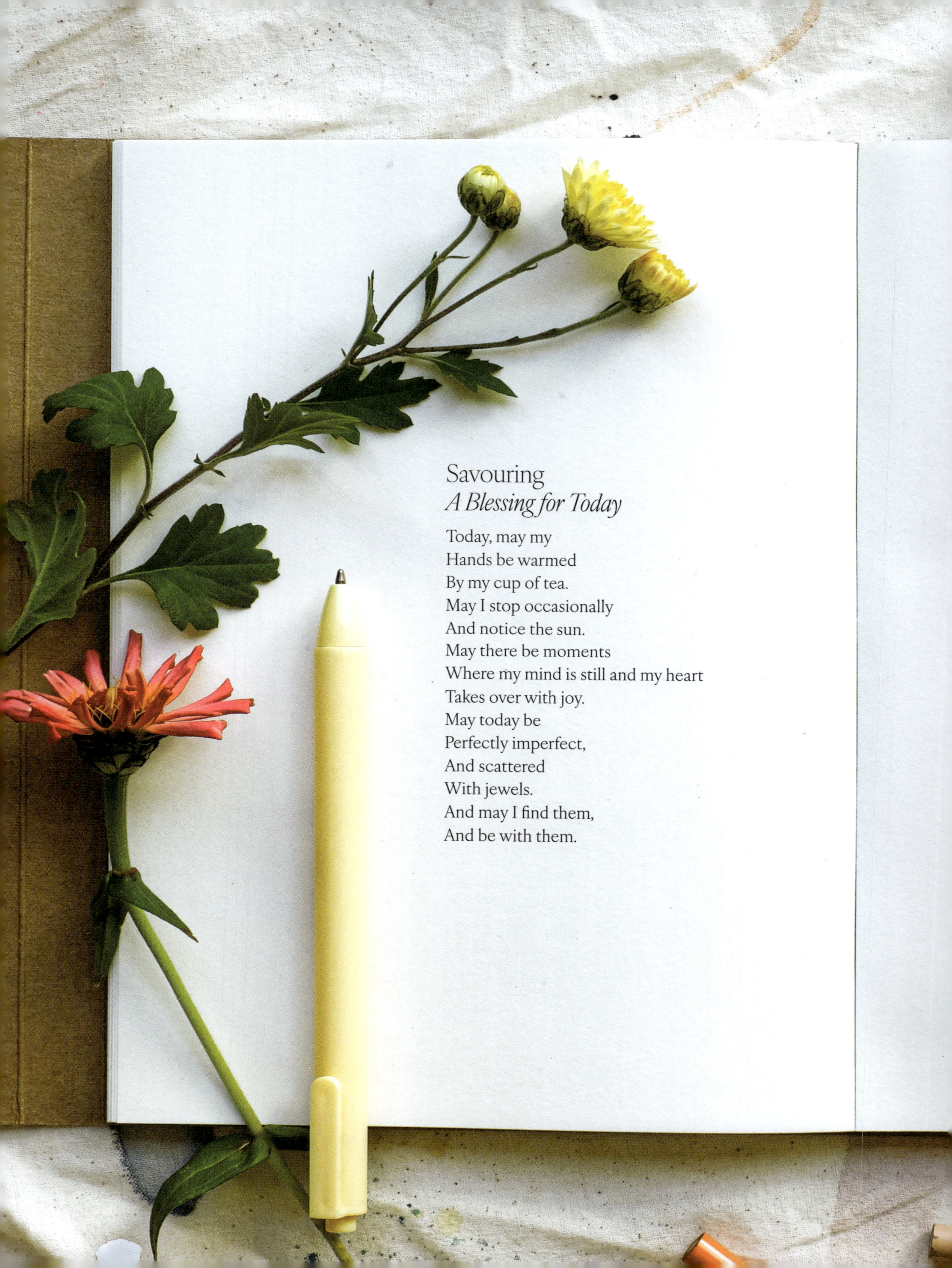

Savouring

A Blessing for Today

Today, may my
Hands be warmed
By my cup of tea.
May I stop occasionally
And notice the sun.
May there be moments
Where my mind is still and my heart
Takes over with joy.
May today be
Perfectly imperfect,
And scattered
With jewels.
And may I find them,
And be with them.

Double down on beautiful moments

We hold on so firmly to our worries. We squeeze them tightly in our minds and weave them between every thought until they colour everything. Worried that letting them go would somehow give them more power, we cling tightly to our worries – not realising that by holding on so fiercely, we're allowing them to take over.

What if we developed a practice of holding onto joy with just as much passion and fervour? We can train our brains to do this with the practice of 'savouring'. By savouring joyful moments, we can colour our view with joy instead of pain – with golden light instead of cold, grey darkness.

We are all aware of what the word 'savour' means and often use it to describe wanting to enjoy a particularly delicious meal. In positive psychology, savouring takes on a deeper, more practical meaning. Fred Bryant and Joseph Veroff (both US psychology professors) created the model. They define it as follows: *'noticing and appreciating the positive aspects of life – the positive counterpart to coping. Savoring is more than pleasure – it also involves mindfulness and "conscious attention to the experience of pleasure."'*

To do this, we need to be aware of a beautiful moment – big or small – and focus on it with *intention* rather than being distracted away from it by the world around us. This way, rather than letting it pass by in a second, we can soak it up for a longer period and become involved in it. 'It is like swishing the experience around … in your mind,' says Bryant, author of the 2006 book, *Savoring: A New Model of Positive Experience*.

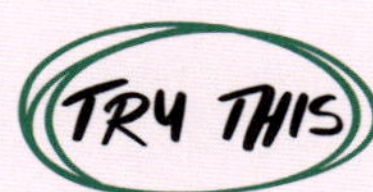

In positive psychology, small acts of noticing and savouring moments of joy can help raise your baseline happiness. These five ideas are inspired by Shawn Achor's 'The Doubler' exercise – a simple but powerful way to train your brain to hold onto the good. Make a beautiful moment last longer and lean into it.

1

If you notice a bird singing outside, focus on it for a few seconds, listen to the song and think about where the bird has been or might be going.

2

If your friend says something kind to you, soak it in, don't bashfully move on to the next topic.

3

While you're doing something pleasurable, be present with it – if you take a bite of a meal, notice the warmth, the texture, the flavour – find details in it that you might not have noticed before. Try to focus on it for a bit longer than you would instinctively do.

4

If you notice a small wonder of nature – a rainbow, a pretty leaf, a ray of light on your bedroom floor – stop and enjoy it, point it out to someone nearby. Be with it for a few minutes.

5

If you have a fantastic night out, or a delicious meal; when you get home, sit for a few minutes and think about it. Remember the details, enjoy it all over again. Feel the joy of joy!

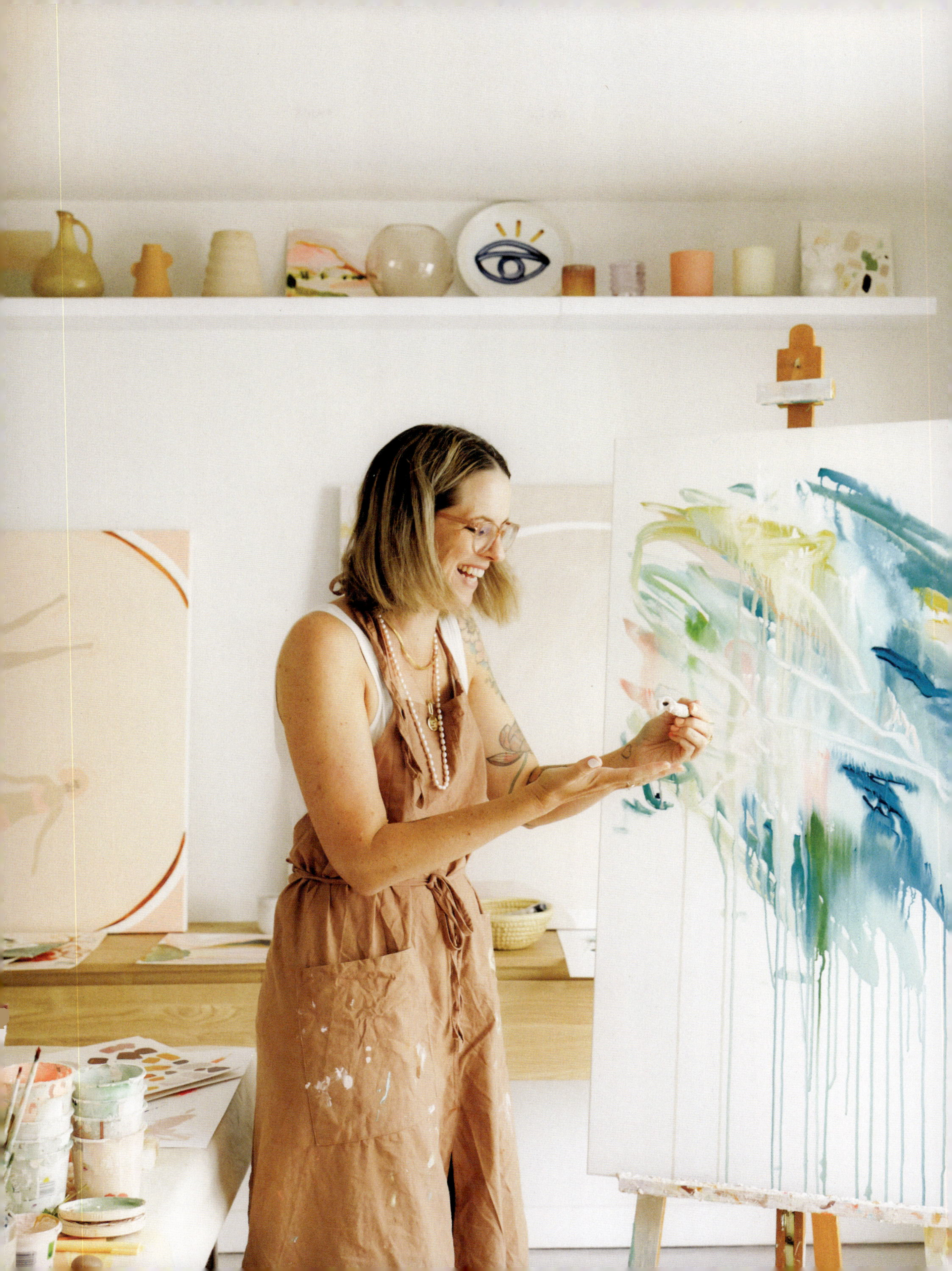

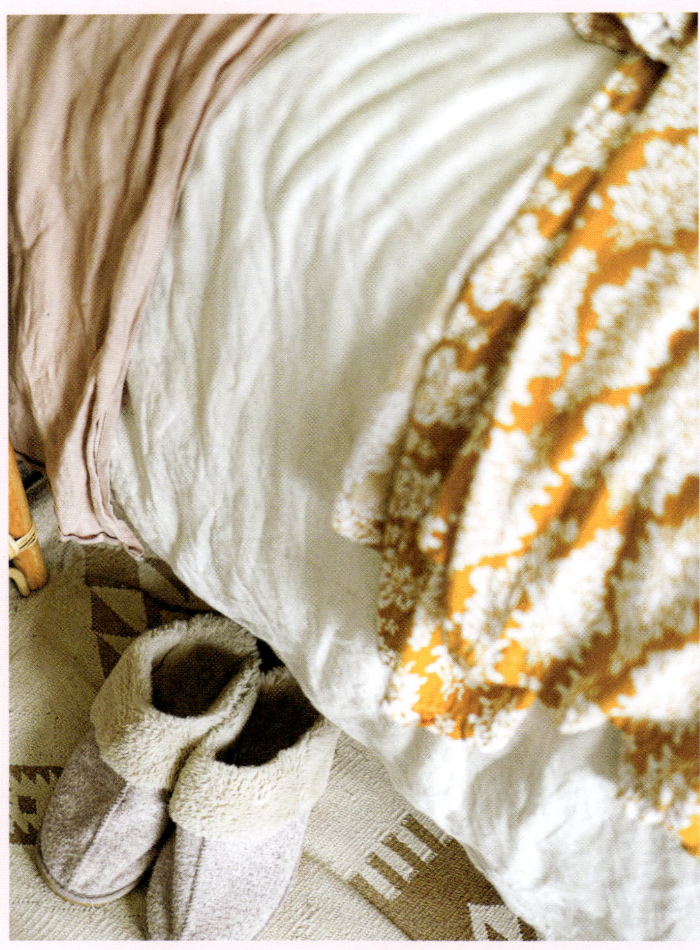

Make it sacred

I've borrowed this title from the wonderful Sarah Blondin (if you want to listen to a voice and heart that soothes your soul, look her up on Podcasts or Insight Timer) who has a beautiful, guided meditation of the same name.

Just those three words – Make it Sacred – bring me into a state of peace and joy. Make it Sacred is the idea of walking through life, even if it's for short moments, with a feeling of reverence and wonder. Seeing your life as a masterpiece and noticing the small but powerful moments of wonder that are everywhere.

This is a beautiful joy practice, and if you get into the habit of doing it, it brings wonder into your day. Like so many of these practices, it works by bringing you into the moment – focusing on the beauty rather than being stuck in your mind.

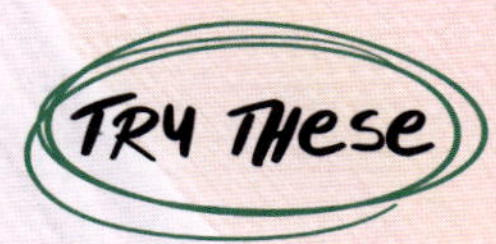

A wonderful way to bring this to life is to create ceremonies out of everyday activities. Find beauty and meaning in simple moments, and transform 'normal' moments by adding a sense of sacredness.

Waking up

Living for another day, each day, must be one of the greatest blessings of all. In the morning, before your head leaves the pillow, take a moment to soak in the joy of being alive. The softness of your bed, the sun waking up outside – feel gratitude for a new day.

Having a shower

Showers can feel like a wonderful metaphor. Use the time to wash off any anxieties or niggles from the day. Picture the water cleaning not only your body but also your soul. Enjoy the sensation of the warm water on your shoulders, and the smell of the soap on your skin.

Serving a meal

Mealtimes can be busy and stressful if you have a family to feed. As you serve the food, be grateful for the ability to nourish yourself and those around you and consider every person that has had a hand in growing, transporting and packaging your food before it got to you.

Lighting a candle

I will find any excuse to light a candle, it just makes everything feel more special. Find reasons to light a candle. The kids have all gone to bed – light a candle to celebrate. You're home alone for a little while – a candle and beautiful music make the time more memorable. As you light it, wonder at the fact that we now have fire at our fingertips, and how its gentle glow changes the ambiance of a room.

Making a cup of tea

Select the perfect cup, feel its coolness on your hands. While the water boils, don't rush off to another task. Wait nearby and take a few breaths with your hand on your heart. Listen to the sound of the water as you pour it into the cup and look for wisps of steam, enjoy the sound of the spoon stirring. Feel the warmth of the cup, and savour the first sip.

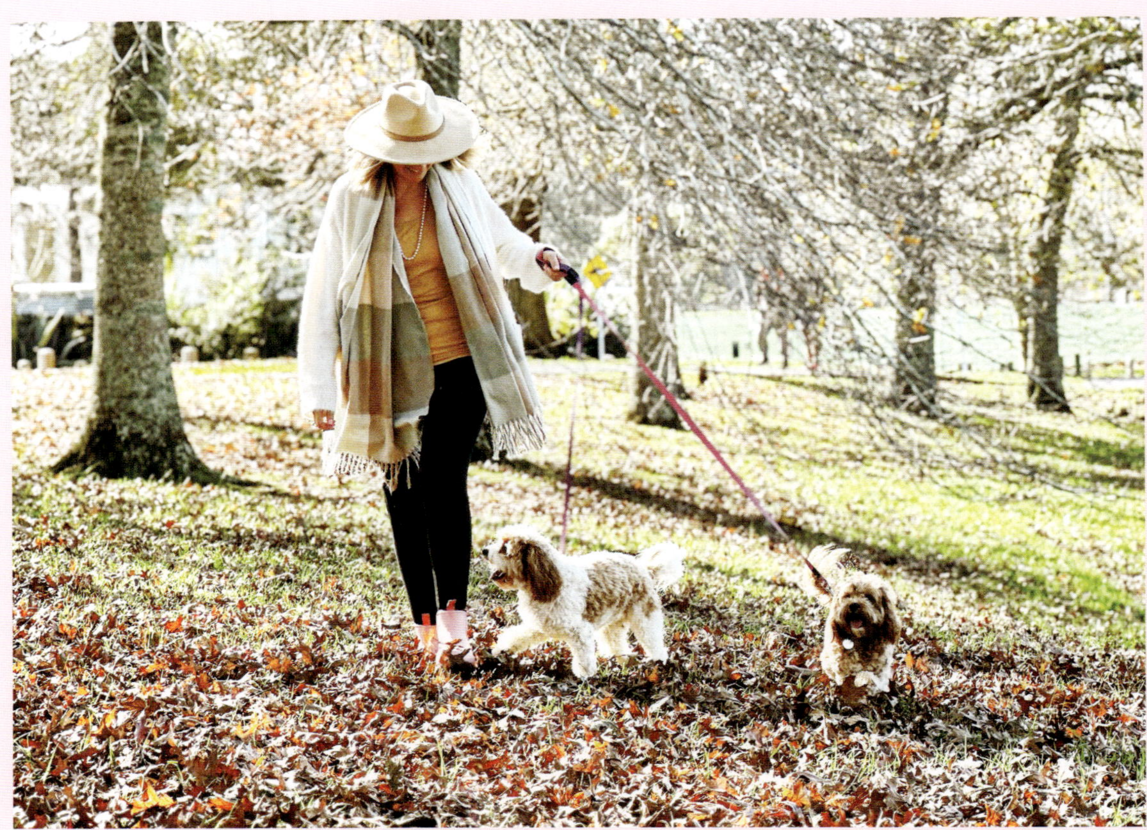

NOTHING FEELS QUITE AS DELIGHTFUL AS CRUNCHING THROUGH THE AUTUMN LEAVES WITH PEACHES AND BEAN.

Delight as a practice

One of my favourite practices is DELIGHT! I've written this word in capitals with an exclamation mark because that's how doing this practice feels to me. I discovered it in a book by Ross Gay, called *The Book of Delights*. Before I read it, I had heard him speak on a few podcasts about how the idea for this practice came to him, and I'm so glad I heard him talk about this because he is an absolute delight himself.

Ross explains that he suspected that delight was like a muscle: the more he looked for moments of delight, the stronger his ability to find it would get, and the more delight he'd experience daily. To test this, he decided to write a mini-essay at the end of each day for one year about things that delighted him.

And what came of this? Well, it turned out Ross was right: delight is a muscle, and the more he looked for it, the more it showed up. In the process, he accidentally invented a joyful daily practice that's available to all of us. One where we look for the good, and find more of it everywhere.

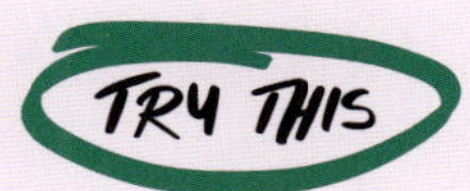

This is a simple practice, and you can decide whether you'd like to keep a written list (there's something so romantic about carrying around a tiny notebook in your car or your bag for this exact reason!), or type them into the notes in your phone. The easiest version, however, is to just say the word 'DELIGHT!' in your head or out loud whenever you notice something delightful.

+

The very first day I heard Ross talk about this concept, I went for a walk (with my rather delightful little dogs) and noticed possibly the most delightful thing I'd ever seen: two elderly women walking towards me pushing their elderly dogs in baby strollers – the front-facing kind.

+

Watching them walk toward me, with their slightly dishevelled but grinning little dogs in strollers, it was all I could do not to shout the word 'DELIGHT!' right in their faces. Since then, I've seen them several times at the same park. Their dogs love getting out but can't keep going for very long, so when they tire, the ladies pop them into baby strollers so they can still enjoy the sights, sounds and smells of the park without their tiny little legs getting too tired.

+

One of the most beautiful aspects of this practice is when it's turned into a shared experience with someone special in your life. It's easily understood and appreciated by all ages, and sharing this practice with others makes it even better. You can simply point out delightful things to your friends and family. Or, you might decide to make a pact with a friend to send each other a picture of something that delights you every day for a month – to build those delight muscles. We light each other up when we share these things. Even if the thing that delights them doesn't delight us – their enjoyment of it will!

An incomplete list of recent delights

+ My dogs' sweet little smiling faces.

+ Just the right cup for my coffee.

+ Colours so subtle that they are almost white – whispering joy.

+ Paintings done by children.

+ The word 'held'.

+ Cleverly named books and paintings.

+ Laughing until I can't stop.

+ Walking with friends.

+ Way too many house plants.

+ Cinnamon.

+ Light streaming into my room in the late afternoon.

+ Evenings that are warm enough to sit outside.

+ A new leaf unfurling on my monstera.

+ My daughter mastering a new trick on the trampoline.

+ Clear, turquoise water in a pool or a tropical sea.

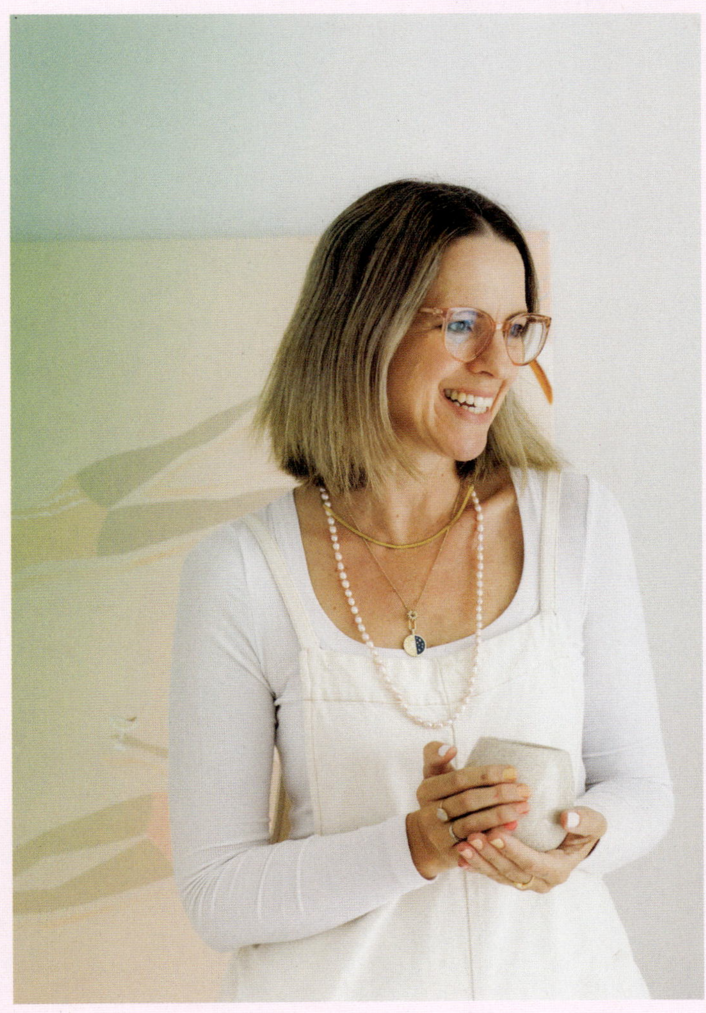

Using 'I love' as an inroad to delight

If delight seems like too much of an emotional leap, particularly on a day when thoughts are busy and twisting up my mind, I use a simple strategy to get myself into 'delight mode'. It might sound silly, but it works – especially when I'm on the move in the car, on a walk, or strolling around a supermarket.

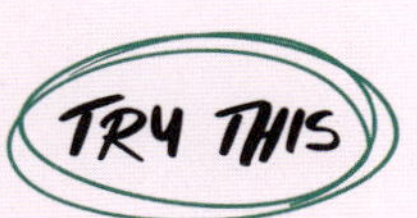

Start the statement 'I love ...', then look around for something to love. Some random results can come out (like 'I love how the sunlight is shining on that car's side mirror', or 'I love the colour of that rice packaging'). But keep going – like a stream of consciousness – repeating 'I love ...' with a corresponding thing in your vicinity to love, over and over for a few minutes.

+

This exercise might sound silly, and you might be tempted to discard it as nonsense, but I urge you to try it once or twice. See how long you can keep up the stream of 'I love' before your busy thoughts creep back in, and see how you feel afterwards. It's another way of being in the moment, delighting in ordinary life, and reminding yourself that you're filled with love and the world is filled with unexpected things just waiting to be appreciated.

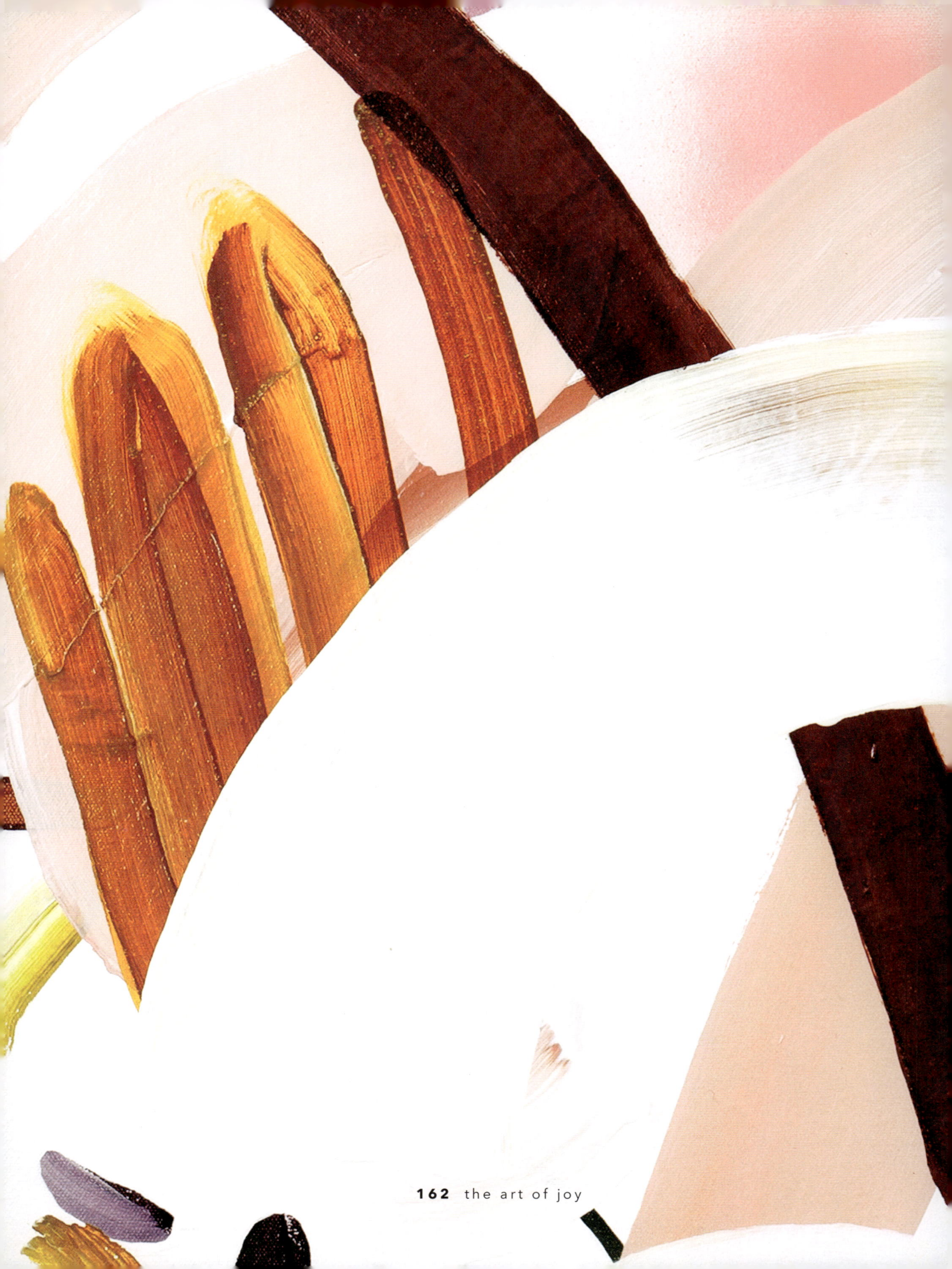

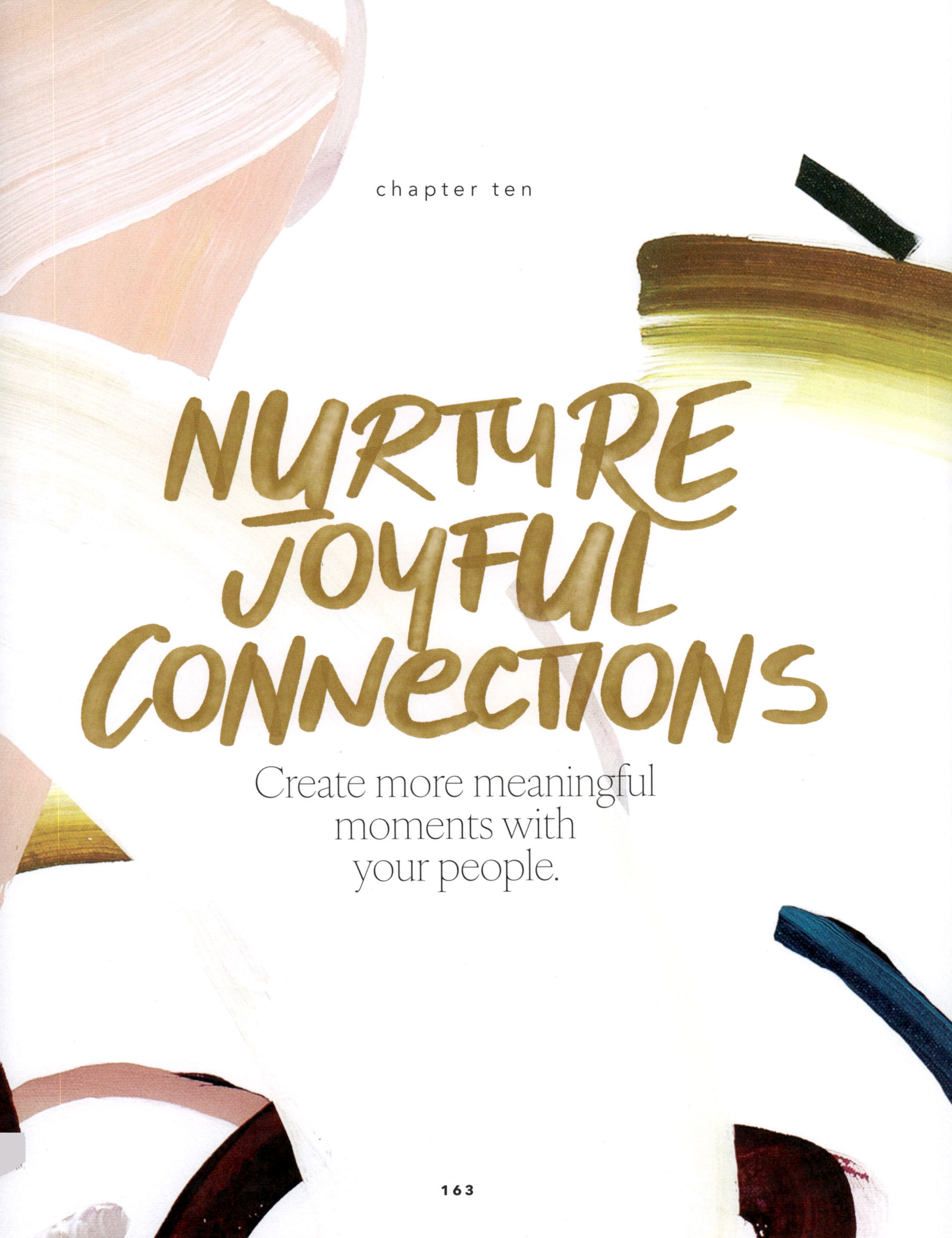

chapter ten

NURTURE JOYFUL CONNECTIONS

Create more meaningful moments with your people.

A book about joy would not be complete without a chapter about connecting with those around us, as connection is absolutely the most important aspect of being alive on this crazy planet. Connections run deep and spread wide. The way our world is organised means that we're connected to people we have never met in offices, factories and farms that we'll never see. Being aware of those connections creates a sense of compassion and love for everyone around us.

Fostering connections with others is one of the keys to a happier, more fulfilling life. It's also one of the six ways to increase baseline happiness that we spoke about on page 78. Our connections are a deep, true joy that must be tended to. Studies have shown that one of the greatest causes of sadness is loneliness, and not only does it affect our mental health, but our physical health too. Social isolation and loneliness have been shown to have similar mortality risks to alcohol consumption, smoking, inactivity and obesity. It is not only our minds and hearts, but our flesh-and-bone bodies that need connection to thrive. We have evolved to live in community with others.

In an ever-increasingly isolated lifestyle – where screens take precedence over physical contact – we need to create and nurture relationships with people intentionally. Undeniably, we are intrinsically connected – tuning into, savouring, and growing those connections is where the magic lies.

Whether we're sharing in joy, pain, or in the necessary but mundane tasks that keep us alive, doing it with other humans makes every experience richer and more beautiful.

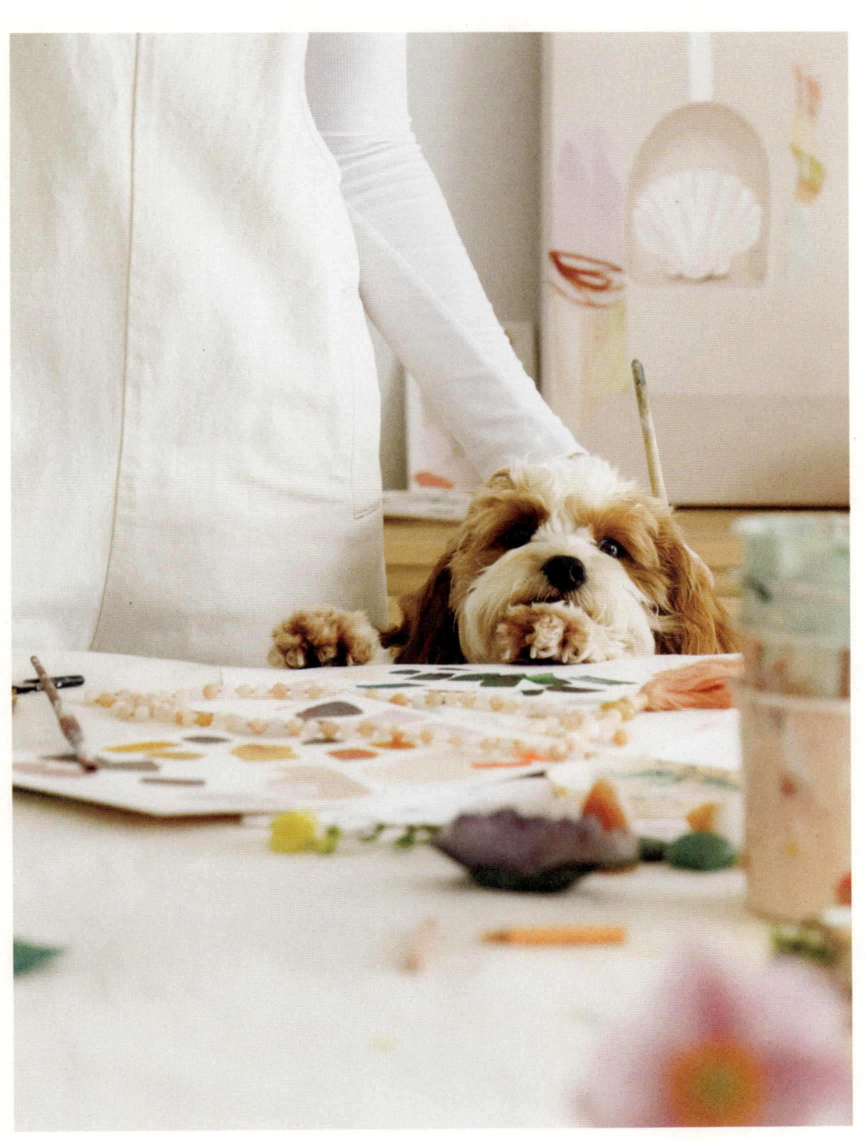

Connecting with family

Isn't it funny that we can live in the same house or apartment as a group of people, day after day, and still forget to connect? It's understandable, I guess. Life gets quite chaotic, and in a sea of tasks, chores and schedules, it might not feel like there is time for much else. But we can (and should) find small moments, in between the necessary chaos, for warmth and connection.

During a rocky patch with my own daughter, I was reminded that this precious connection needed nurturing. I realised that 90 per cent of our communication involved me asking her to do something, or telling her not do something!

Noticing this was an eye-opener because that's certainly not the type of parent I set out to be. If this sounds like a confession, that's because it is. I couldn't deny that the sweetness with which I treated her as a baby and a young child had slowly eroded in the torrent of endless tasks, requests, messy bedrooms, snacks, screen-time warnings and distractions.

Since then, I've become more intentional about how I connect with her in the 'nothing moments' – those in-between times, like when she's eating a snack and I'm cleaning the kitchen, or in the car on the way to school. Rather than retreating into my own mind and chewing on a business challenge or coming up with a new creative idea, I revel in her presence. I remind myself what a privilege it is to have this magical human be such an integral part of my life. I ask her questions, and give her answers my full attention. I smile when I talk to her and look her in the eye. I come up behind her and tickle her (one of her favourite things) and try to inject more playful conversation into our interactions. I should have been doing these things all along; I probably thought I *was* doing them, but I'm definitely doing them now, and we are both so much happier for it.

Since our day-to-day responsibilities aren't going anywhere, it's up to us to nuture our close relationships, and infuse our busy days with connection, love and play. We each have different ways of showing and receiving love, and on page 168, you'll find a guide to five 'love languages'. If you want to connect with someone, it will be much more effective if you relate to them in *their* love language. So, ask your person what their love languages are, and show them love in those ways.

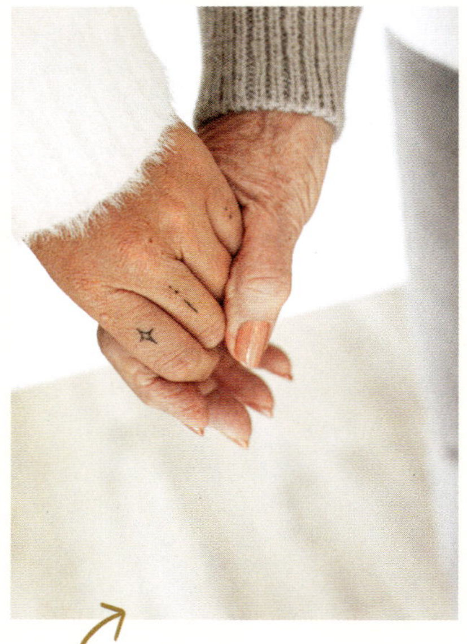

A WAY TO FIND OUT ANOTHER'S LOVE LANGUAGE IS TO ASK: 'WHEN DO YOU FEEL THE MOST LOVED BY ME?' I FEEL LOVED WHEN HOLDING MY MUM'S HAND.

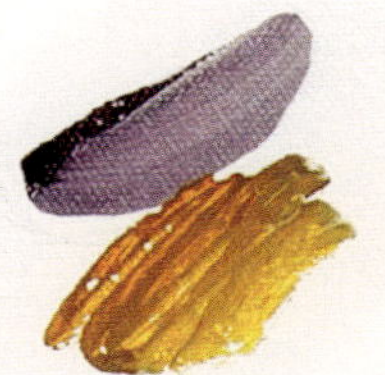

Connection exercise #1:
3 questions

If dinner conversations have become transactional, try asking more interesting questions, ideally ones that align with your values or intentions for your family. For example, I might ask my daughter, 'What kind act did you do or see today?' Since I value kindness, I want to move it up on the priority list of topics. Ask the same question of each person at the table before moving on to another.

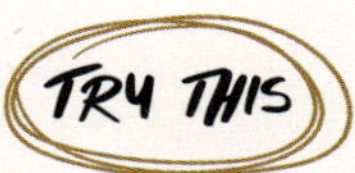

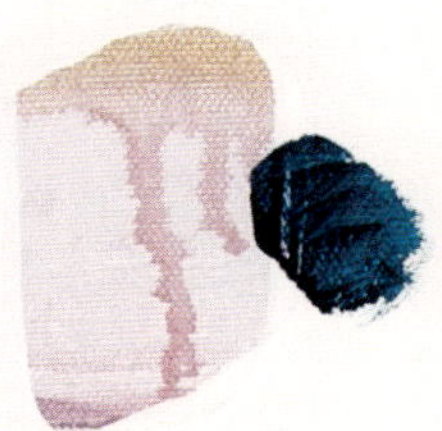

Questions can be meaningful or playful. They can relate to the day or have a broader view. There's no set formula, the point is to connect. Here are some ideas to get you started.

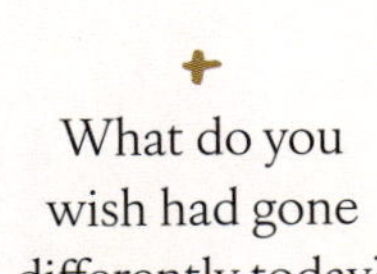

+ What do you wish had gone differently today?

+ What is your favourite thing about the person to your right?

+ What is the most beautiful thing you have ever seen?

+ What made you laugh today?

+ If you could pick any superpower, what would it be, and why?

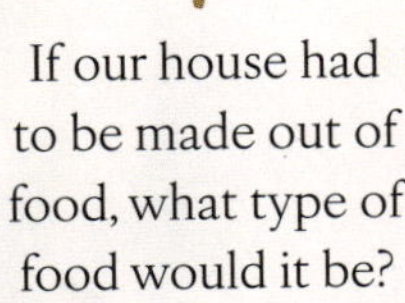

+ If our house had to be made out of food, what type of food would it be?

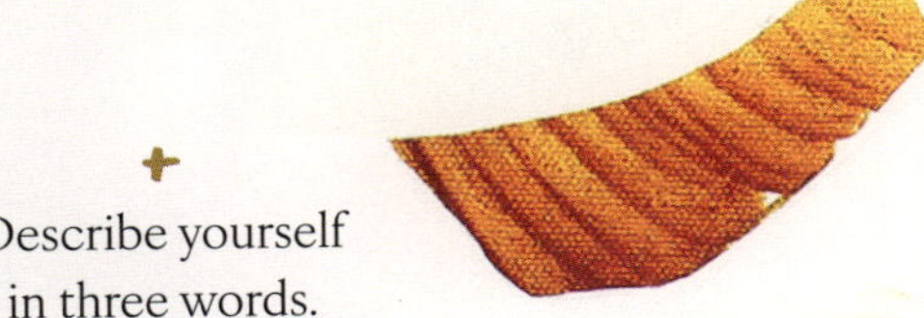

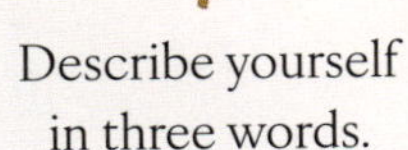

+ Describe yourself in three words.

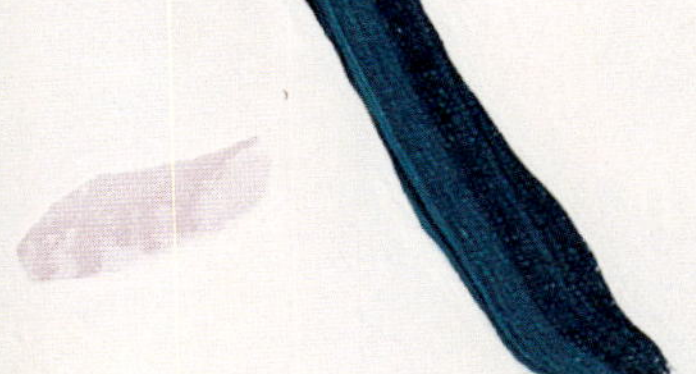

Chapman's five love languages

The concept of love languages was developed by Dr Gary Chapman and outlined in his book *The 5 Love Languages*. According to Chapman, these are the five primary ways people express and experience love, which he calls 'languages'. These are:

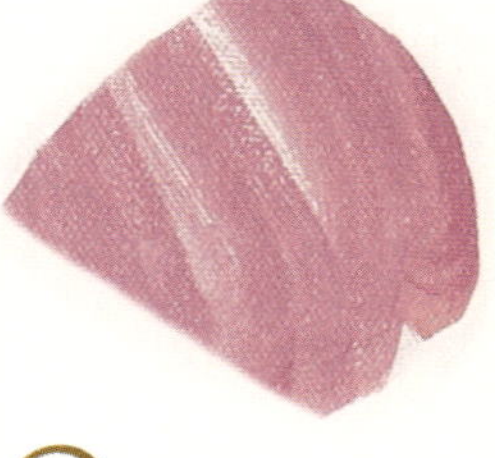

1
Words of affirmation

This language uses words to affirm other people, expressing love, appreciation, and positive affirmations through verbal acknowledgment, compliments, or words of appreciation.

Example: A little note tucked into a lunchbox, a lipstick kiss on the bathroom mirror with *You've got this* written underneath. A spontaneous text telling them what you admire about them.

2
Acts of service

For these individuals, actions speak louder than words. They feel loved and express love through acts of service, which could be anything from doing household chores, cooking a meal, or any other task that can help or ease the responsibilities of their loved ones.

Example: Making them a cup of tea without being asked to. Folding the washing, or handling a task they've been dreading to ease their load.

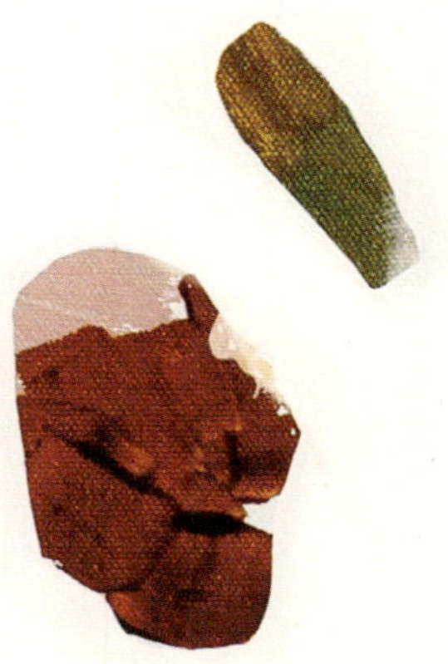

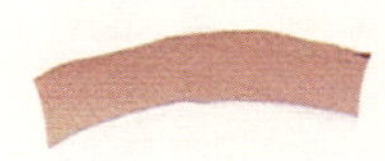

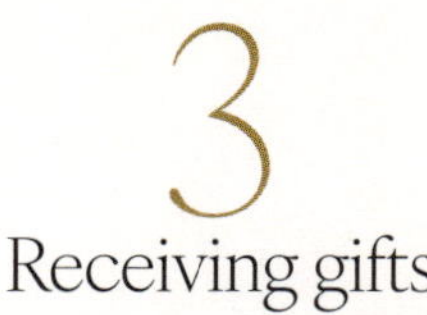

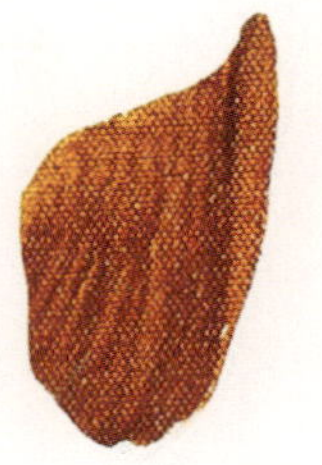

3
Receiving gifts

This love language is about giving and receiving tangible tokens of love and affection. It's not necessarily about the monetary value of the gift but more about the thoughtfulness behind the gesture and the fact that the gift is a physical symbol of love.

+

Example: Bringing home their favourite pastry just because. Leaving a flower on their pillow, or gifting a tiny trinket that reminds you of a joke you both share.

4
Quality time

Spending meaningful time with them or giving them your undivided attention is essential if your loved one identifies with this language. Quality time might involve conversations, shared activities, or simply being together in a way that fosters connection and understanding.

+

Example: Going for a walk together without your phone. Taking time to have a proper chat over breakfast. Planning a date night that's just the two of you, even if it's on the couch.

5
Physical touch

For individuals who feel loved through physical touch, physical expressions of love, such as hugs, kisses, holding hands, and other forms of physical closeness are vital. This love language emphasises the warmth and comfort that comes from physical proximity.

+

Example: Reaching for their hand when you walk side by side. Giving them a long hug at the end of a busy day, or a back rub while you're watching TV.

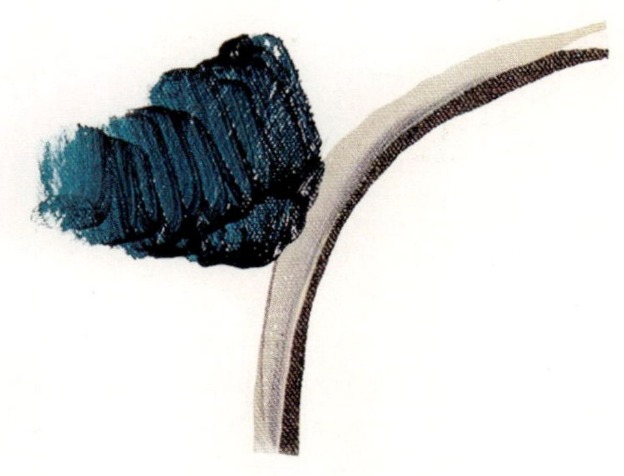

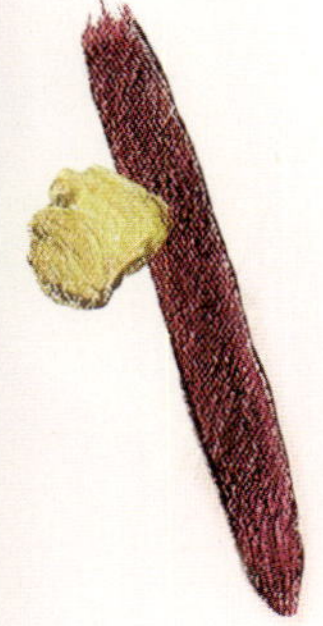

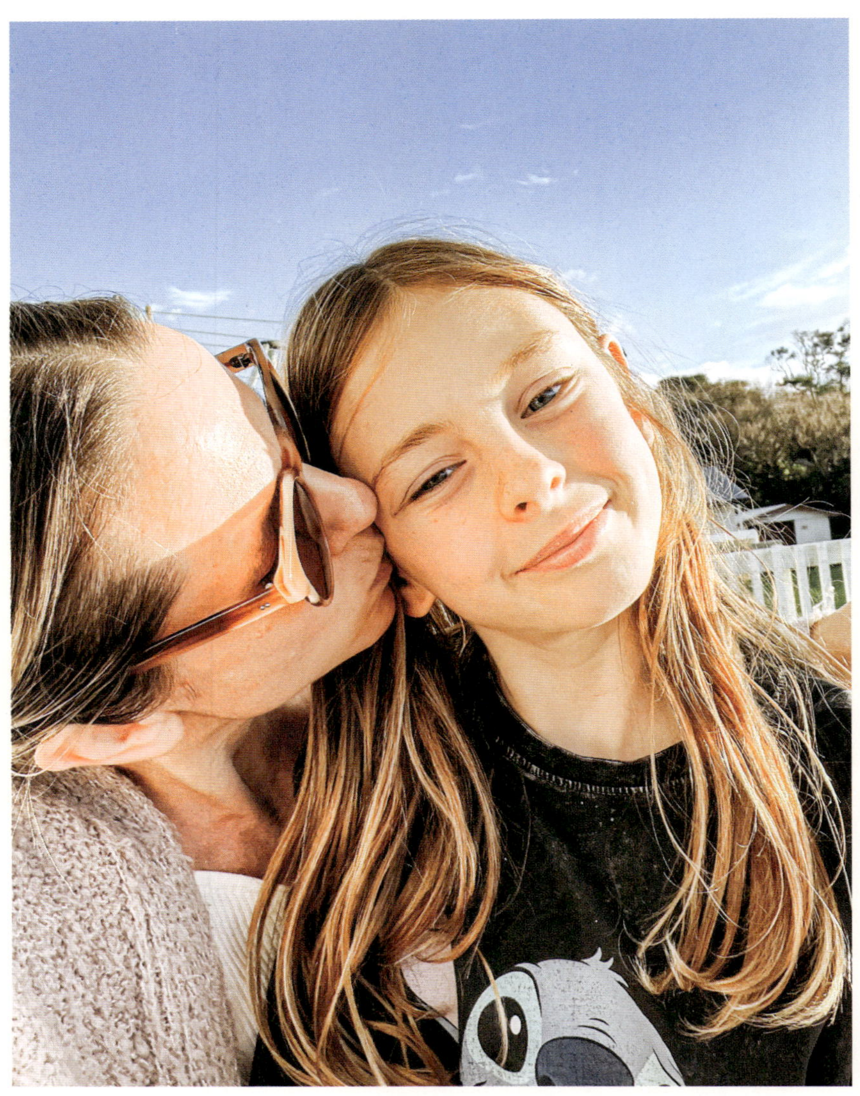

Connection exercise #2: Meet them where they are

To connect with people, it is important to know what they need from you in the moment. I heard a phrase that frames this idea succinctly: If someone comes to you with a problem, you need to find out if they want to be *Heard, Hugged or Helped*. I have a tendency to jump straight into helping, but often a child, friend, or partner just wants to be heard.

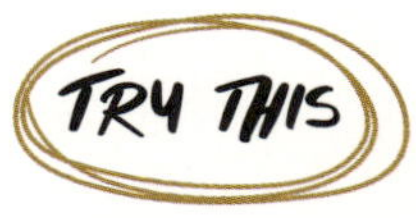

Next time someone comes to you with an issue or a gripe, ask them: 'Do you want to be Heard, Hugged or Helped?' Then be with them in the way that they need.

Connection exercise #3: Tiny moments of belonging

Not everyone has someone on-hand 24/7 to offer them a hug or a listening ear. Thankfully, we can experience moments of connection in other ways. Simply being out in the world among other people can boost our mood as well as our sense of belonging. You don't always need a long conversation to feel connected. Sometimes, just being near another life is enough. Animals, too, can be an incredible source of comfort and co-regulation. Small moments of warmth matter deeply. Such as:

TRY THIS

- Saying good morning to someone walking past.
- A brief chat with a barista.
- People-watching in the park.
- Having your cat curl up in your lap.
- Giving a genuine compliment to a stranger (their shoes, their dog, their energy!).
- Letting someone go ahead of you in a queue.
- Sharing a knowing smile with a fellow shopper when the line is long.
- Stroking your dog's fur.

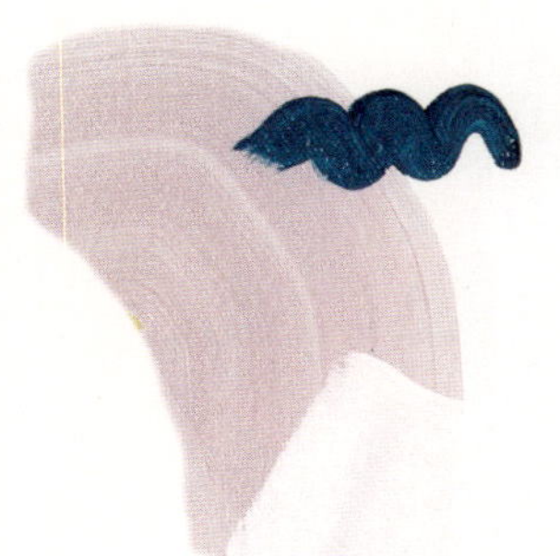

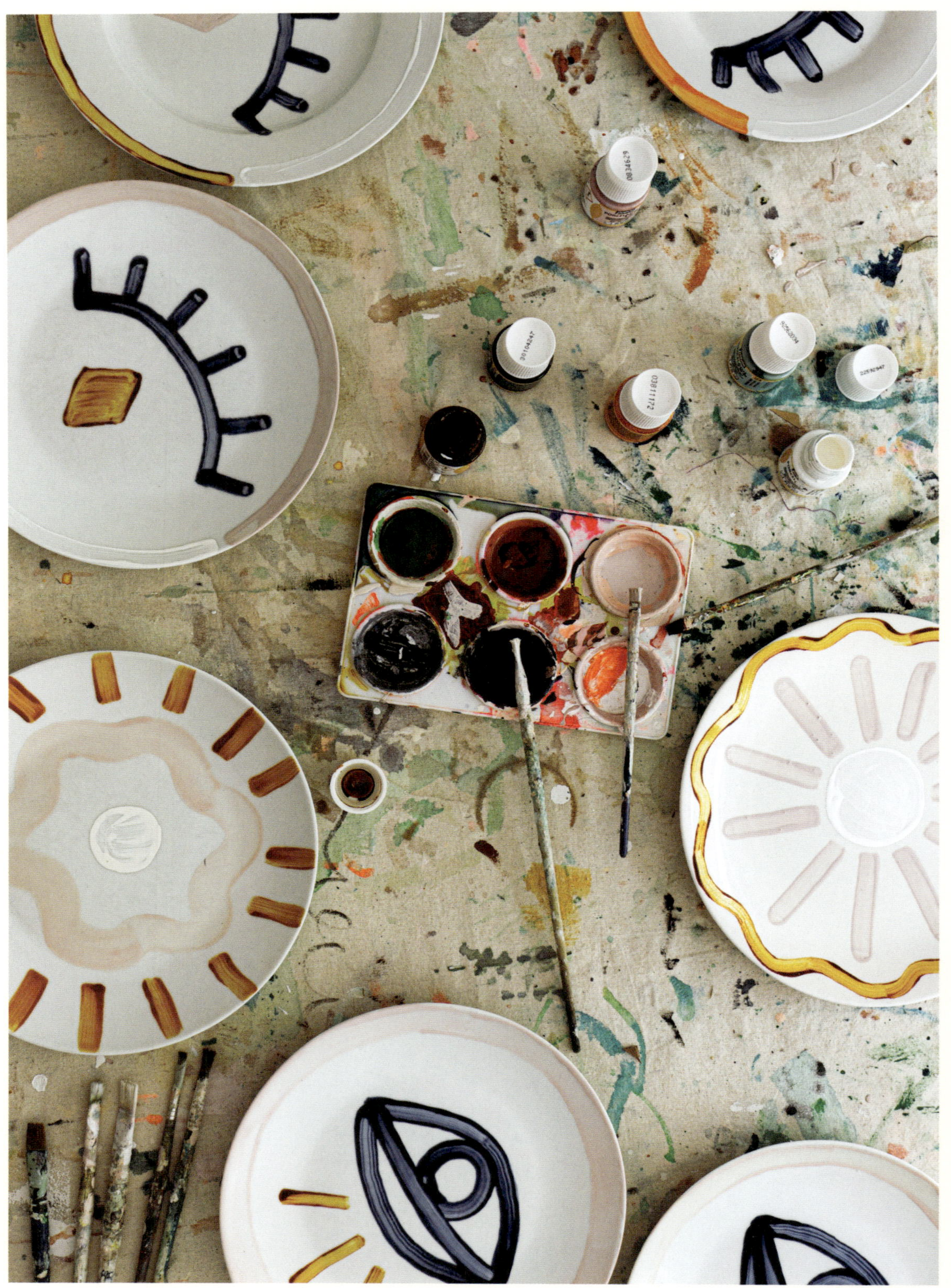

Connecting with friends

My friends are an integral part of my life. Since my husband and I separated in 2022, they've become even more so. Their support and companionship have kept me alive and provided countless moments of joy.

Lately, I've been experimenting with creating 'intentional gatherings'. I first heard about these on an episode of Glennon Doyle's podcast, *We Can Do Hard Things*, where Priya Parker was a guest. She wrote *The Art of Gathering: How We Meet and Why it Matters*, and in it, she highlights that while many of us are good at making time to spend with people we love, we don't always do it with intention.

Think about it; other than a few key events such as weddings, 21st birthdays and funerals, our gatherings can be a bit random and unintentional. We get together, eat, drink, play and chat, and this is great fun, but could some of these gatherings be more meaningful? At all of the milestone events I just mentioned, we are there for a reason that we all understand, and we are usually celebrating the people involved. People feel special and connected. Why can't we bring this feeling into our gatherings more often? The answer is, we can.

What if we plan gatherings more intentionally? This doesn't mean they can't be big or elaborate, it just means that there is an idea behind them – something that connects the guests to each other and makes them feel seen, understood and appreciated. Start with a purpose and, as the host, communicate that to the guests. Use that intention to inform who you invite, where you will gather, and what types of things you'll do. If you're drawn to this idea, I urge you to listen to the podcast episode or visit Priya's website.

I hosted my first intentional gathering in April 2024. I'm not one for half measures, so I went all out on this one, planning for months in advance – but you can create your own on a simpler scale if it works better for you. I found immense joy in expressing myself through this event, so much so that I considered the planning of it one of my 'play' activities.

THIS WAS SOME PREP FOR MY SPECIAL GATHERING. THESE DETAILS MADE IT MAGICAL.

My goddess party

Not too long ago, I had a dinner party for my closest girlfriends. I called it a 'Modern Goddess Dinner'. I've always been fascinated with the idea of goddesses, and even did an entire art series and exhibition of goddess archetypes in 2019. The table was adorned with an eclectic mix of candles, flowers, a scattering of crystals and some hand-painted, goddess-themed plates (I'm always looking for an excuse to paint something).

I spent evenings writing notes about each of my friends, highlighting what makes them exceptional and unique: their goddess qualities. Each one started with a headline/goddess title. For example, there was *Abby: The Goddess Whose Smile is Made of the Sun; Hayley: Goddess of Making Things Beautiful; Keah: Goddess of the Vast, Warm, Open Heart*. Their titles were followed by a paragraph or two describing their best qualities, and what they mean to me. At the dinner, I read them all out – creating a space where each guest got to know each other on a deeper level, and more importantly, felt special and seen.

Each guest was told to dress as their unique goddess self. We ate, drank, laughed, and some of my closest friends who didn't know each other formed brand new bonds. We celebrated the wonder of being a woman, and a Modern Goddess.

My guests all felt the love and intention that was infused into the evening. We all remarked that we need to spend more time telling each other how wonderful we are, rather than wait for our funerals! It even inspired a few of them to create their own intentional gatherings, which warms my heart.

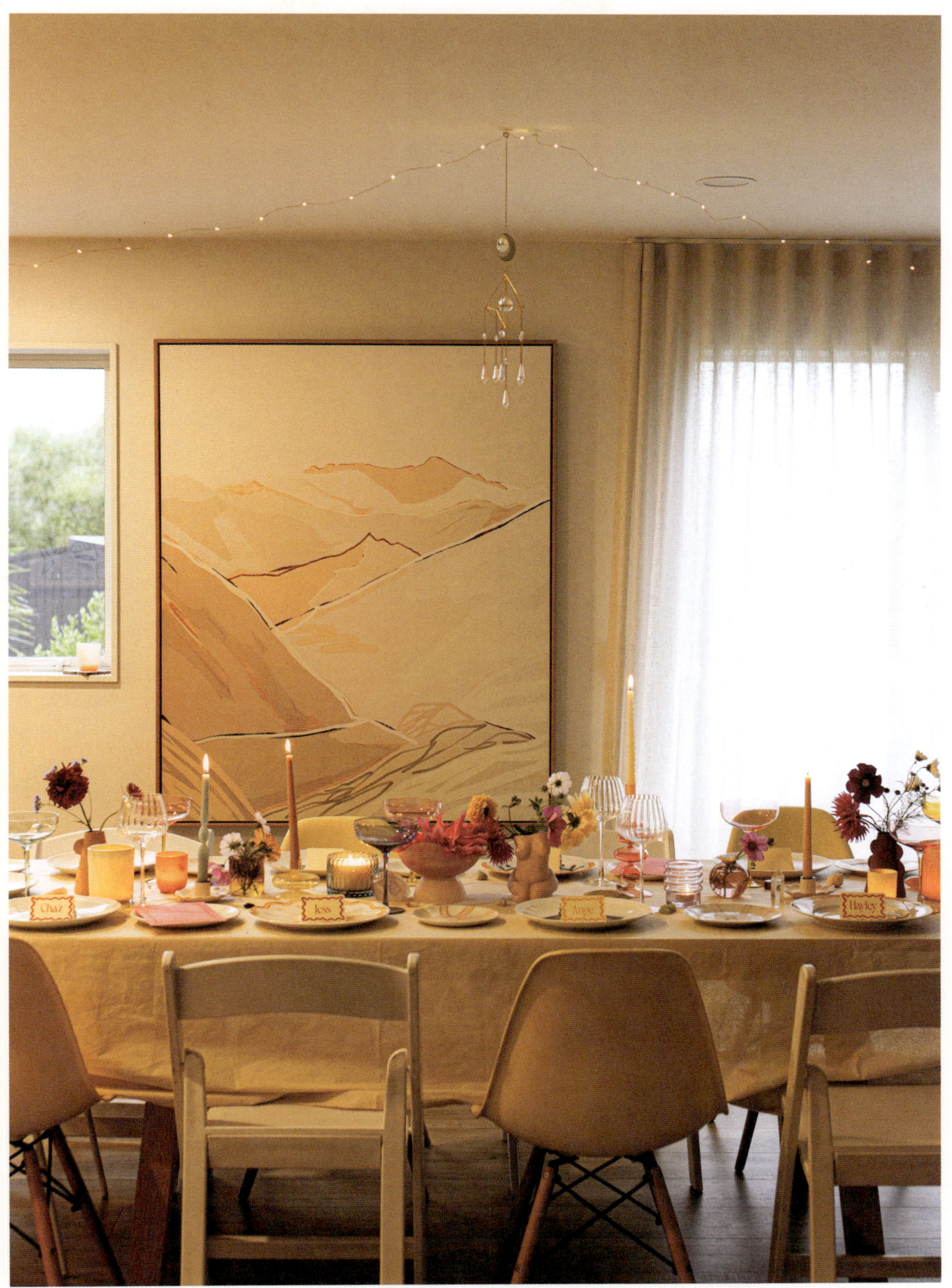
Chaz
Jess
Ange
Hayley

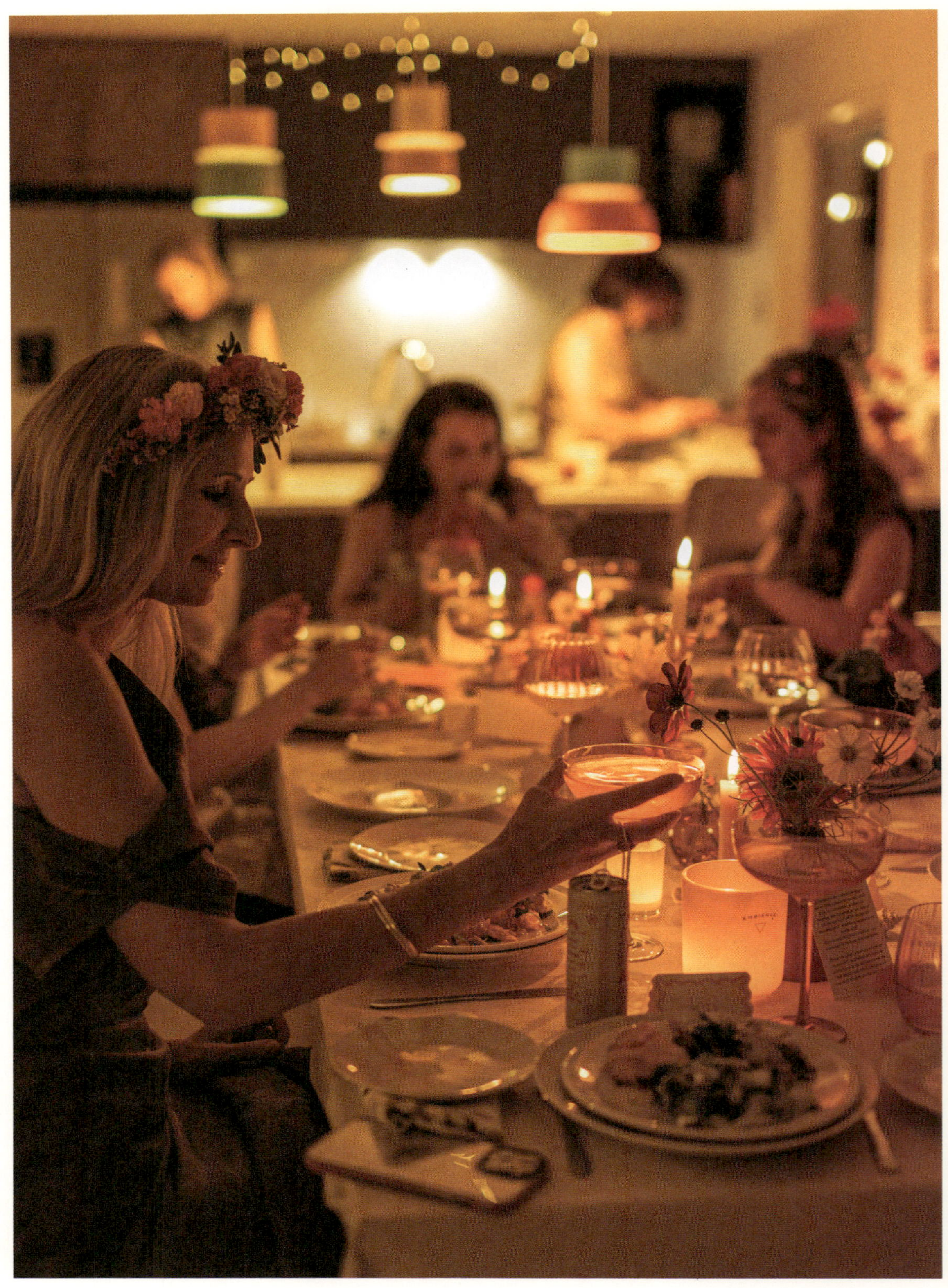

Connection exercise #4: Plan your own intentional event

To create an intentional gathering of your own you can go large, like I did, or start small. It doesn't need to cost much or take much planning. The key is *specificity*. Tell your guests the purpose of the gathering and inject some meaning into it. The possibilities are endless, and this can be extended to work and family gatherings too.

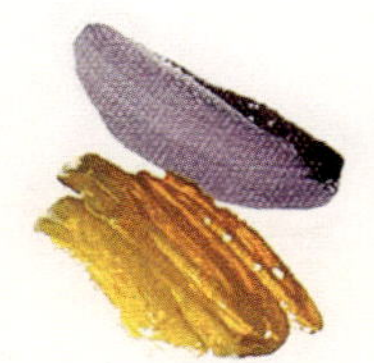

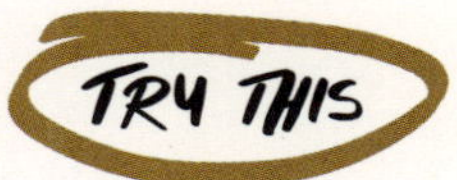

Stuck for ideas? Here are a few suggestions.

1
The question dinner

Host a meal where each course comes with a question. Use prompts like 'What brought you joy this week?' or 'What risk are you glad you took?'

2
The swap brunch

Everyone brings an item - something meaningful they're ready to part with. Share the story behind it, then swap. This is a gentle way to let go and connect.

3
Bring a chapter

Ask guests to bring a short book excerpt that moved them. Read that aloud and share why it mattered. This gives a peek into each other's inner world.

4
Intentional walk and talk

Go for a walk and give the conversation a theme, like *What I want to let go of*. Take turns sharing. Movement helps open up deeper conversation.

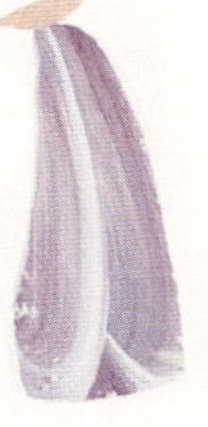

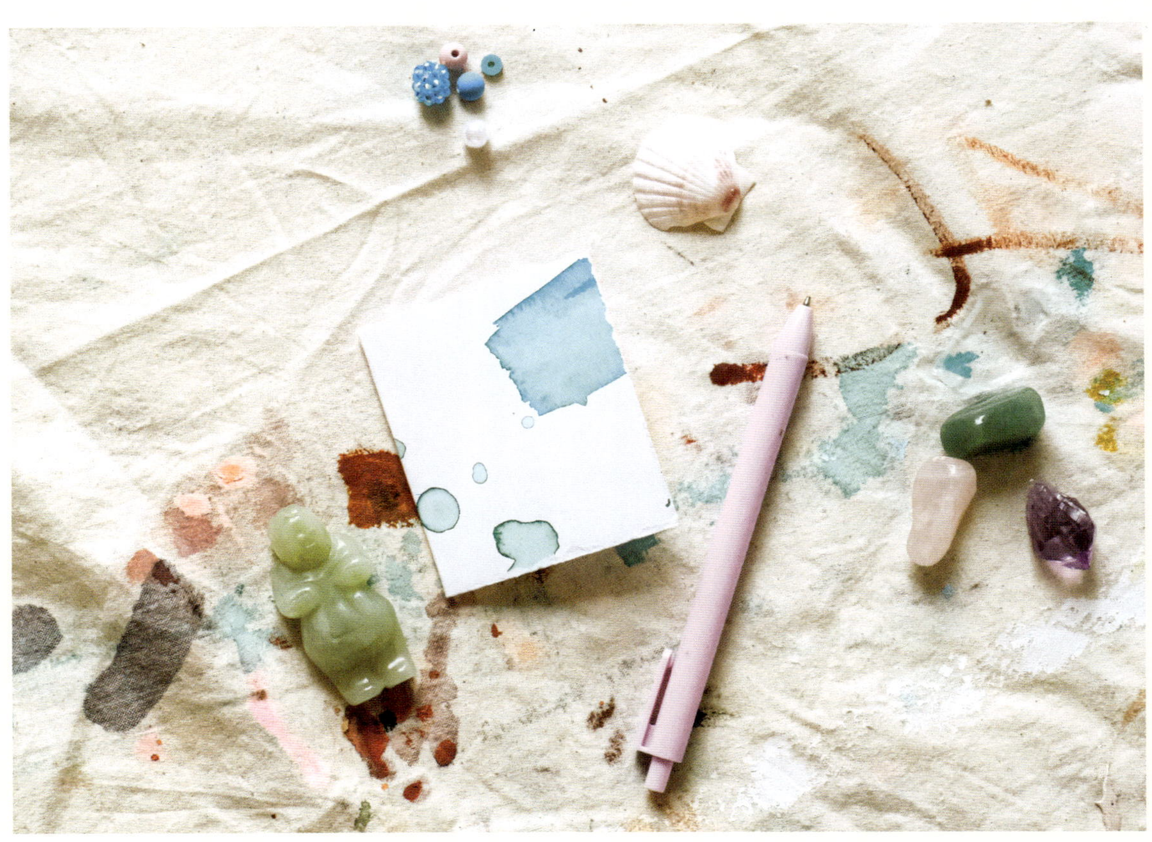

Connecting with kindness

A few years ago, in about 2019, I did a 'metta' meditation. No, this has nothing to do with the company formerly known as Facebook. There are two 't's in this metta, it has been around for a lot longer, and does a lot more good.

Metta is the Buddhist concept of loving-kindness. A metta meditation is a wonderful, heart-opening practice that focuses on extending goodwill to yourself, those around you and then those further away. I had done metta meditations quite a few times, but for some reason, on that specific day, the meaning and feeling behind it really sank in – it was the rather un-illustrious setting of a quick guided meditation on an app while I drove to work (still concentrating on the road).

Guided by the friendly voice on the app, I spent six minutes picturing the face of a complete stranger and repeating the words, 'I wish you well; I hope you stay happy. I wish you well; I hope you stay happy.' I randomly picked the face of the man who works at the petrol station I usually go to. A simple thing. An act of kindness, expecting nothing in return. The most amazing thing happened in that six minutes. It left me on a complete high – so much so that I repeated the exercise at various points in the day with different faces in my head.

I realised then that I had experienced a phenomenon that I'd been reading into – the 'Helper's High'. One simple act of kindness starts a chain reaction of delicious hormones and endorphins, scientifically proven to make us feel joy. It is such a real thing that scientists gave it its rather enticing nickname (the Helper's High). First – the endorphins rush in, producing a small natural high. Next, oxytocin increases. Oxytocin is known as the love hormone because it boosts your sense of connection, love, trust and optimism. Then, your serotonin levels increase. This leaves you feeling calm and helps your body to heal. And as if that hormonal cocktail isn't enough, your cortisol levels decrease – so you feel considerably less stressed.

'Kind' is a word that has lost its power over time. A word that disappears into the realms of 'nice' and 'sweet'. It's a quiet sort of virtue bestowed on people who might lack more charismatic traits. But, kindness is one of the most powerful tools we have at our disposal to create a more loving world, and to improve our feelings of joy.

On a deeper level, kindness helps us achieve one of life's most important goals – connection. Kind acts are outwardly focused; by definition, they connect you to the world around you. A meaningful connection to people, animals or the natural world brings about a sense of enormous wellbeing. It removes you from your obsession over your own self-narrative and gives your life meaning and purpose.

It has been proven over and over again that being kind makes you happy. But that is only one side of this fantastically double-edged lightsaber of joy. The real magic comes when you start to spread it. It is like a super beneficial virus. If you are kind, it encourages others to be kind. It gives people hope and taps into their sense of connection and community. It is powerful and has the potential to change society – little old kindness packs a big punch.

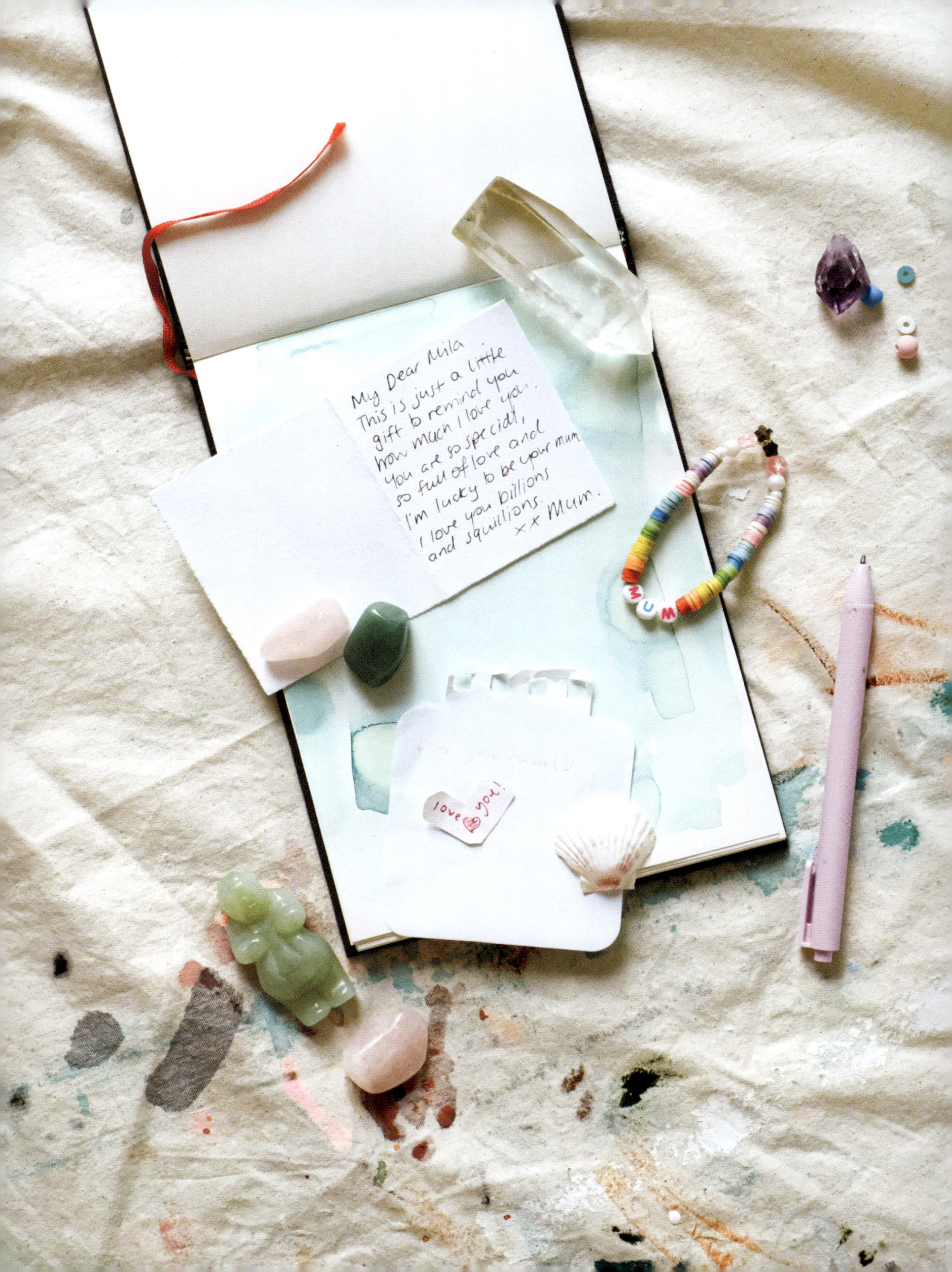
My Dear Mila
This is just a little
gift to remind you
how much I love you.
You are so special,
so full of love and
I'm lucky to be your mum.
I love you billions
and squillions.
xx Mum.
love you!
MUM

Connection exercise #5:
Tiny acts of kindness

Tiny acts of kindness can shift someone's day, as well as your own. They remind us that connection doesn't need to be big to be meaningful. A kind word or small gesture can ripple outwards in ways you may never see. The more you notice opportunities to be kind, the more they seem to appear. I have a few ideas you can start with, but I believe you'll think of many more things as you go. It becomes quite exciting once you get into it.

Hug someone.
Leave random positive notes on people's cars.
Write someone a thank you letter.
Do the dishes/laundry/ anything when it's not your turn.
Listen. Really listen.
Say thank you with meaning and eye contact.
TRY THESE
Compliment someone to their boss.
In busy traffic, let other drivers in front of you.
Donate an old piece of clothing each time you get a new one.
Smile at strangers (particularly ones you're annoyed with).
Save a bug instead of squishing it.
Put your phone down and connect.
Make a meal for a new mum.
Give your time to a child to play a game of their choice.

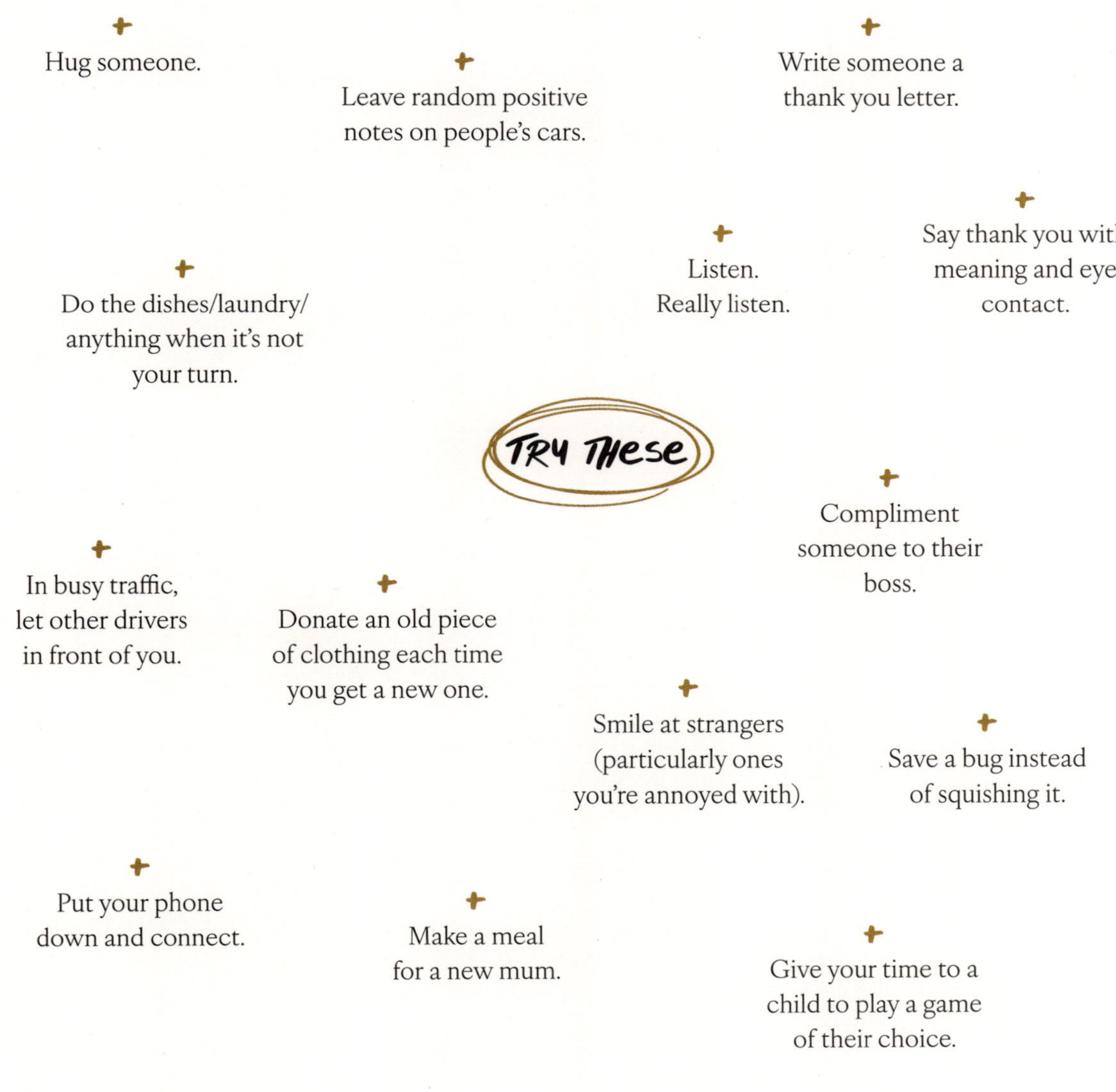

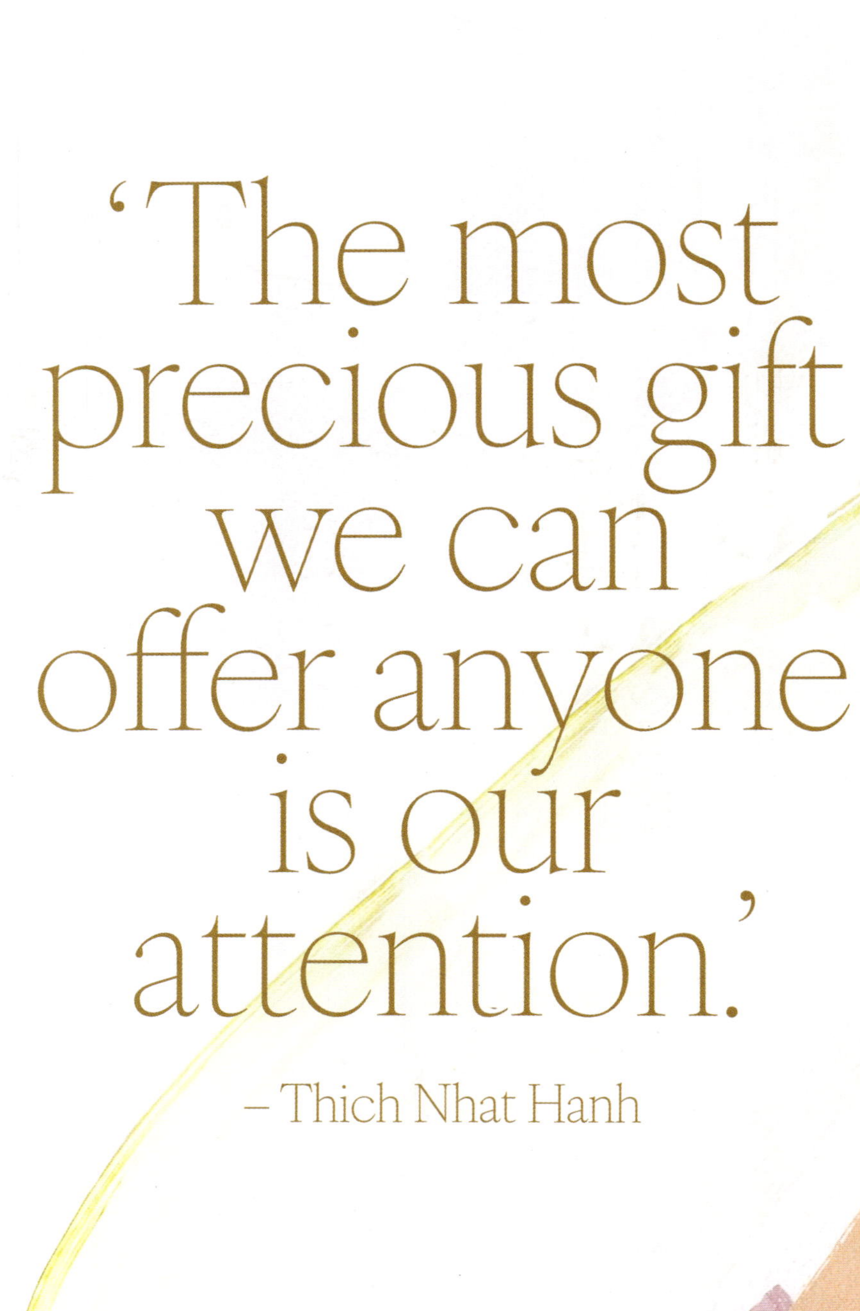
‘The most
precious gift
we can
offer anyone
is our
attention.’
– Thich Nhat Hanh

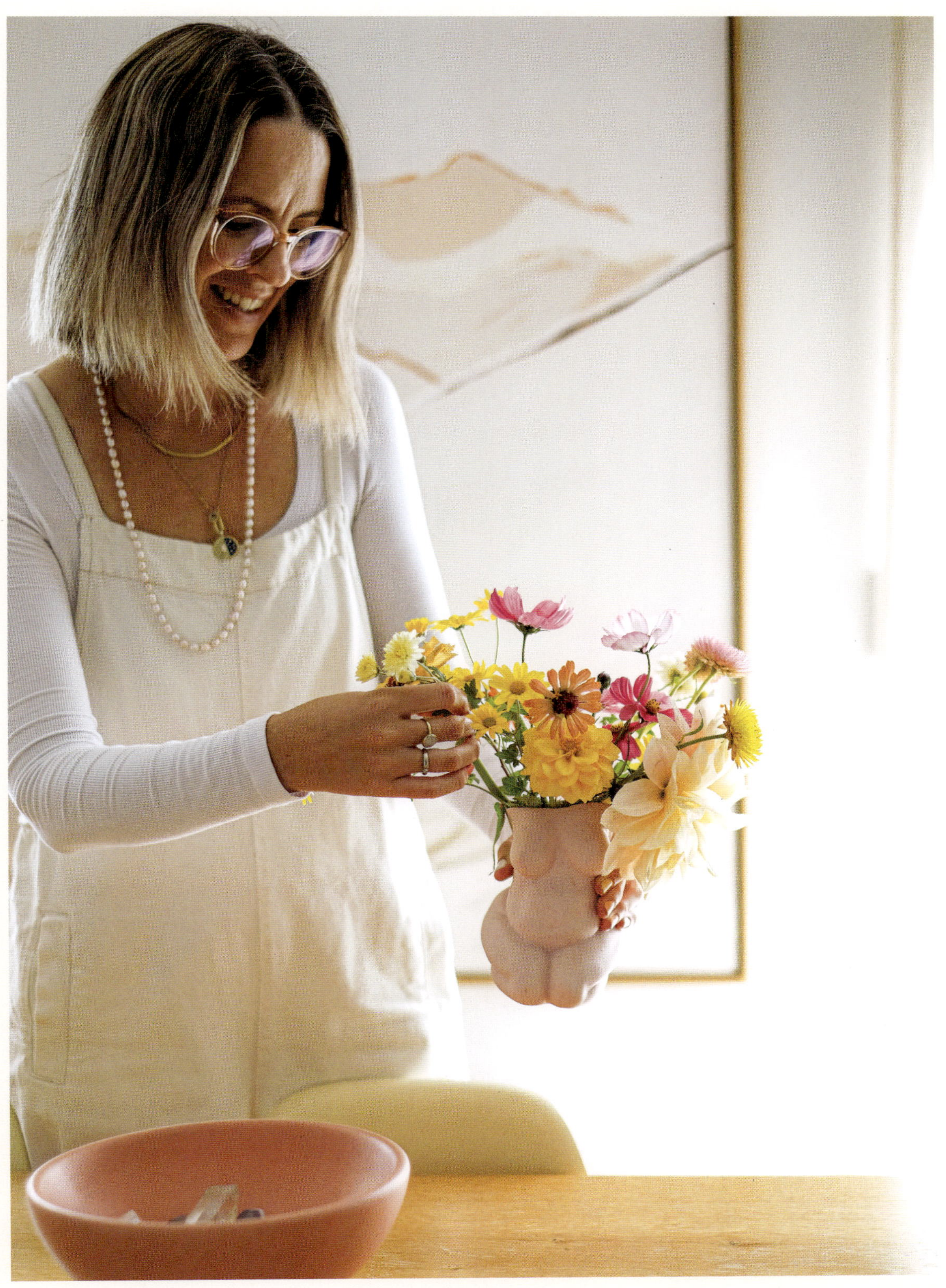

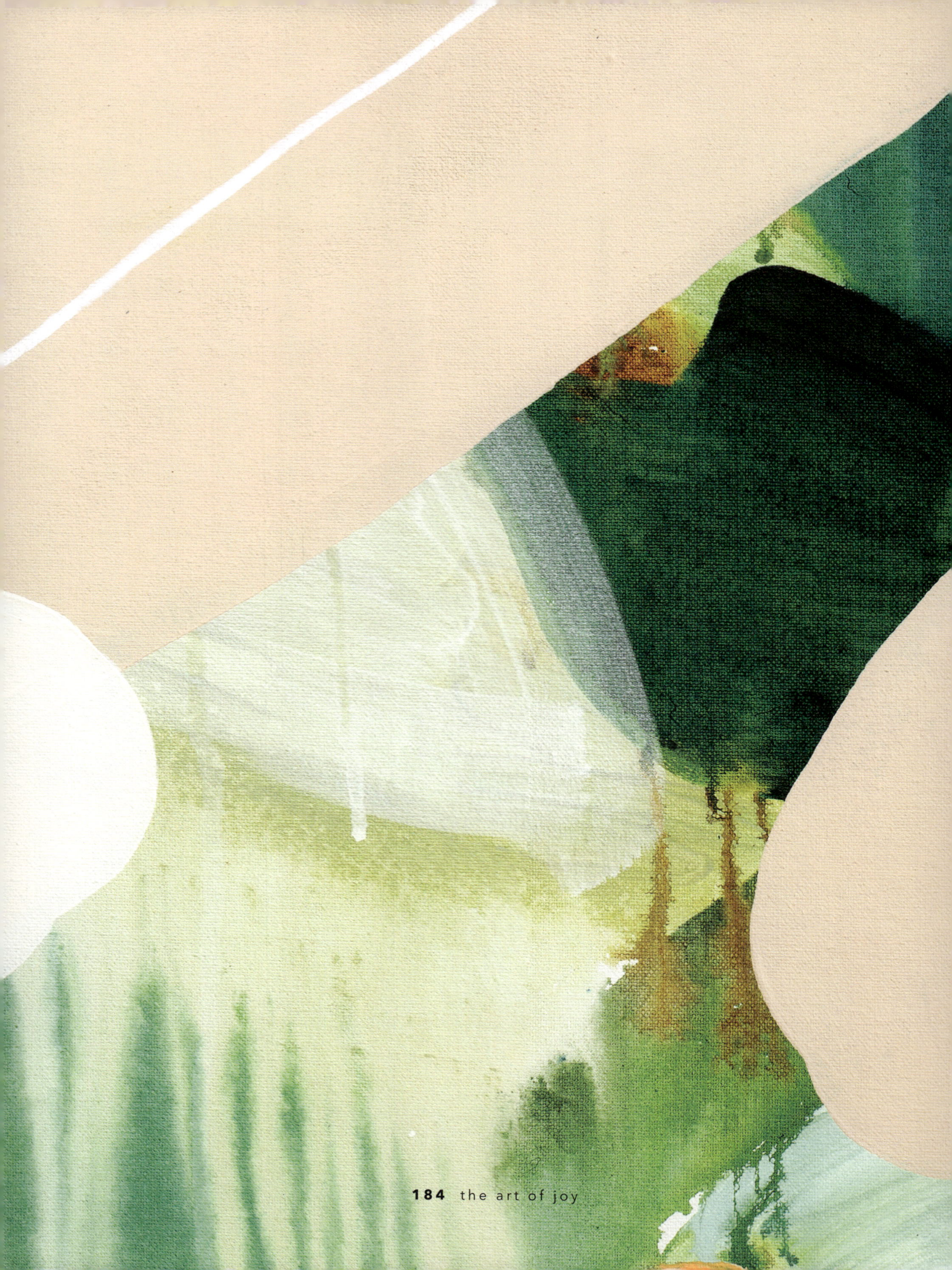

chapter eleven

MAKE HOME A HAVEN

Decorating and arranging for joy.

I'VE TRANSFORMED MY 'WHITE BOX' INTO A WARM, INVITING HOME. MY HAVEN. AFTERNOONS IN MY BEDROOM ARE FILLED WITH THIS GLORIOUS LIGHT.

When I moved into my current home I was nervous. Previously, I'd lived in character-filled (aka old) homes with interesting nooks, mismatched details and lived-in charm. Having recently separated from my husband, this was also the first home I had ever moved into without a partner, so moving into a new build seemed like a sensible idea – avoiding constant problems and repairs. The downside to new is that my home was a big, shiny, white box. There was zero character or soul – although, in a different light, I could see it as a blank canvas. Something I'm quite fond of for its potential.

For the first time, I was given the opportunity to create a home infused with my own energy and intention – without worrying that I was pushing it too far or stepping on anyone else's toes. As the only adult in the home, it was my own creative project.

I have learned a few things while feathering this particular nest over the last little while. As a disclaimer, even though I create art for beautiful homes, I am not an interior designer. The way I have approached the interior of my home is not based on any specific principles or style; it has been guided by delight. During this process, I have often wondered how many people forgo the idea of a personalised, joyful home to match what they have seen in a magazine or on Instagram. The ideas I am sharing here might not guarantee that you will have a cohesive, perfectly designed home. In fact, I can almost guarantee that they won't, but they will encourage you to be surrounded by a nourishing, joyful space that is created for you and the others living in it. A home that brings moments of joy to every day.

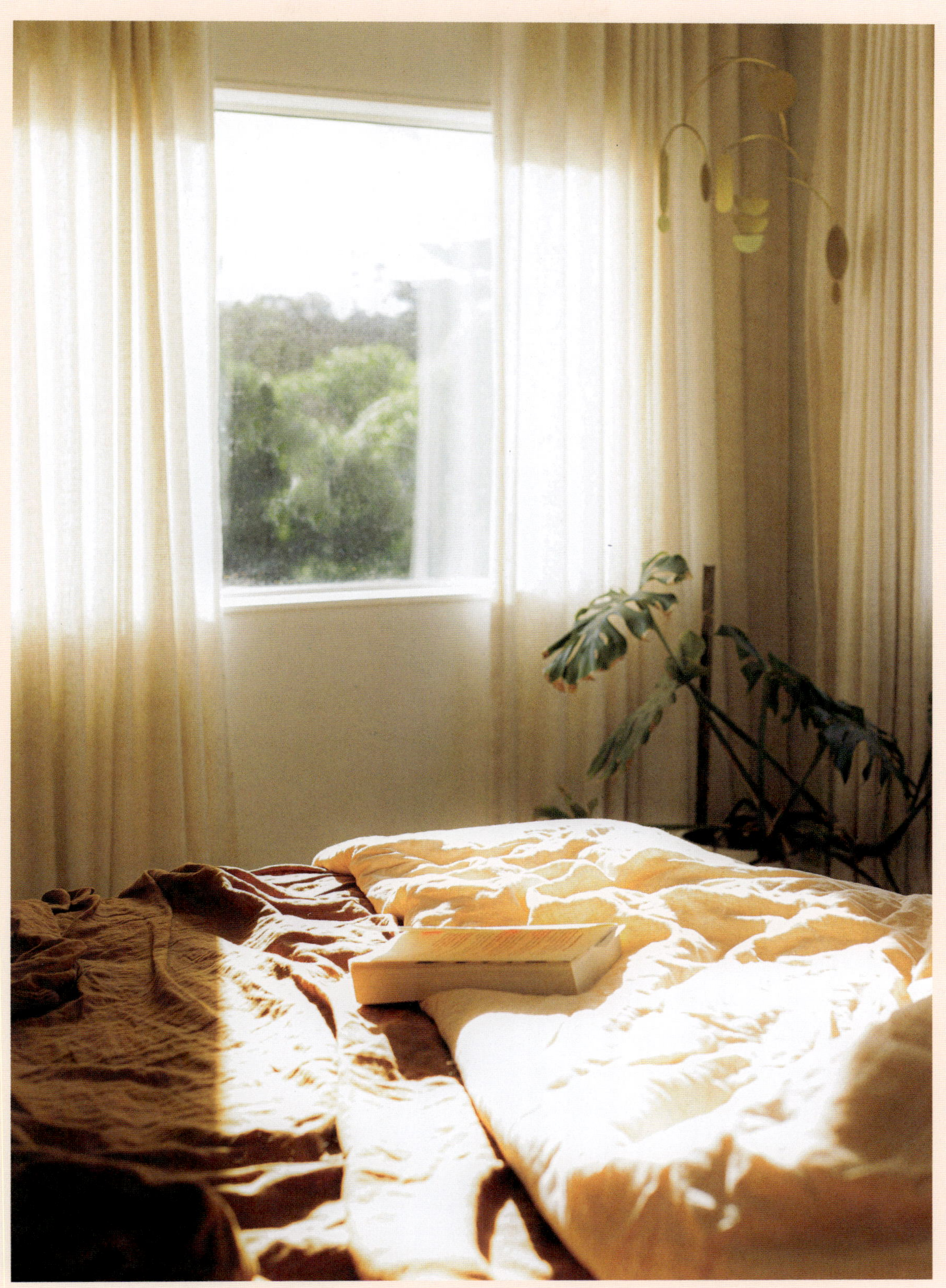

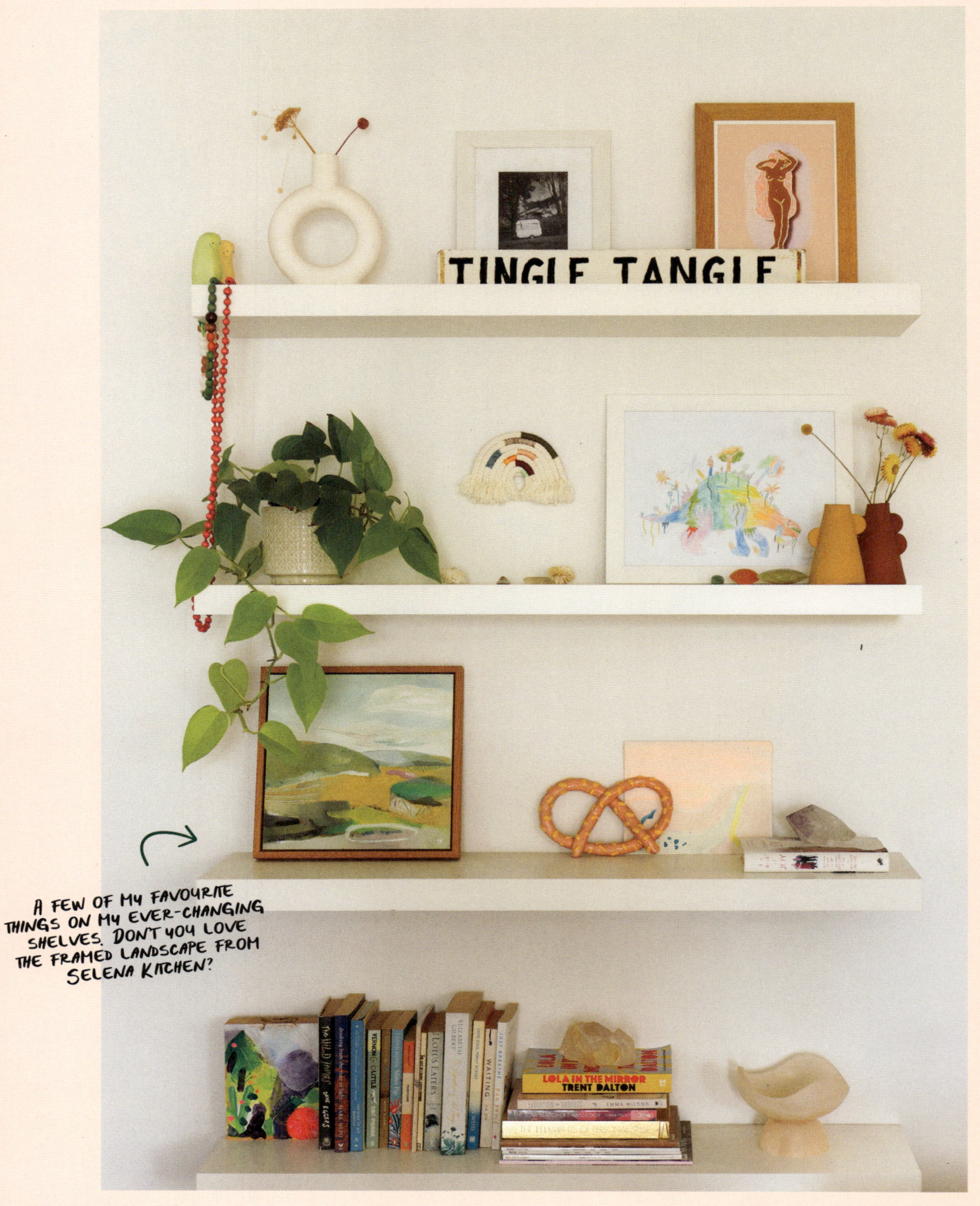

A FEW OF MY FAVOURITE THINGS ON MY EVER-CHANGING SHELVES. DON'T YOU LOVE THE FRAMED LANDSCAPE FROM SELENA KITCHEN?

Clusters of delight

My favourite trick in creating a more joyful home is forming clusters of delight for my eyes to land on. I like to have a balance of space and things, and in the areas where there are objects, I aim to make them as delightful as possible.

What is delightful to you will be different to what is delightful to me. The trick is to move past the shiny Instagram profiles and Pinterest boards that tell us what we're *supposed* to have, and find out what truly brings us joy. Below are some of the things that bring me an immense amount of joy in my own home.

Children's art

I give this the same priority as adult art. I have a few of my daughter's old paintings hanging in my kitchen and entryway and a rainbow-coloured drawing of a dinosaur by my best friend's son (and one of my favourite humans) in my living area. They hang alongside artworks and objects by respected artists and, of course, me!

Paintings and prints

I have a growing collection of artworks, mostly small, from a few outstanding female artists in New Zealand, Australia, and one from Rarotonga. I choose art based on how it makes me feel, and a lot of how it makes me feel is based on the colour palette.

Art objects

My Pete Cromer budgies, a pretzel by Alice Berry, two small vases from Formantics and a macramé rainbow made by Fleur Woods are some of the sweet little objects that make my heart sing.

Trinkets

Little treasures that make me smile such as my crystals, vases, candles, and sentimental souvenirs from travels or everyday life. These small pieces may not match, but each one holds a happy memory.

Natural touches

I love including small elements from nature in my everyday spaces. That could be a leaf picked up on a walk, a feather found on a pavement, or smooth stones collected with my daughter. These grounding details connect me back to nature and the present moment.

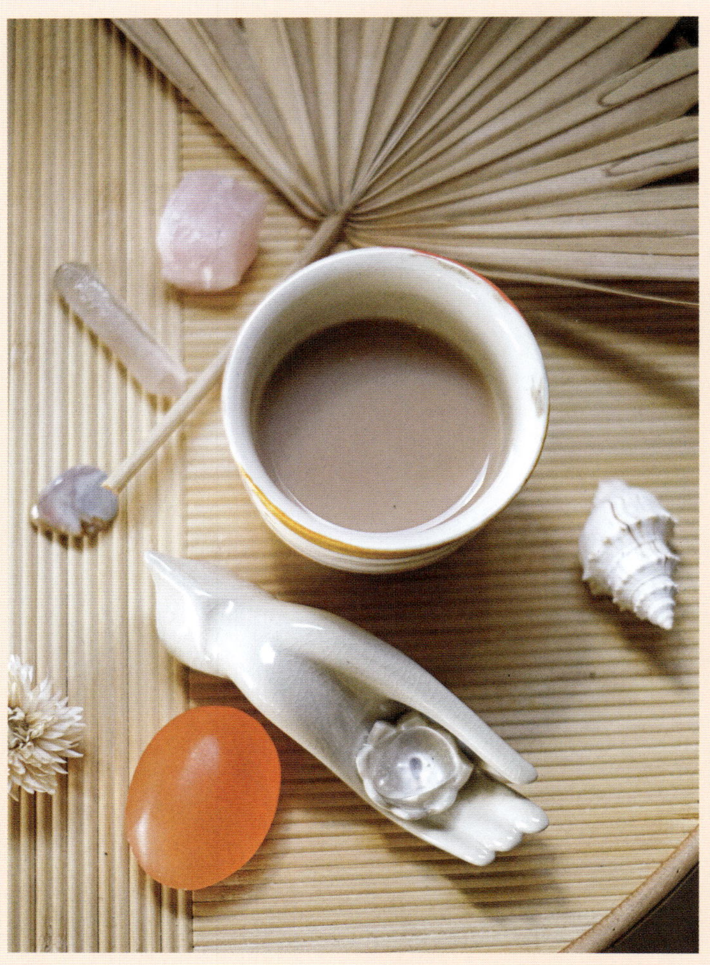

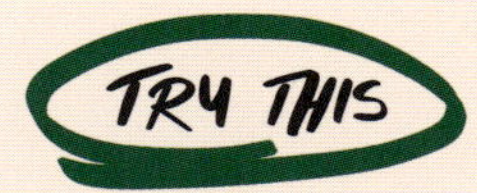

Create a cluster of objects in your home, prioritising how they make you feel. Don't question why they make you feel good, there doesn't need to be a reason. You can start by looking through drawers for old keepsakes that haven't been displayed, or pull out a small vase and collect some wildflowers from a local green area as a centrepiece.

+

Allow yourself to play – try combinations of things until they make you smile. This is a very low-commitment exercise. If you decide in 10 minutes that you don't like what you have picked, move it and try again another time. The key is to focus on how it makes you feel – prioritise that.

Why clusters?

I think what makes my clusters joyful to me is the random pairings of things that are together purely for aesthetic reasons – happy places for my eyes to rest. Such as a beaded necklace that my daughter and I made together when she was in preschool that adds a touch of playfulness to my shelves, and a sun catcher that I bought at a music festival that randomly projects rainbows onto my table, walls and floor at certain times of the day.

ARRANGING BEAUTIFUL THINGS CAN TURN A CUP OF TEA INTO A SPECIAL MOMENT TO SAVOUR.

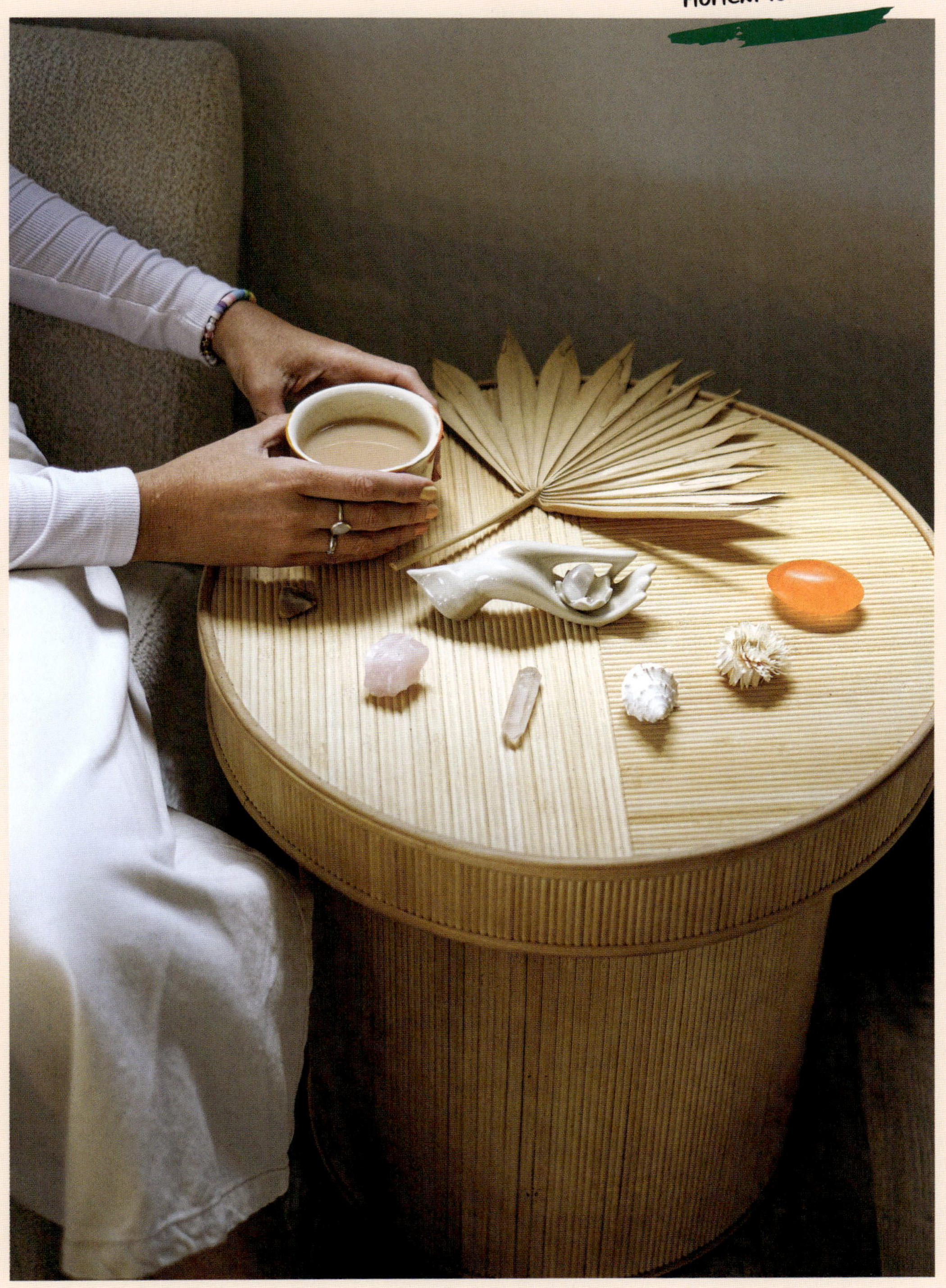

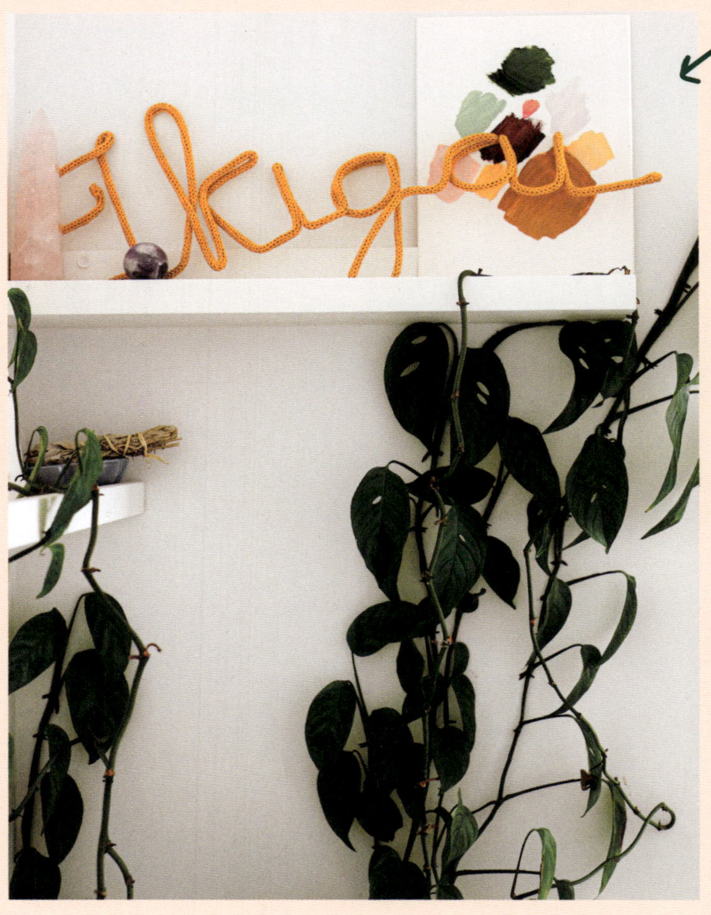

THE KNITTED WIRE WORD SPELLS 'IKIGAI' WHICH IS THE JAPANESE CONCEPT OF FINDING YOUR PURPOSE IN THE INTERSECTION OF WHAT BRINGS YOU JOY, WHAT YOU'RE GOOD AT, WHAT PEOPLE NEED AND WHAT YOU CAN BE PAID FOR. I HAVE IT IN MY STUDIO AS A DAILY REMINDER ABOUT WHY I'M HERE – TO CREATE JOY.

Embrace every shade of green

The work-vs-reward ratio on plants is unimaginably good. Let's just take a moment to appreciate the magic of them. These lush green beings that adorn our homes started their lives as tiny seeds, little specks of nothing. A few months or years later they are sometimes huge, always exquisite, living, growing things that help us to breathe and make us feel so darn good. We get to watch them silently sprout new leaves (if you ever want to marvel at that, get a monstera) and even flowers. If we stop to look at them for just a moment and consider each vein on every leaf, we can't help but be in awe, all for the measly price of regular water and a spot with the right amount of sun.

Studies have also shown that plants reduce cortisol levels (reducing stress), improve air quality, increase focus, help with healing time, and make us feel generally happier. They truly are magic little bursts of green.

Experiment with styles

Think of your home as your playground – try to make space and allowance for everyone to find ways to play with it. I have an empty area in my living space – between the dining room and lounge – where I can dance. I love to dance.

My daughter's room is a bit of a free-for-all. I have resigned myself to the fact that there is Blu Tack on the walls and a lot more chaos than I would have in my own space. I also let her regularly move things around and make little hideouts out of blankets and cushions. She has an alarmingly large collection of plushies that stare, smiling at us while I put her to bed at night. It's definitely not my idea of a calm, beautiful space – but that's not what she's into right now. Her room is an expression of herself, and I have had to let go of some aesthetic values to allow it to develop. I do walk in and feel a complete sense of *her*, and for a 10-year-old girl, I think that's priceless.

In contrast, my room is a haven of tranquility and light. It inspires wonder and joy in me, which is my favourite type of play.

Adapt rooms to suit your needs

When I started painting again, I had all of my paints in a big plastic box, and in the evenings I would throw a drop sheet over my dining table and unpack them. Claiming that as my temporary creative home gave my practice room to grow. It didn't take long for me to carve out a dedicated art space in the garage instead. That space grew as my art got bigger and more prolific. Eventually, cars weren't allowed in that garage, and the lawnmower was moved to the shed. By the time I went full-time as an artist, we had partitioned a tiny room for tools and whatnot, and the rest of the garage was renovated into the perfect studio.

The garage doors were replaced with glass bi-folds, overlooking our sweeping view of the city and harbour. This story illustrates that if you start with a tiny space for what you love, it might grow into something extraordinary. Your home isn't supposed to be a static space – the best ones change and evolve as you do.

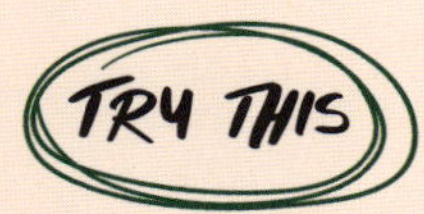

Could you carve out a small space in your home for something you love? If you're the crafty type, maybe there is a corner of your home (even if it's in the garage) that you can pretty-up and use to create.

+

If you don't have the space for a permanent play area, you could have a designated temporary space and a box of tricks to unleash on it regularly. If you love to sing or play an instrument, create a zone where you can do that regularly. Having an area dedicated to your passion will remind you to do what lights you up.

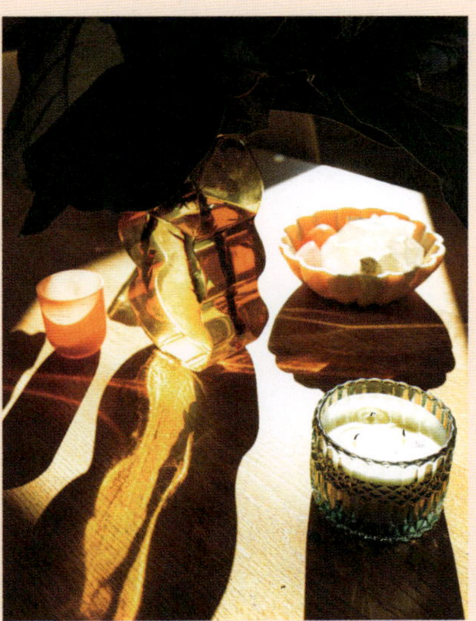

I LOVE THIS SPACE FOR HOW IT CATCHES THE SUNLIGHT – I USE IT FOR VISUAL PLAY.

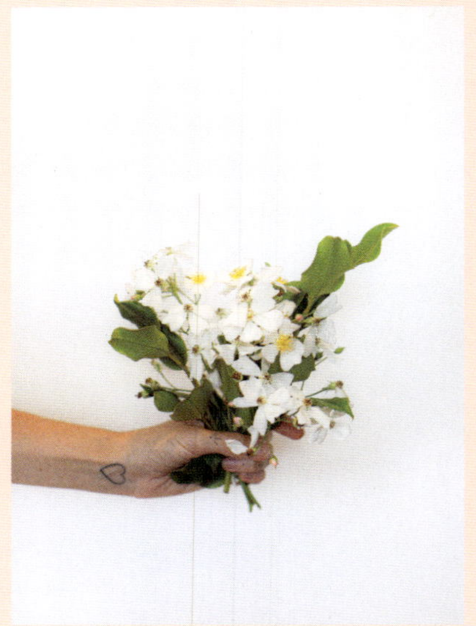

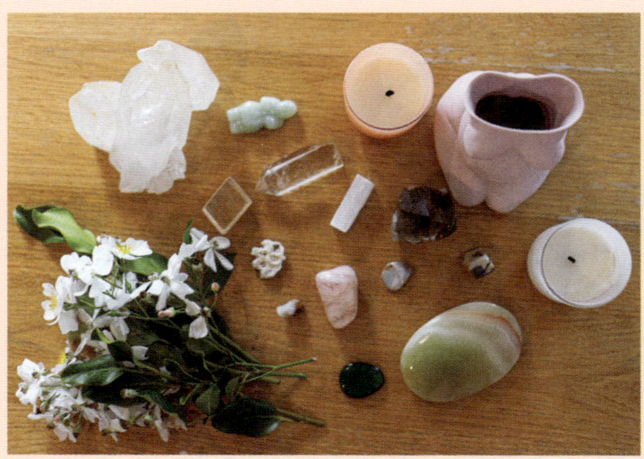

Rearranging will awaken your eyes!

Once we have lived with things in a certain way, they become invisible. Objects put there to bring us joy eventually become part of the furniture and no longer bring us out of our thoughts and into the moment. To counter this, I like to rearrange things often. The furniture and bigger things stay in one place most of the time, but I have plenty of areas in my space that allow small things to be moved and rearranged.

Rearranging them is a joy in itself, and then noticing the objects again in their new places brings me back into the delight of the moment. Two of my favourite places for this are my shelves and my dining table.

My shelves are a visual feast. They're right in my living area and visible from most angles of the open-plan space. I take great joy in playing with the clusters of objects on these shelves. Sometimes I rearrange the small collection of books or move objects off the shelves completely to make space for things that I'd forgotten about. I like creating moments that make me smile – like my Pete Cromer budgies draped in the beaded necklaces, with my lush green little plant underneath them.

My dining table is a wonderful playground. I have somehow turned it into a secular altar – a place for my crystals, candles and sacred objects. I do my Letters from Love and most of my writing at this table, so it helps me to have a space that feels special, and one that changes often, to keep it alive and noticed.

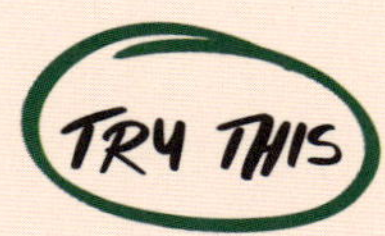

Find an area in your home where you can play with rearranging. Create a few clusters of objects in the area, then set a reminder on your phone to change it in two weeks. When you rearrange it, enjoy the process, feel the objects' heaviness or texture in your hands and take in their colours. Engage with the objects and remember to prioritise joy in placing them.

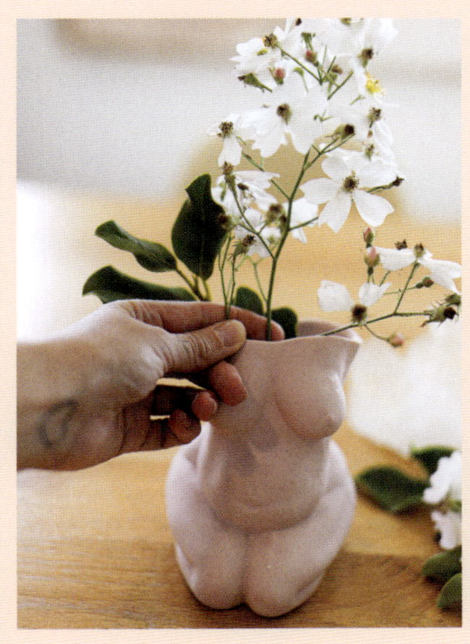

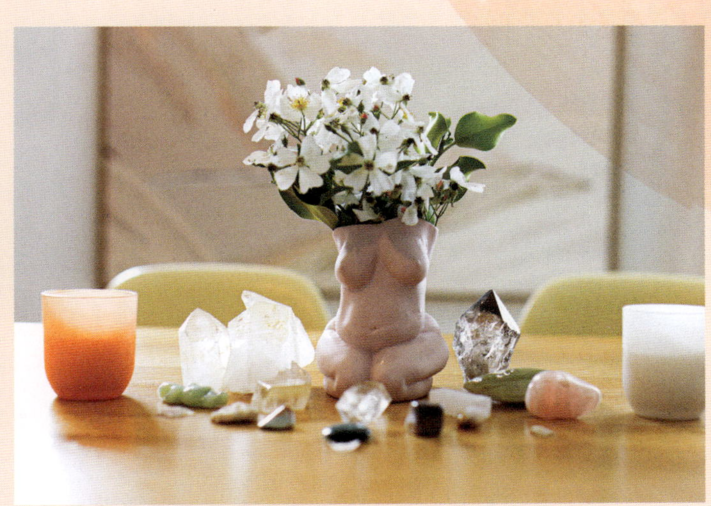

A sacred space

I have a few sacred spaces in my home. By sacred, I don't mean that they are created to worship a deity, but rather, they are made to encourage a feeling of quiet and specialness. These spaces are perfect for my joy practices or even just to show me the beauty of an ordinary moment because of how they feel.

My dining table

As mentioned before, I have turned this space into an altar. I love the act of arranging my crystals, vases and candles on the table when I'm settling down to write. Even just lighting a candle makes everything feel a little bit more sacred. When people come to visit, the children pick up the crystals and ask about them; I encourage them to create their own arrangements and the 'altar' becomes a talking point. Sometimes, it's over the top and extravagant; other times, it's a small candle and a handful of crystals. Every time I sit at the table, it brings me joy.

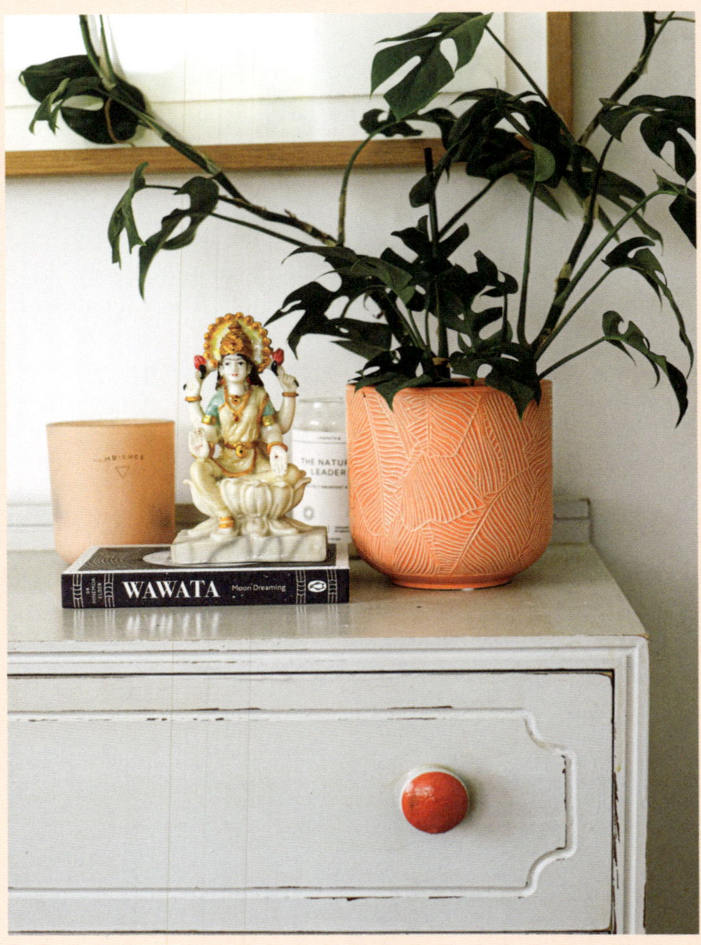

AN EVER-CHANGING SACRED SPACE IN MY BEDROOM.

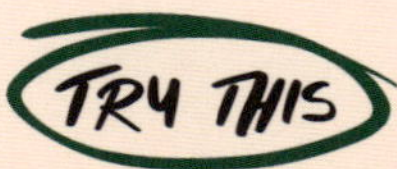

Why not set up an altar space of your own? To help form it, figure out something you'd like to dedicate it to. Mine are often dedicated to feminine energy. You could pick a feeling or quality that you would like more of in your life and dedicate it to that (for example, calm, excitement, connection, creativity). Having a theme helps you to pick your objects and gives you an intention to pour into it while you arrange them.

+

It helps visually to make the arrangement symmetrical. Try putting the tallest object in the centre and work your way down to the smallest. Arrange it in a circle, a diamond or a perfectly spaced straight line. Maybe everything in the arrangement is one colour? Enjoy the process and enlist your children if you think they might enjoy it too. Remember, this is here for the purpose of joy. Play with it.

My bedroom

Every object in my bedroom has been picked to add serenity and beauty to the space. I have a brass mobile hanging in the corner, just where the afternoon light comes in. My monstera and mini monstera bring just the right amount of nature into the bedroom; my semi-sheer curtains add softness and movement to the room. Every artwork is beautiful and feminine and adds moments of colour and delight to quite a neutral space. My linen bedding has been chosen for its perfect colour palette to tie it all together. When I'm in here, I can't help but relax.

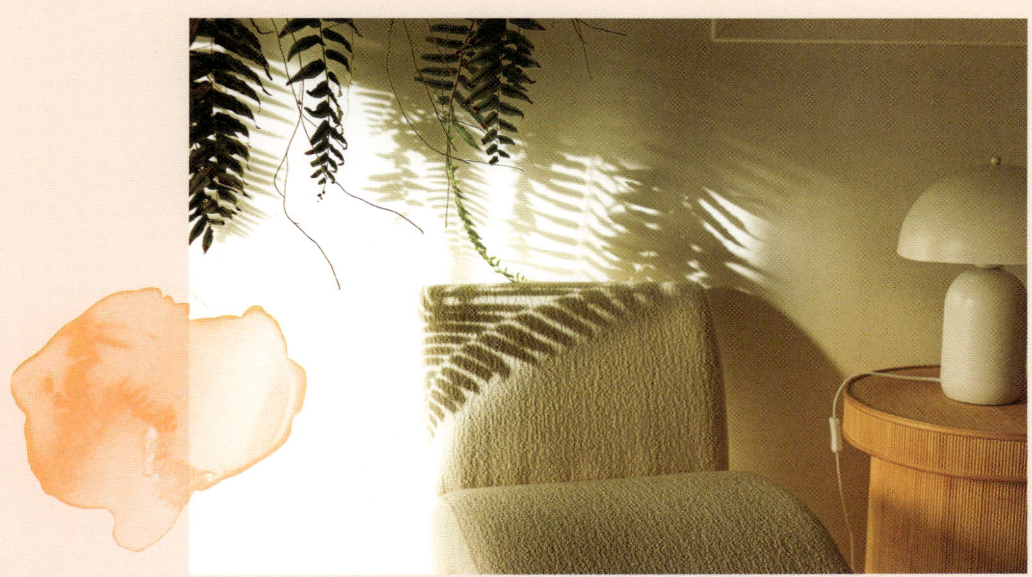

I'M FOREVER PLAYING WITH TINY RAINBOWS FROM MY LIGHT CATCHER.

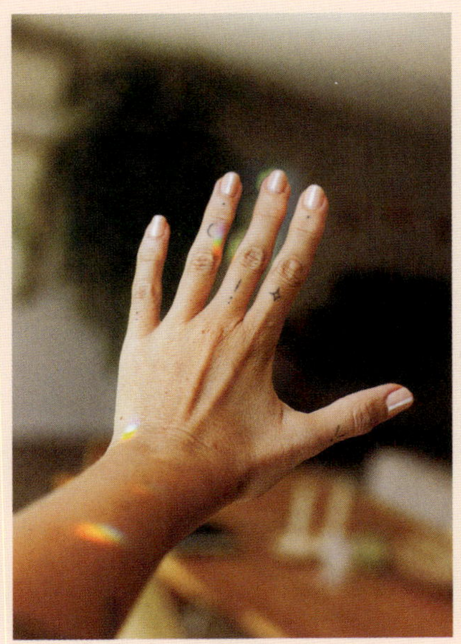

Catching light

A simple and effective way to bring yourself into the wonder of the present is through light. I love a good sunbeam, and positioning things to play with those delicious beams is a great source of joy. Plants are perfect for this. My Boston fern makes the craziest shadows in the late afternoon, and I have been known to spend a few minutes using my phone to photograph the beautiful shapes of my monstera on my carpet in the morning.

I recently bought a sun catcher – one of those faceted crystal balls that hangs in the window, waiting for direct sun to transform into rainbows. I vividly remember Pollyanna (I'm ageing myself with this reference – you might need to google!) seeing the magic of a crystal prism for the first time. The fact that I now own a rainbow-making machine completely blows my mind. I spend a lot more time than I should playing with the rainbows.

The important point of all of these joyful-interior tips is to create ways to slow down and notice the things around you. Interact with your space; when you see a sunbeam, take 30 seconds to be with it. Put your hand through it and watch where your own shadow falls. These tiny moments add up, and there are so many of them there, just waiting to be captured.

Homely project
Make a joyful mobile

There's something quietly magical about making something with your hands – especially when it's colourful, soft, and made with love. This felt mobile is a joyful little project that's easy to customise with colours and shapes that make you smile. Whether you hang it in a nursery, hallway or by your desk, it's a gentle reminder of the joy you can create with a few simple materials and a little creative time.

You will need:

- A wooden ring (approximately 15cm diameter)
- Felt sheets in various/favourite colours
- Large sewing needle
- Embroidery string
- Paints (acrylic or test pot paint)
- Paintbrush
- Scissors

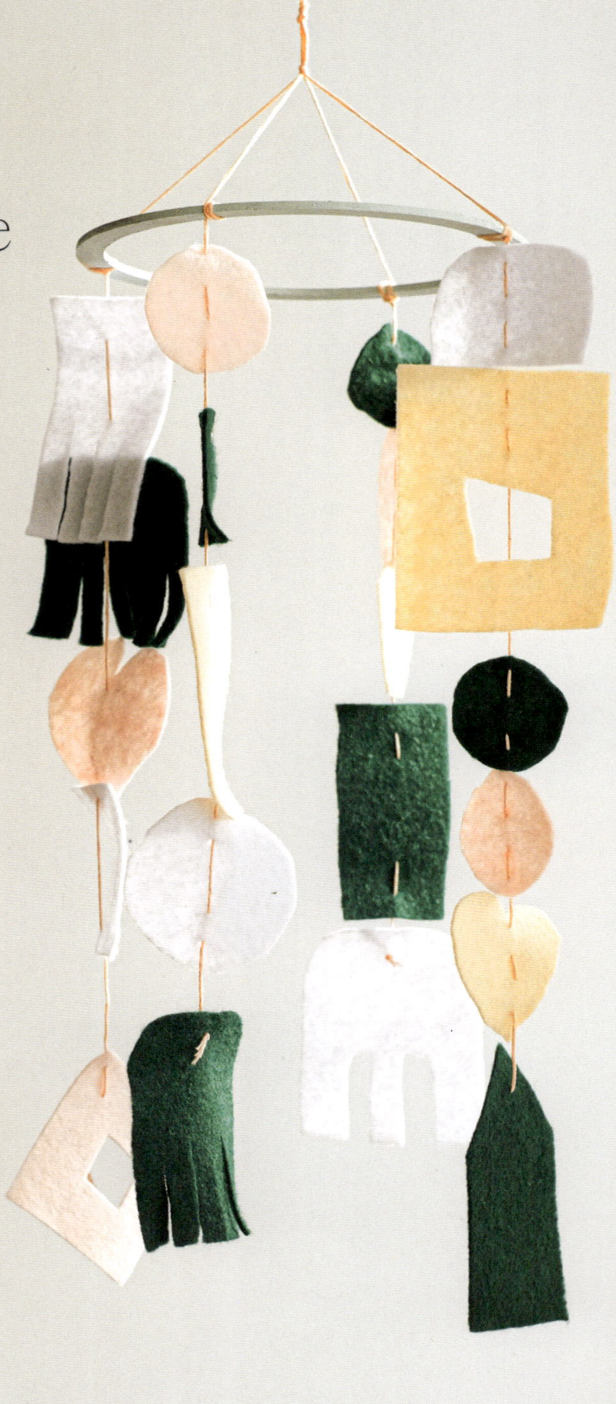

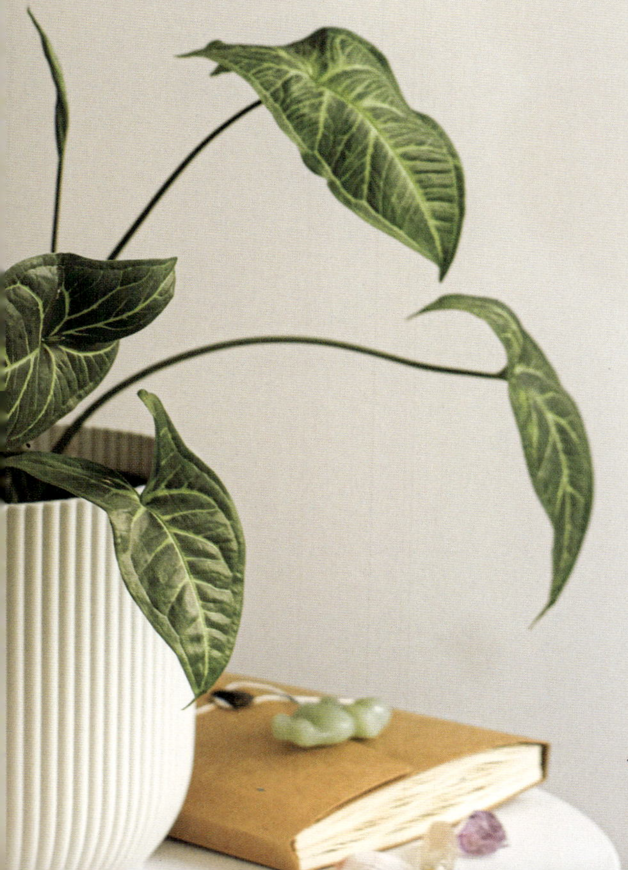

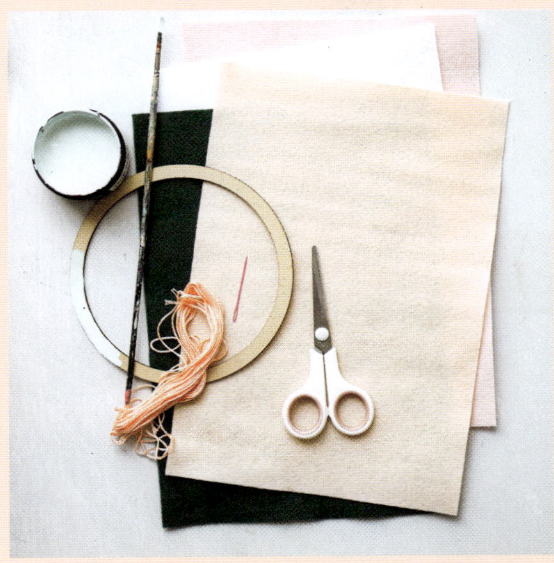

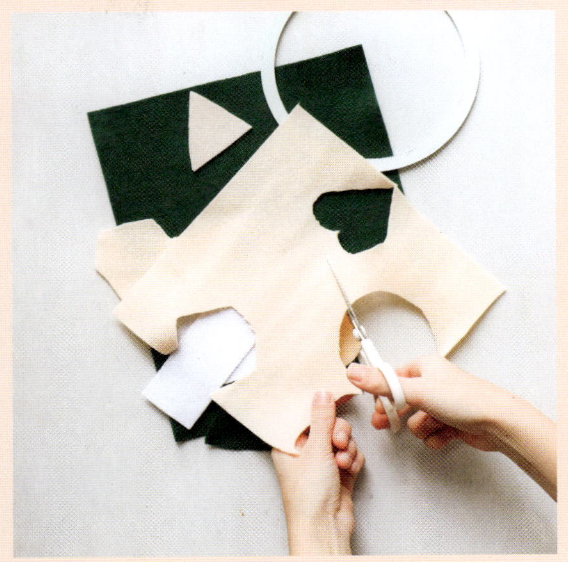

1 Paint the wooden ring in your chosen colour. I like using test pot paints – they give great coverage and dry quickly. While the ring is drying, cut four lengths of thread or string, each about 50cm long.

2 Cut your shapes from the felt sheets. Choose whatever brings you joy – stars, hearts, circles, leaves, or abstract blobs. Aim for a mix of sizes and colours to give your mobile a playful, layered look.

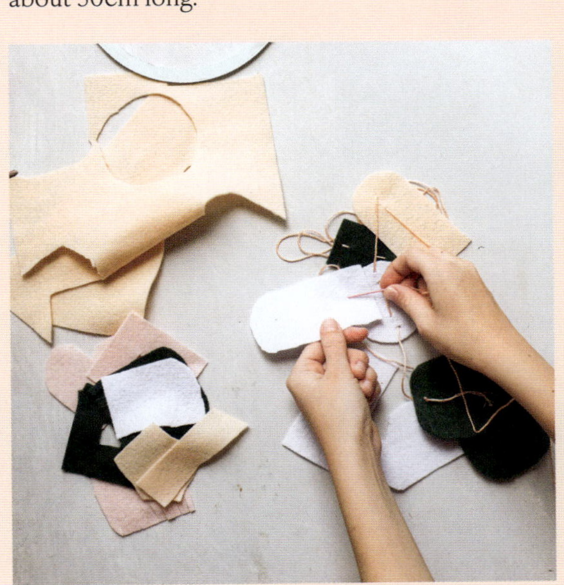

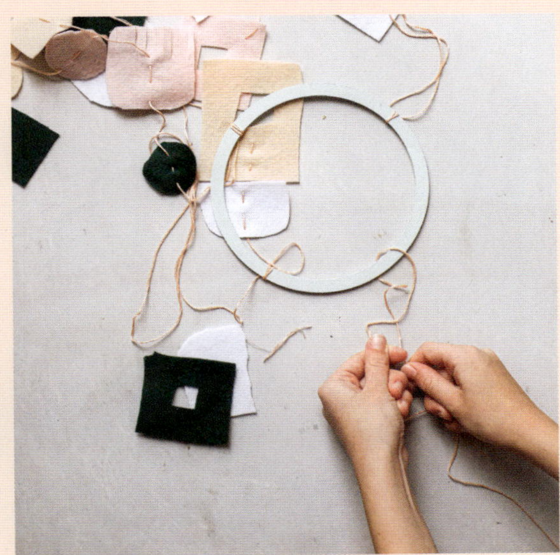

3 Take one length of thread and begin threading your felt shapes onto it. Start from the bottom, knotting under each shape to keep it in place. Repeat with the remaining threads to create four individual hanging strands.

4 Tie each strand to the wooden ring, spacing them out evenly. Leave extra thread at the top so you can tie them all together and create a loop for hanging. Step back, admire your joyful creation, and hang it wherever needs a little magic.

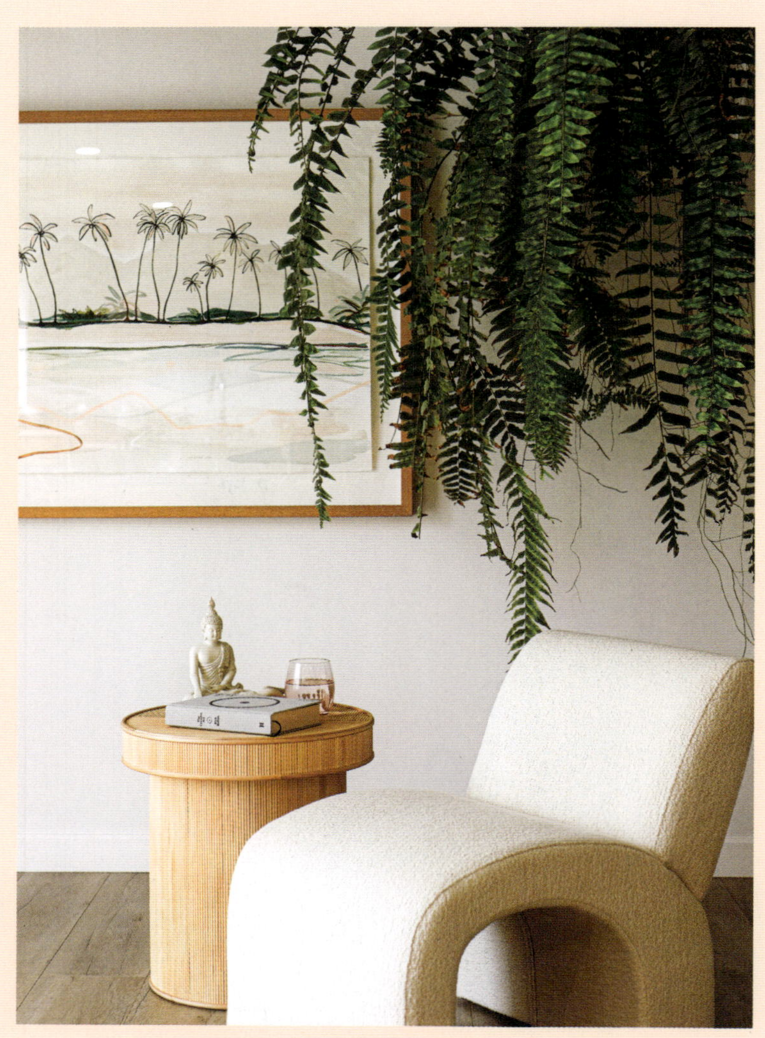

Get plants.
Get lots of
them, be a crazy
plant person,
name them,
speak to them,
make it weird.

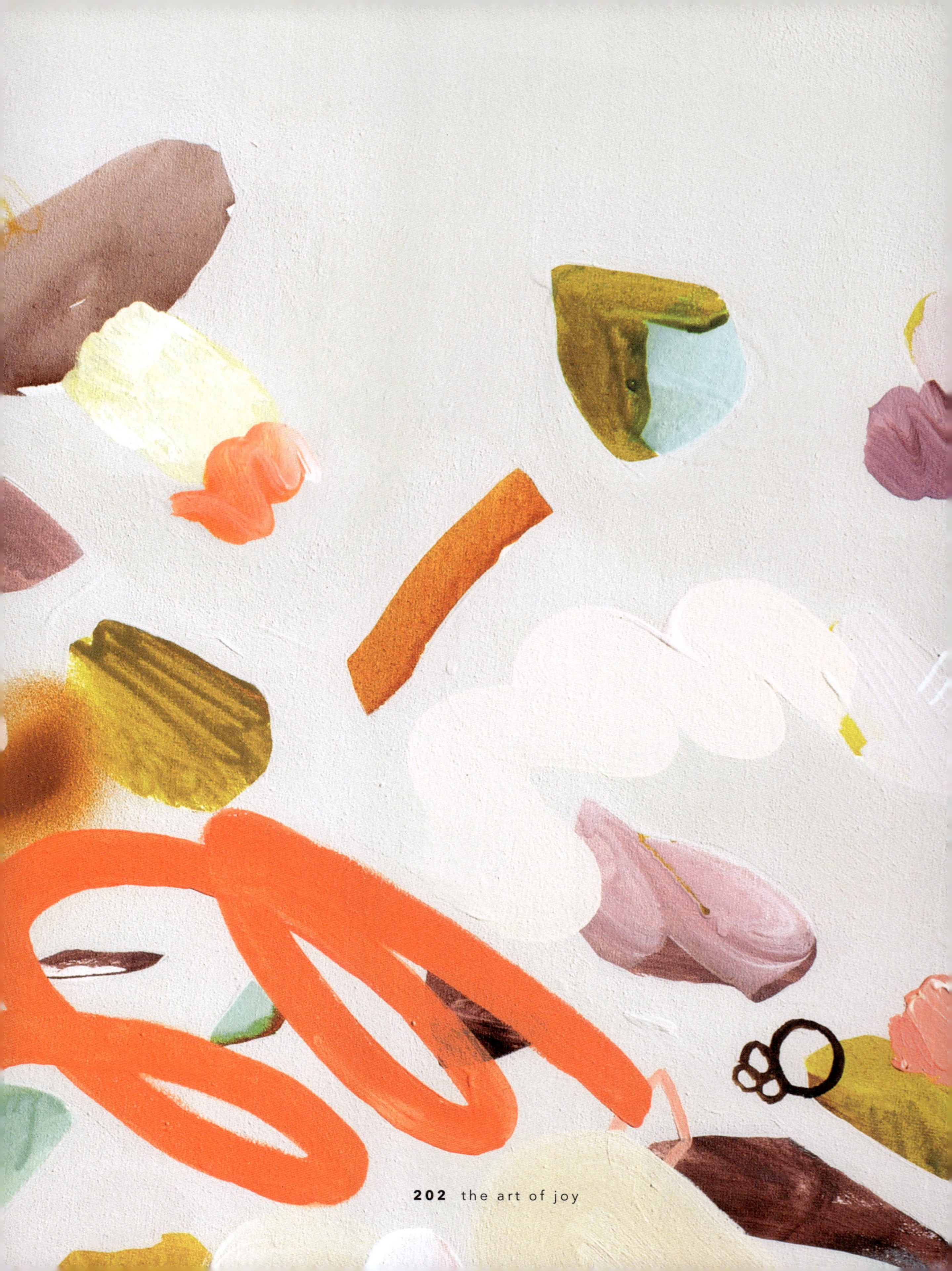

chapter twelve

THE JOY OF COLOUR

Discovering how colour makes you feel and embracing it in your life.

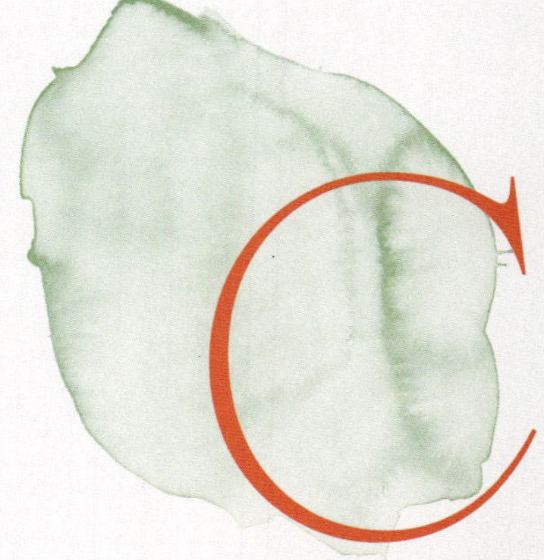

Colour is my happy place, love language and how I best express my joy and wonder. I'm often asked how I pick my colour palettes – where I get my colours from – and on the surface of it, I'm not entirely sure. But if I focus on where I find my colour inspiration, it always comes from a feeling. I love feeling *into* colours rather than sticking to any rules or set ideas, and I believe that if we all approach and use colour with more feeling and intuition, we can create more joy in our lives. You don't have to be an artist to be connected to colour. It's all around you, from your home space to your clothes, down to tiny details like the mug you use for your cup of tea.

The colours I use to paint are colours that I love. I want to spend my days playing with them and watching them become artworks. I adore mixing them, stirring them in a thick pot of ice-cream-coloured beauty. But I wasn't always a colour expert. When I was a graphic designer, I always felt that colour was one of my weaker aspects. I would spend hours on colour selections, but I never really felt like they were quite right. I think that was because when you're designing for a brief, there are so many aspects to consider, so I was stuck in my head – where colour makes less sense.

I opened up to colour when I began painting. The process of finding my creative voice opened my eyes again to the world around me, and I was on a creative treasure hunt every waking hour. I remember driving home on the North Western Motorway on a wet day and falling in love with the swoop of the yellow lines on a curved section of the motorway, with the wet, silvery road reflecting a warm, late afternoon light.

That's the thing: colour is everywhere. I have been inspired by piles of laundry just as viscerally as a walk through an art gallery. Discovering what colours light your soul is an exercise in mindfulness, in being present with the colours you see without judging what the object is. Luckily, we have a wealth of magnificent colours at our fingertips. We can see them in beautiful homes and artworks on Instagram or on a deep dive down the Pinterest rabbit hole. These colour treasure troves are a wonderful place to exercise your colour muscles to discover what colours make you come alive.

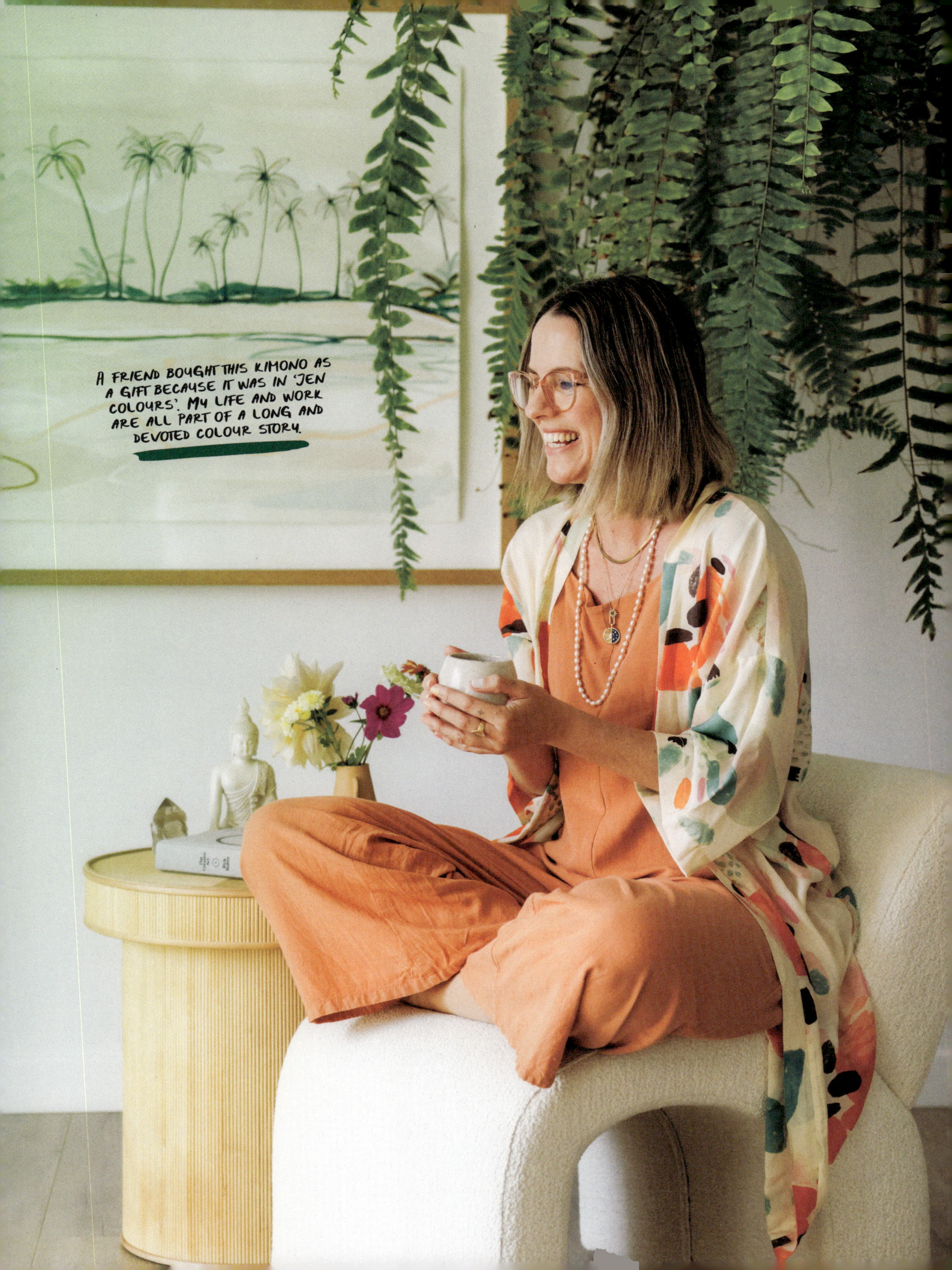
A FRIEND BOUGHT THIS KIMONO AS
A GIFT BECAUSE IT WAS IN 'JEN
COLOURS'. MY LIFE AND WORK
ARE ALL PART OF A LONG AND
DEVOTED COLOUR STORY.

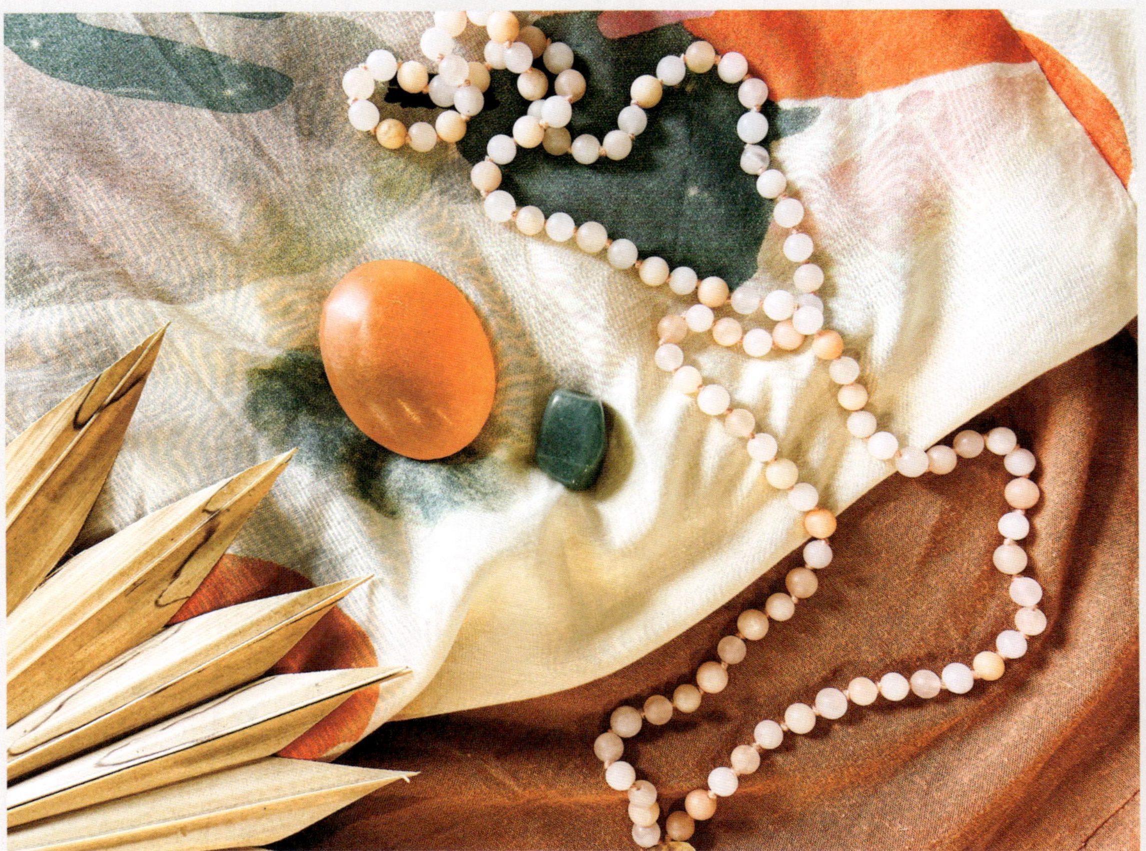

I LOVE TO LAYER TEXTURES AND TONES USING MY FAVOURITE ITEMS OF CLOTHING AND TRINKETS.

Proportions make all the difference

When I'm creating a palette, I often do it on my computer with little blobs of colour in Photoshop. You can do the same if you have access to an app or program with a colour picker. Sometimes, I'll see a colour moment in real life or on a screen that pulls me in. I put it into Photoshop and pick the colours that are catching my eye to use as the start of a palette. The blobs in my palettes are different sizes because proportion matters. Some colours work well in small doses, and others can be washed across a space in large amounts.

If you fall in love with a rich mustard in a Pinterest pic, figure out if you love it as an accent or if you want enough of it for an entire sofa. The outcomes are very different, and you can have too much of a good thing! I learned this the hard way. I still have a mustard sofa, but it's currently in my daughter's bedroom, happily hidden under her ridiculously large collection of Squishmallows.

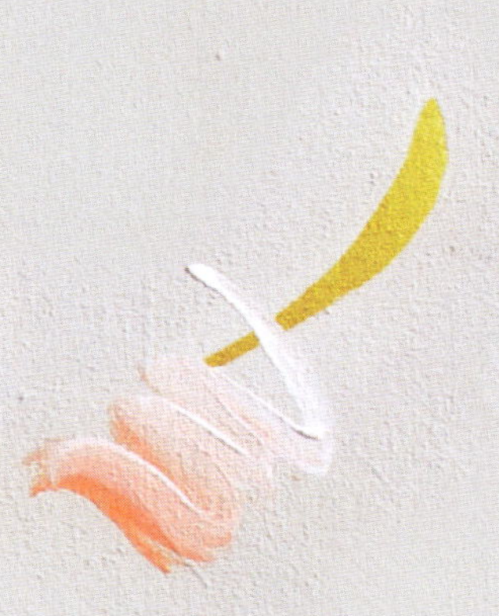

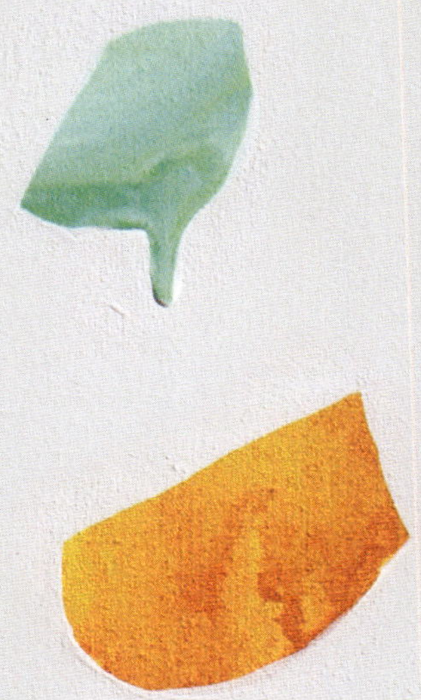

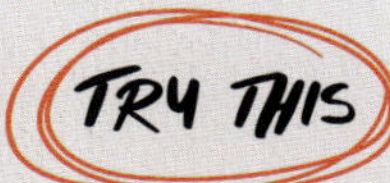

Spend some time on Instagram or Pinterest looking at just colours. Don't search for the term 'colour', just scroll through your usual feed, and rather than reading posts, looking at faces, or turning your attention to what brand of shoes someone has just bought, soften your focus a little and see each post as a colour palette.

+

While you do this, notice if any of the palettes stand out to you. They may make you feel warm and happy or excited. Conversely, some might make you annoyed or uncomfortable or just plain bored. Screenshot (or Pin) the ones that you're drawn to.

Once you're done, look at all the images together (Pinterest is great for this, you can have a dedicated colour board) and see if there are common threads or recurring colour stories that you're drawn to. Look around your home – are these colours represented in your space and in your wardrobe? Or have you chosen safer, more expected options?

+

You don't need to throw away all of your furniture and clothes, but next time you need to buy something new, start bringing in some of your joy colours. Slowly, your life will evolve to express more of your personal joy.

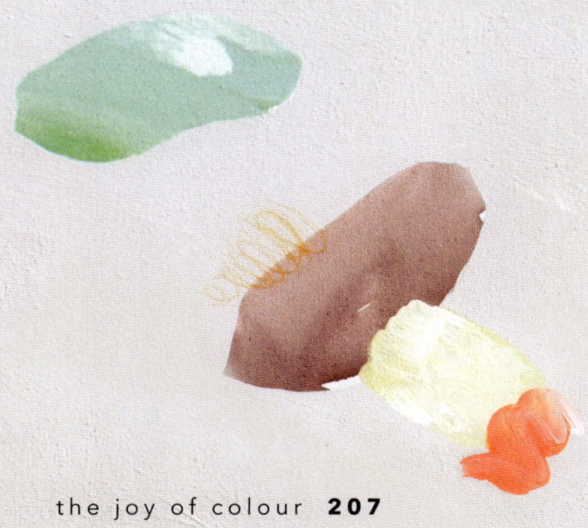

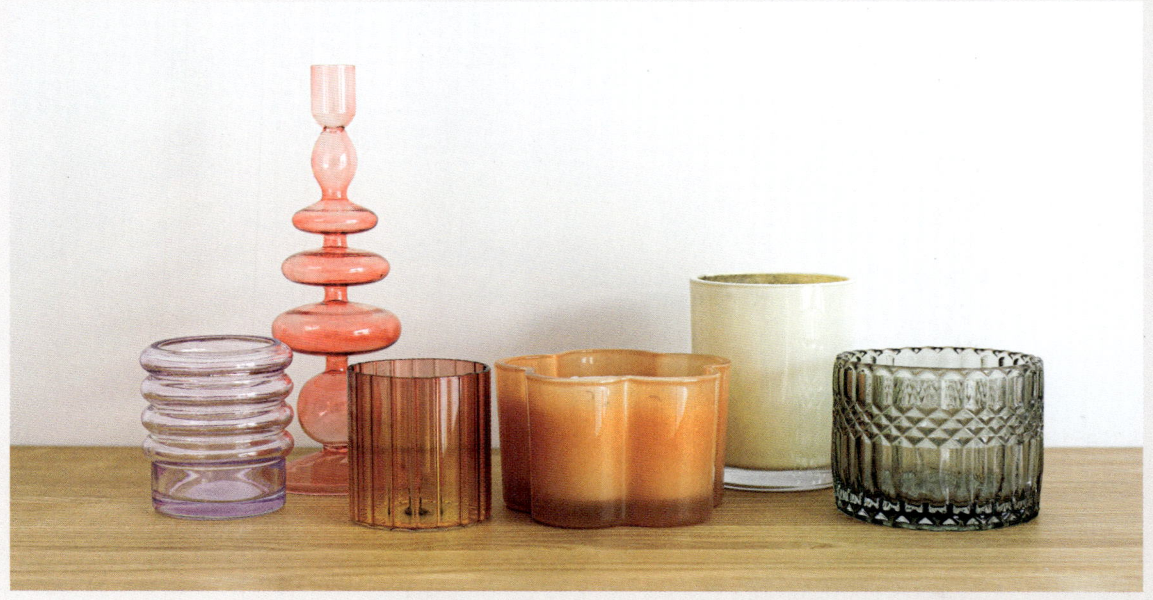

Don't be scared, it's only colour

Some are nervous about colour and stick to something safe because they're not entirely sure if two colours will work together well – so we often pick bland or boring colours to lower the risk of getting it wrong (think of every blue-grey office space you've ever seen). Being colour-conservative dulls your life and misses the opportunity for self-expression. I'm not saying everyone should have a maximalist house and a wardrobe like Iris Apfel (RIP, what an icon), although that is undoubtedly a joyful possibility. Remember, your colour love is personal. I opt for soft colours with delicious neutrals and pops of playfulness. I love gentleness in my home but with moments of surprise.

You might prefer strength and excitement or the blissful calm of a tonal space. All I ask is that it makes you happy. Seeing it on Instagram is a start; it's a place to test what you love, but don't let it dictate you into a style because you feel like you're supposed to – choose from a place of joy.

Colour gradients

I'm obsessed with gradients. They are a fabulous way of arranging things that can otherwise feel cluttered and disorganised. Think of a box of coloured pencils – first, imagine them arranged in a mess, and then in a satisfying rainbow gradient. Which makes you feel better?

EVERYTHING LOOKS BETTER IN A GRADIENT, EVEN A ROW OF WELL-WORN SHOES.

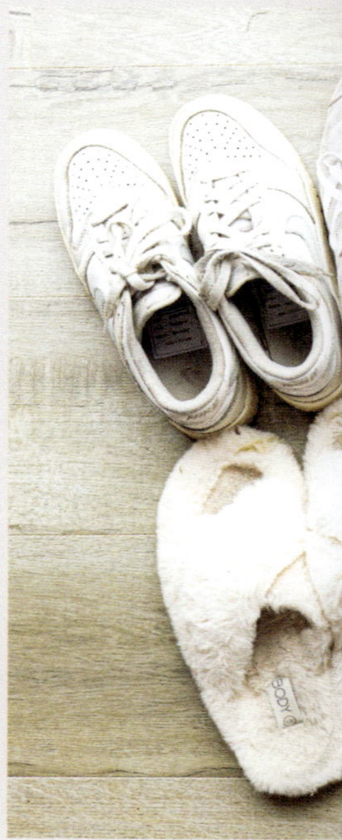

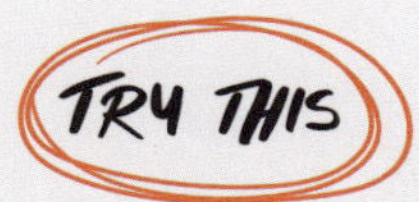

A classic use of gradients is for bookshelves – arranging them in a rainbow gradient is an instant burst of delight for your eyes. Try the same with a messy wardrobe of clothes.

+

Colour gradients work well within a limited palette too – you don't need the full rainbow to make it work – arrange similarly coloured objects near each other from dark to light and feel the calm. Arranging colours to softly transition adds depth and interest and feels so wonderful to look at. If you're repainting an area, consider using two or three similar tones, rather than just one.

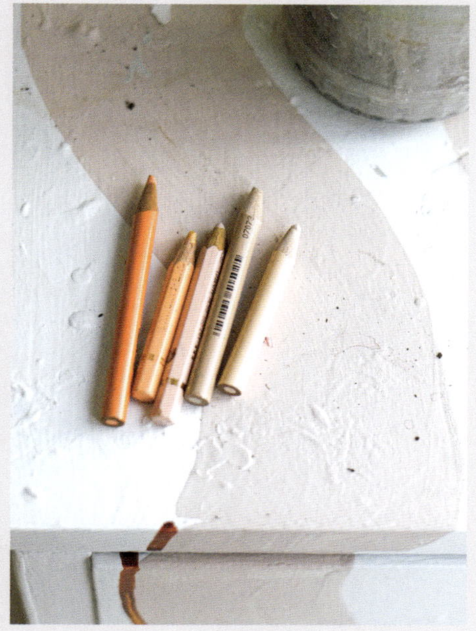

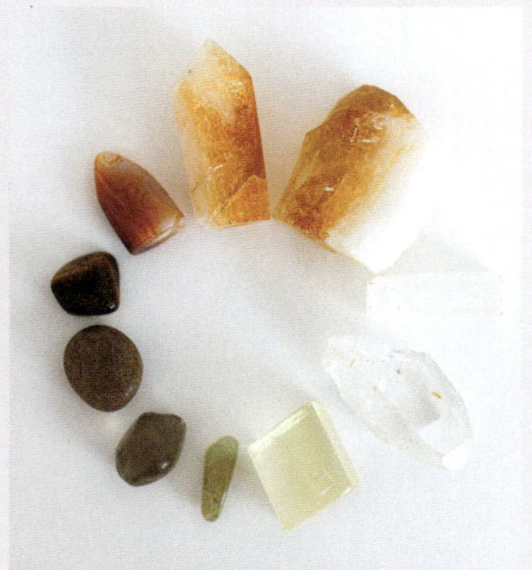

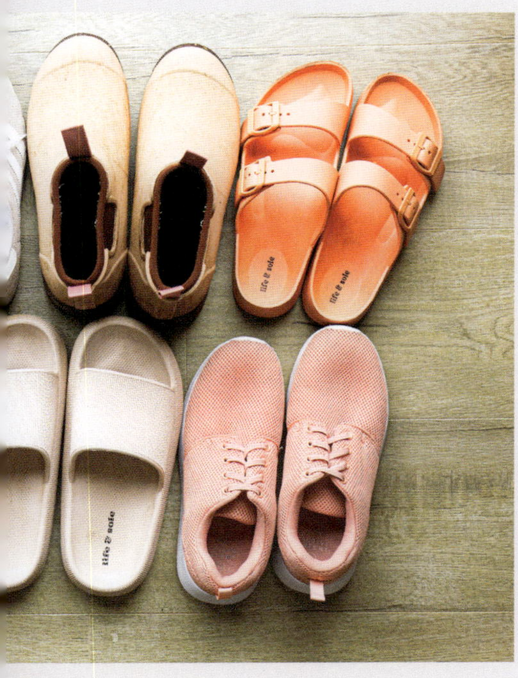

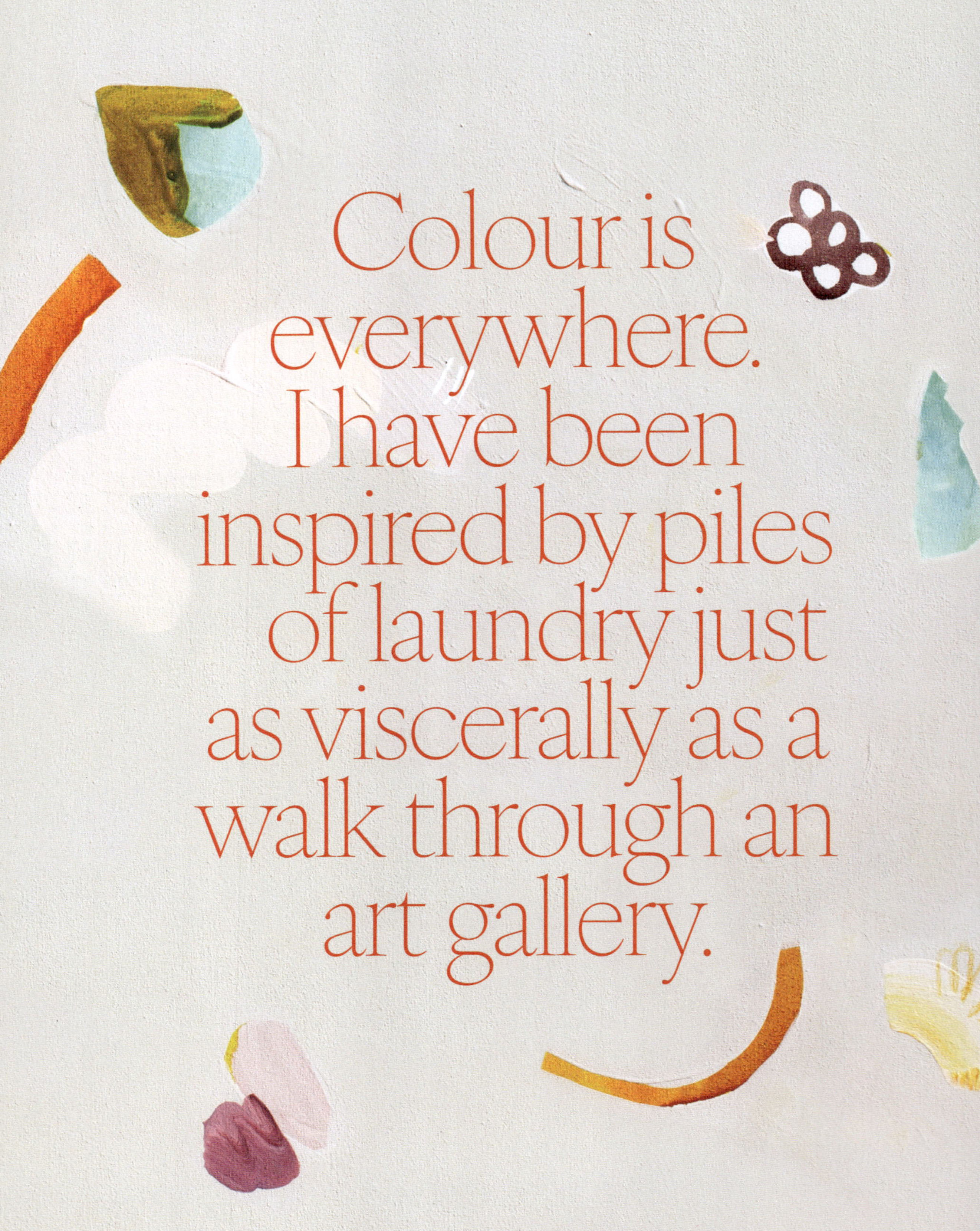

Colour is everywhere. I have been inspired by piles of laundry just as viscerally as a walk through an art gallery.

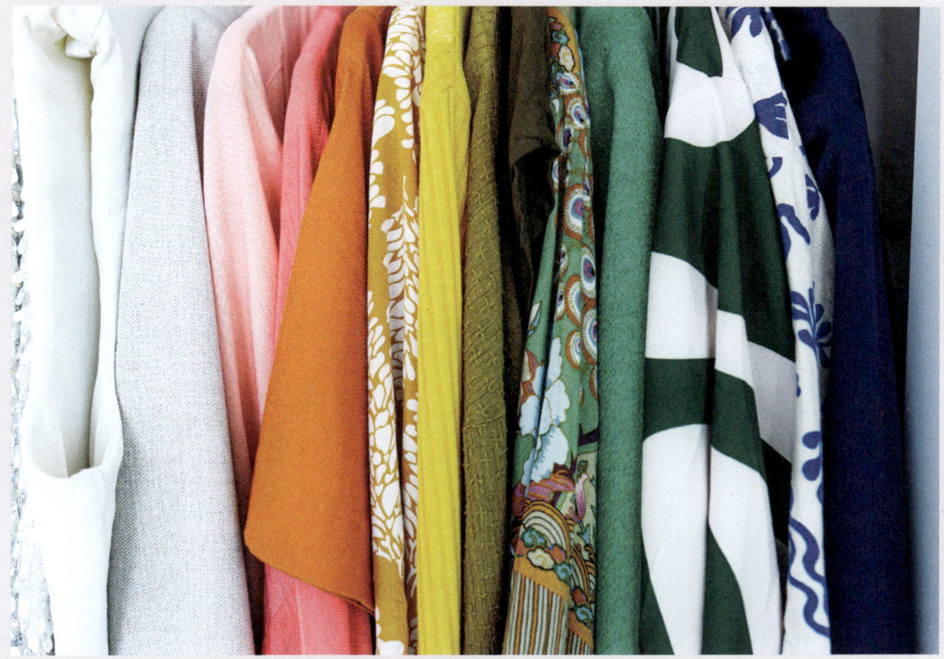

Using colour for joy in your own life

Surrounding yourself with colours that make you feel good is a great start. Remember, you don't need to throw everything out and start from scratch. You can slowly build your colour story, or even find things you already own and give them more importance in your space. You can inject colours into your space in small, inexpensive ways – cushions, tea towels, mugs or books that you didn't enjoy but have a lovely coloured cover! Create little joy-clusters with them so that they catch your eye and your heart. Or you can go large and buy an artwork that brings all of your colour dreams to life in one go – then use this as a starting point to build on.

Colour doesn't need to be permanent and based in objects that you have bought. You can engage in colour play (see over) to soak in the benefits of being around colours you love. From page 214 onwards, I'll show you how I use palettes as a starting point for my work.

THERE ARE SO MANY EASY WAYS TO MESS AROUND WITH COLOUR...

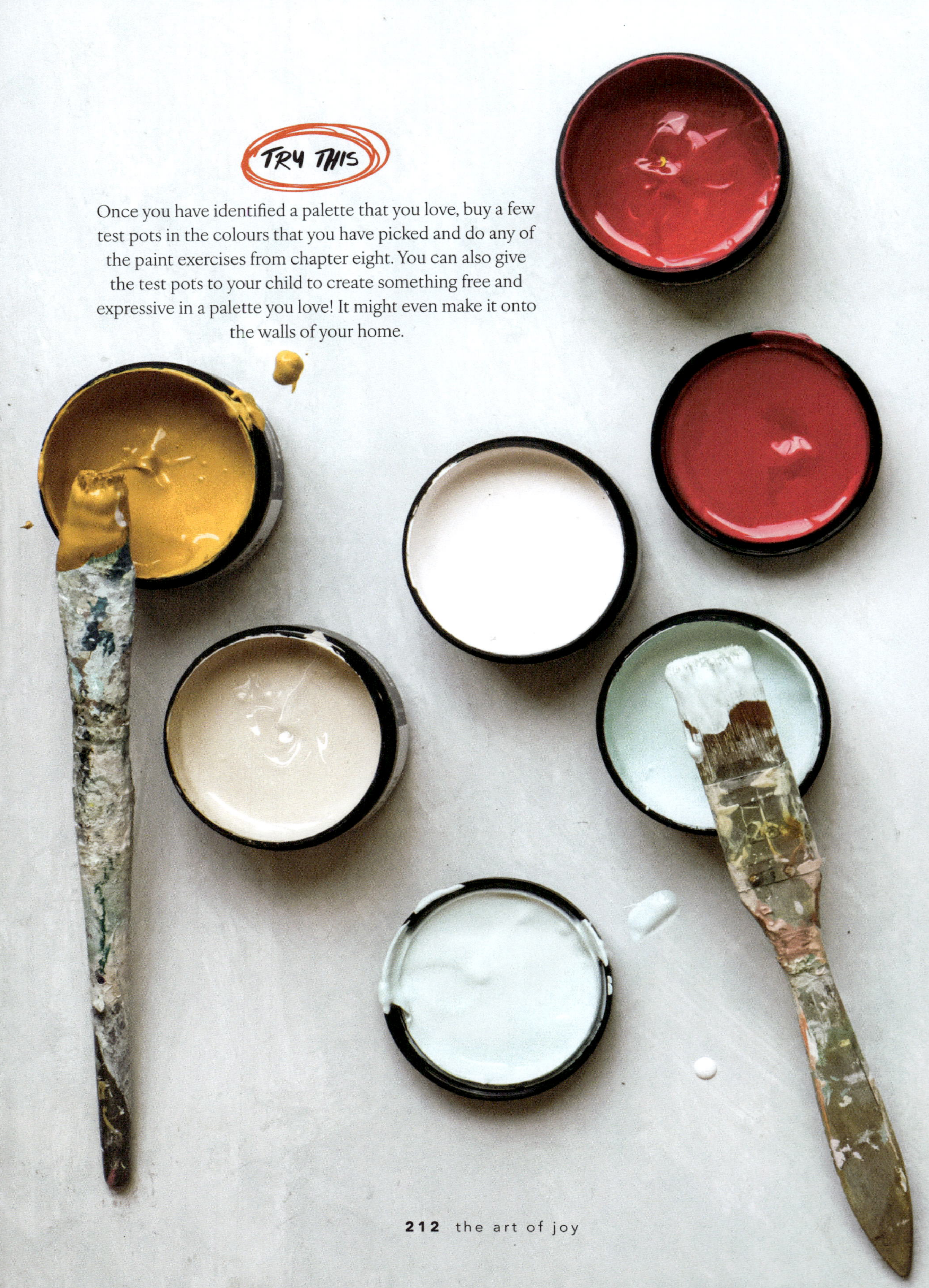

TRY THIS

Once you have identified a palette that you love, buy a few test pots in the colours that you have picked and do any of the paint exercises from chapter eight. You can also give the test pots to your child to create something free and expressive in a palette you love! It might even make it onto the walls of your home.

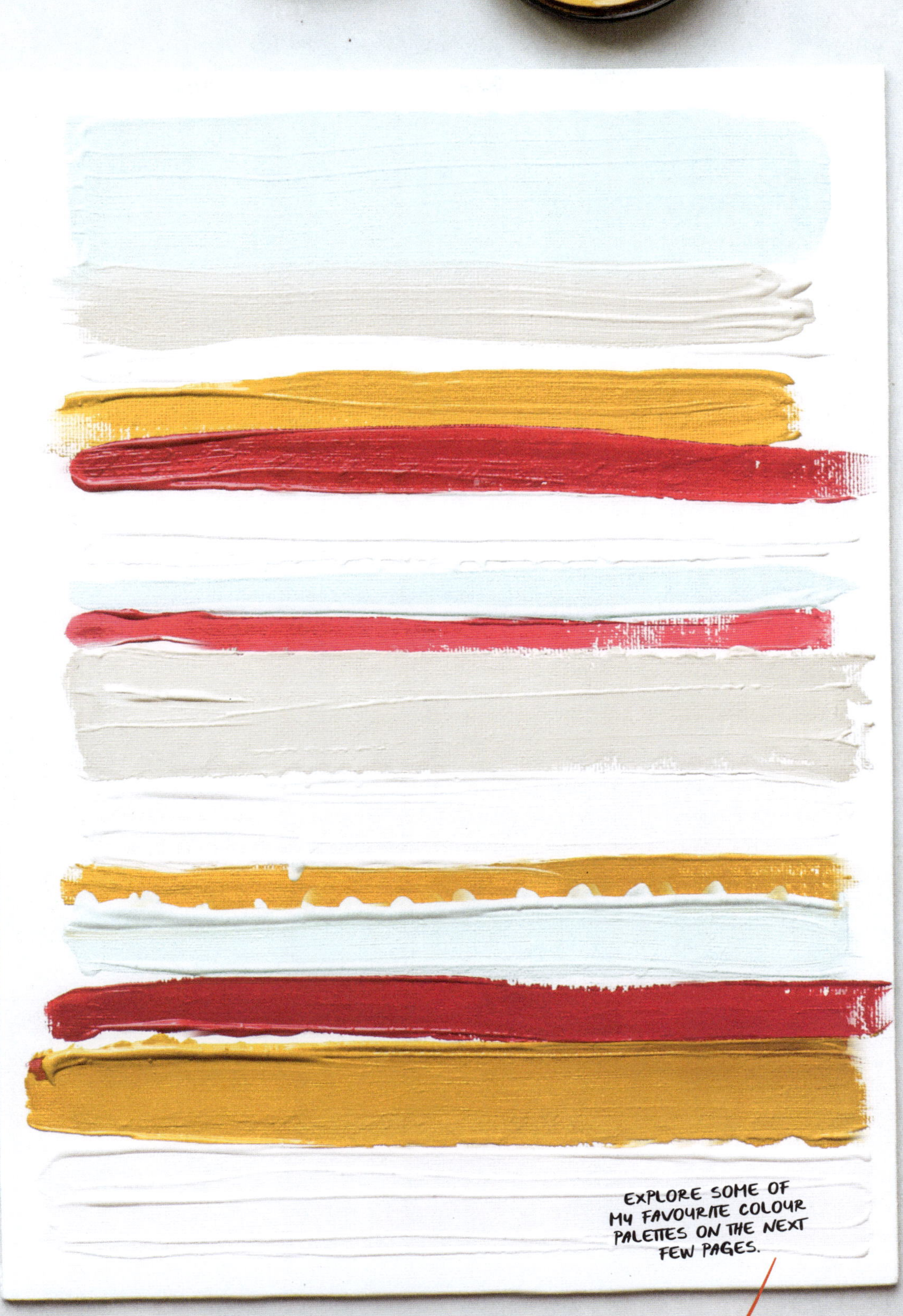
EXPLORE SOME OF
MY FAVOURITE COLOUR
PALETTES ON THE NEXT
FEW PAGES.

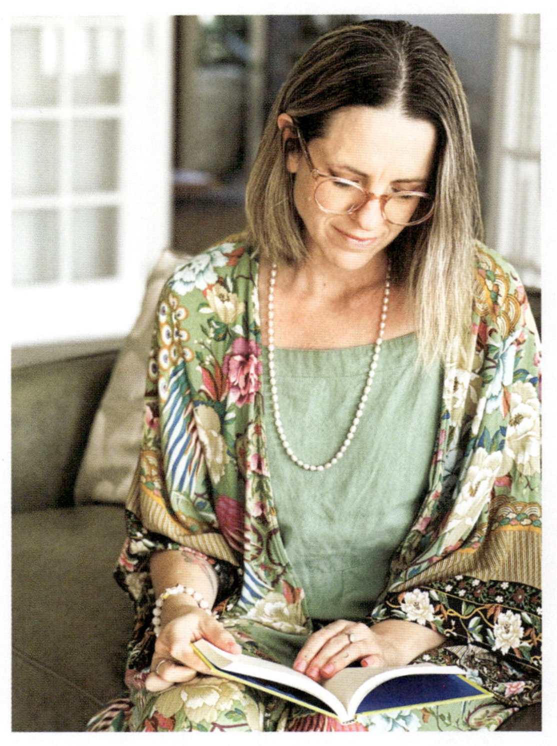

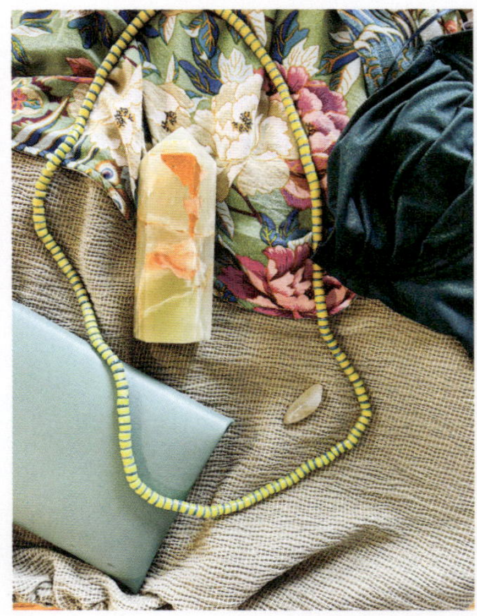

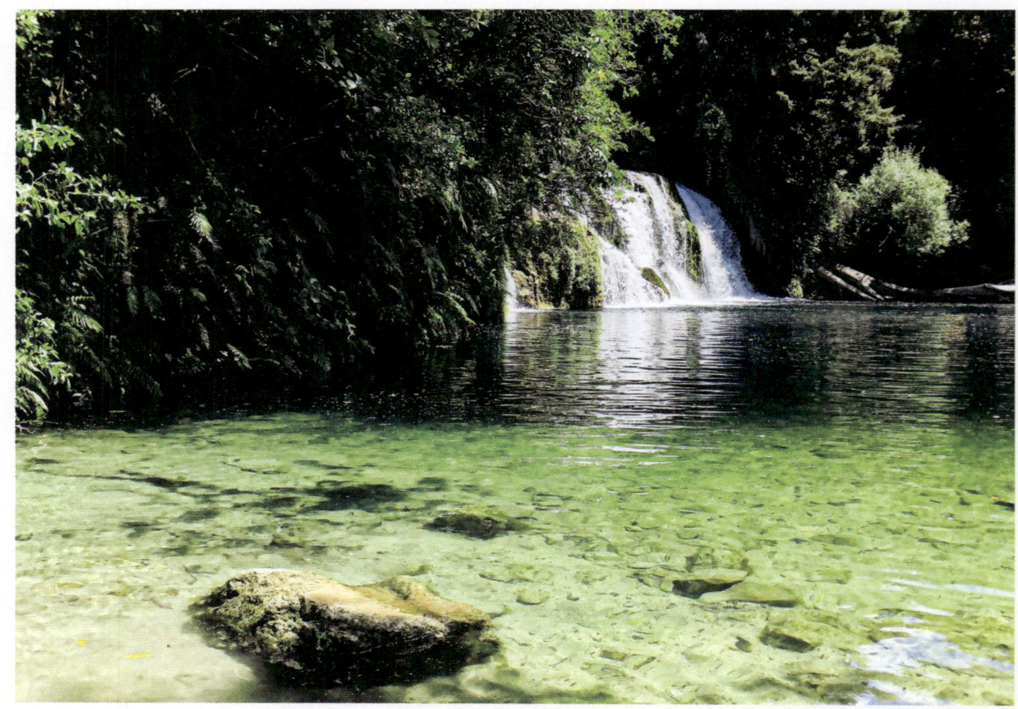

Palette #1

Turquoise waters, rich foliage and pops of pinks – this palette originated at a waterfall in Hawke's Bay but was translated into a more tropical setting. See the artwork on the next page.

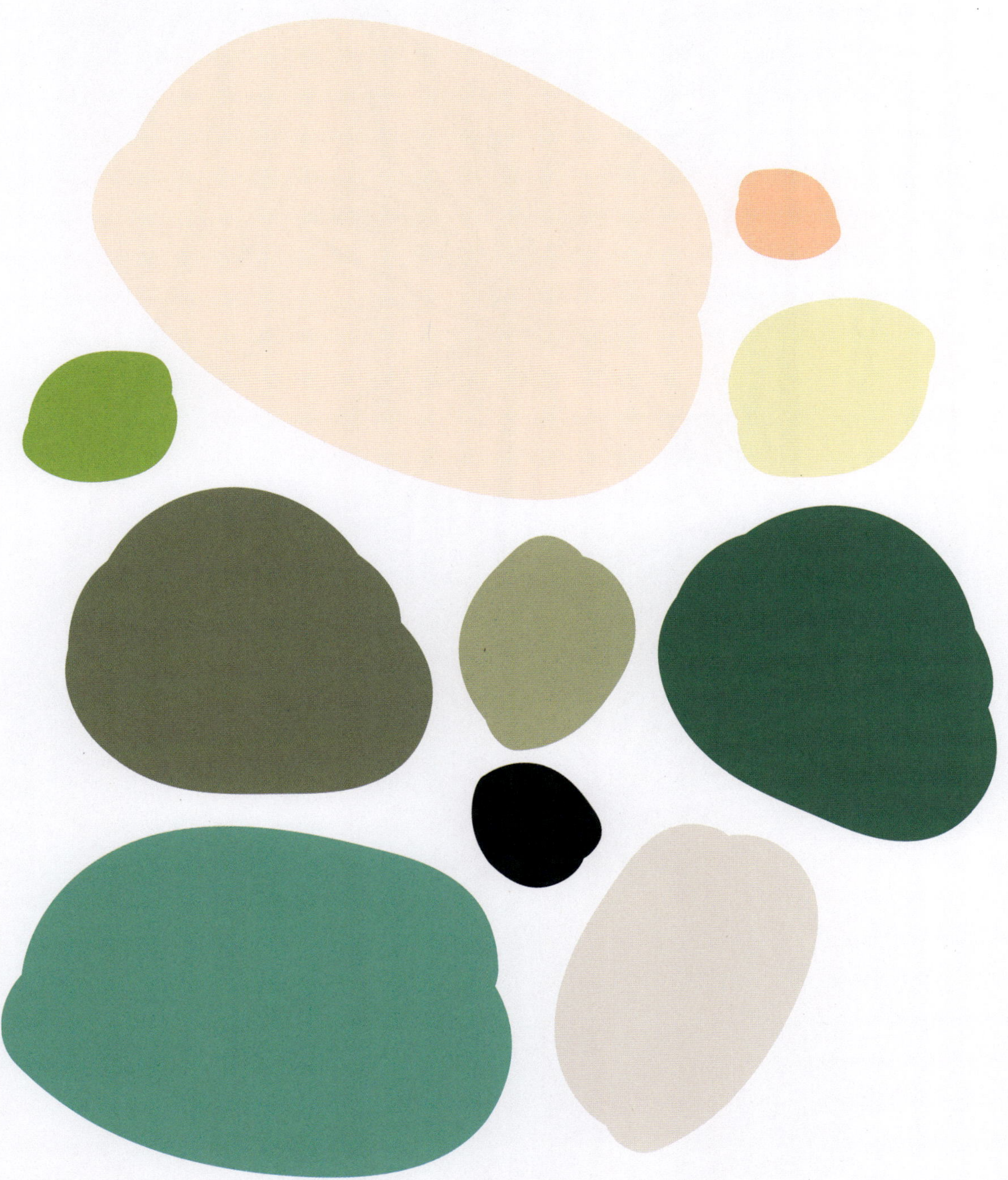

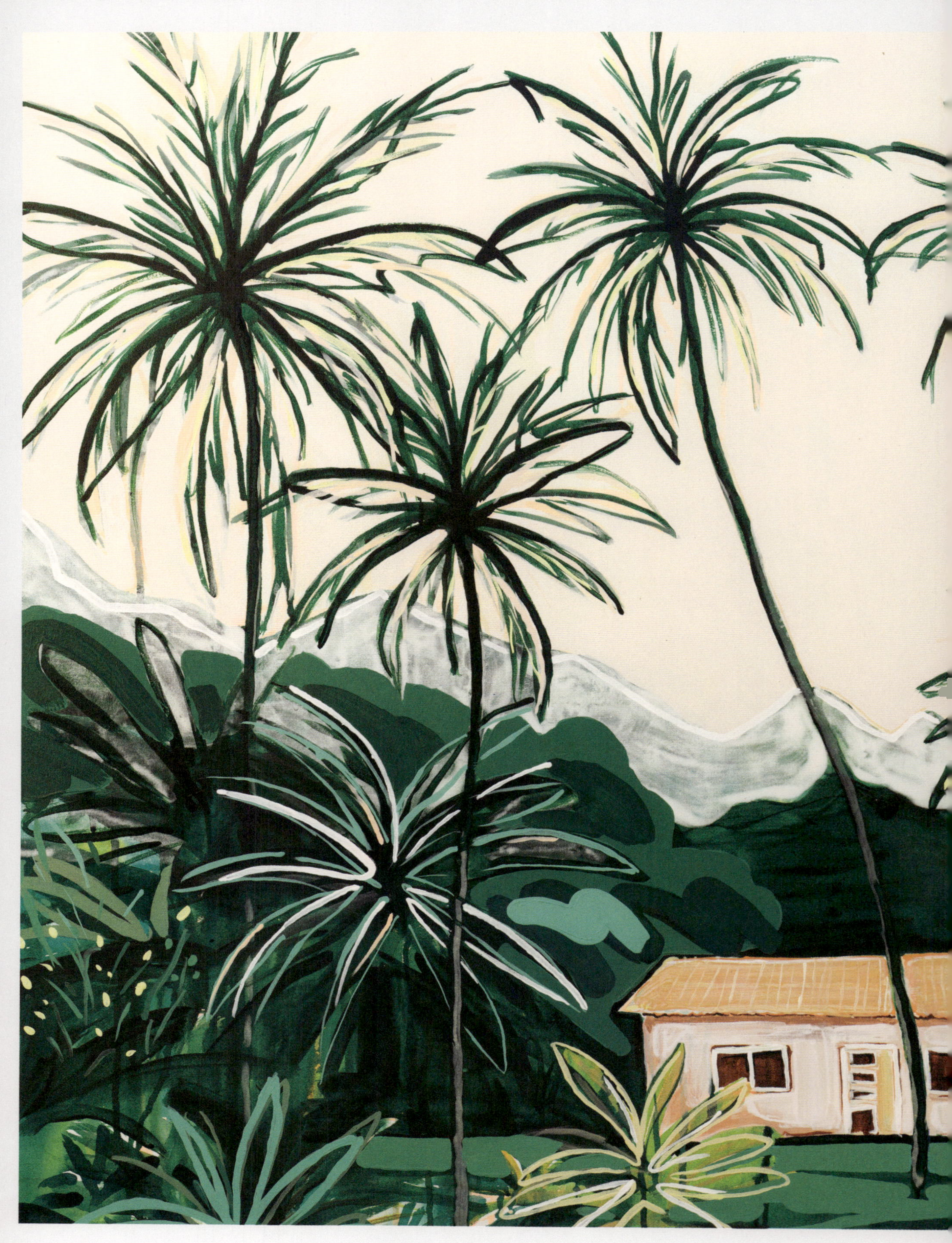

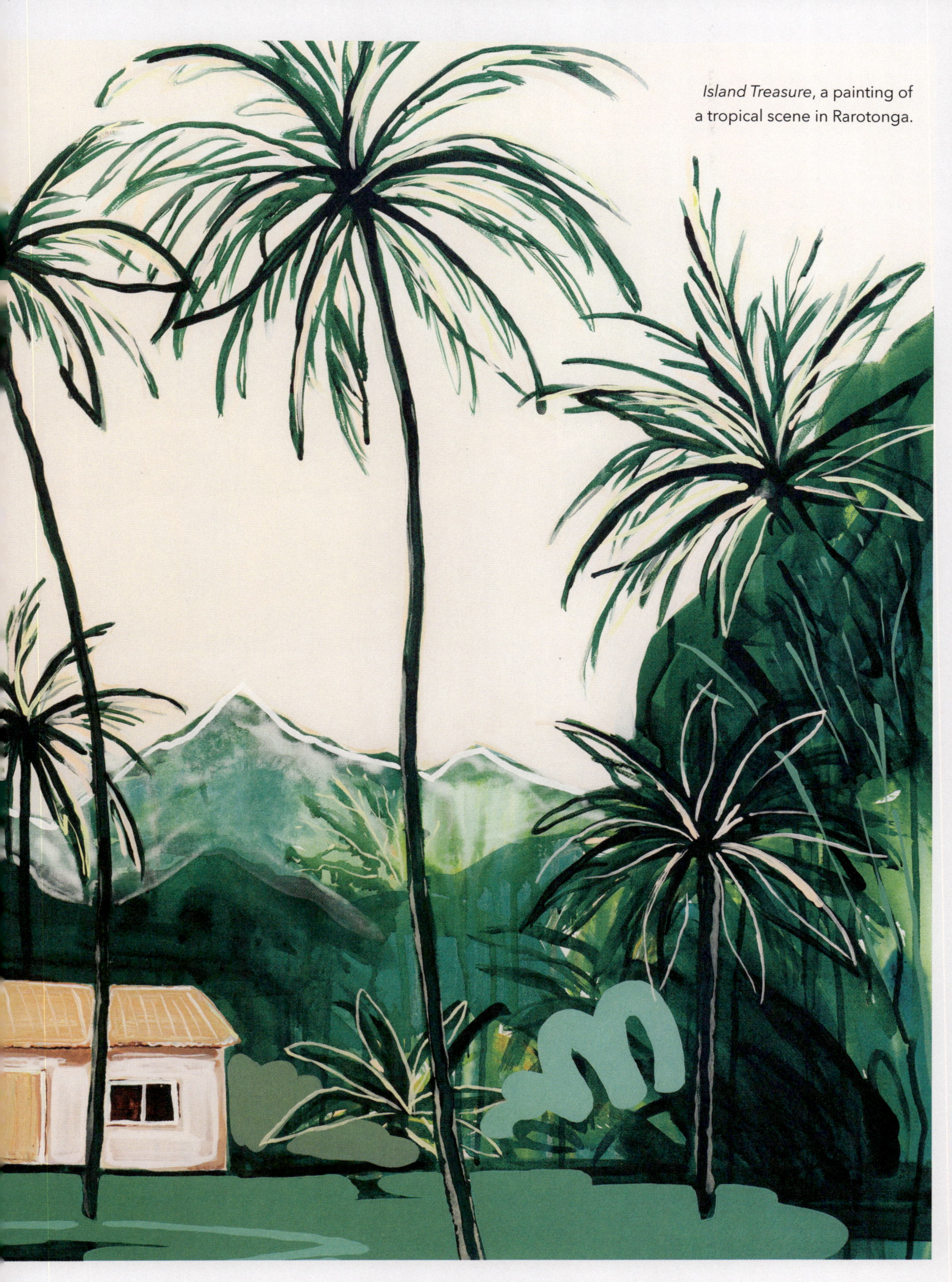

Island Treasure, a painting of a tropical scene in Rarotonga.

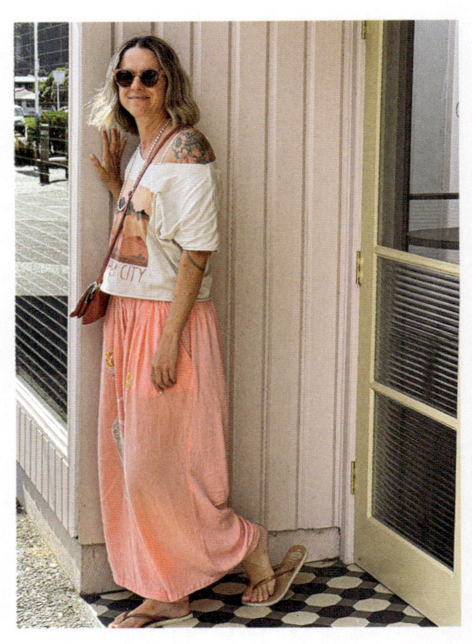

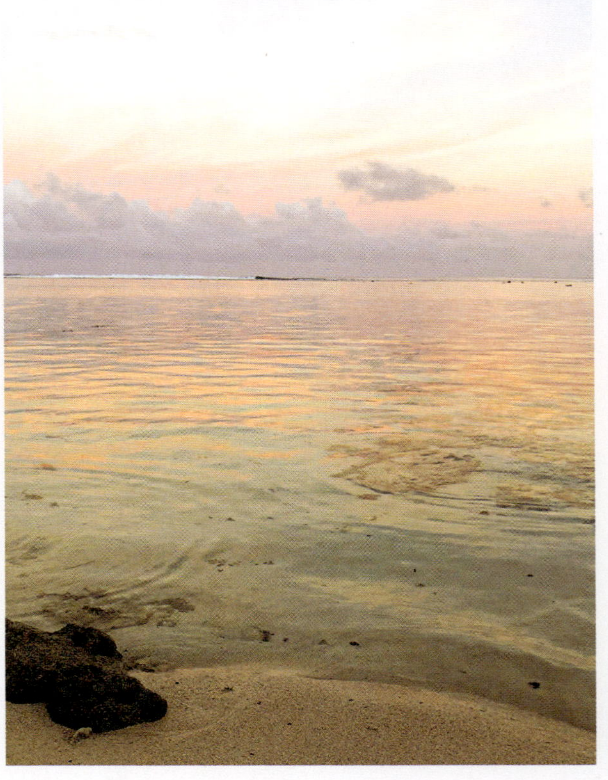

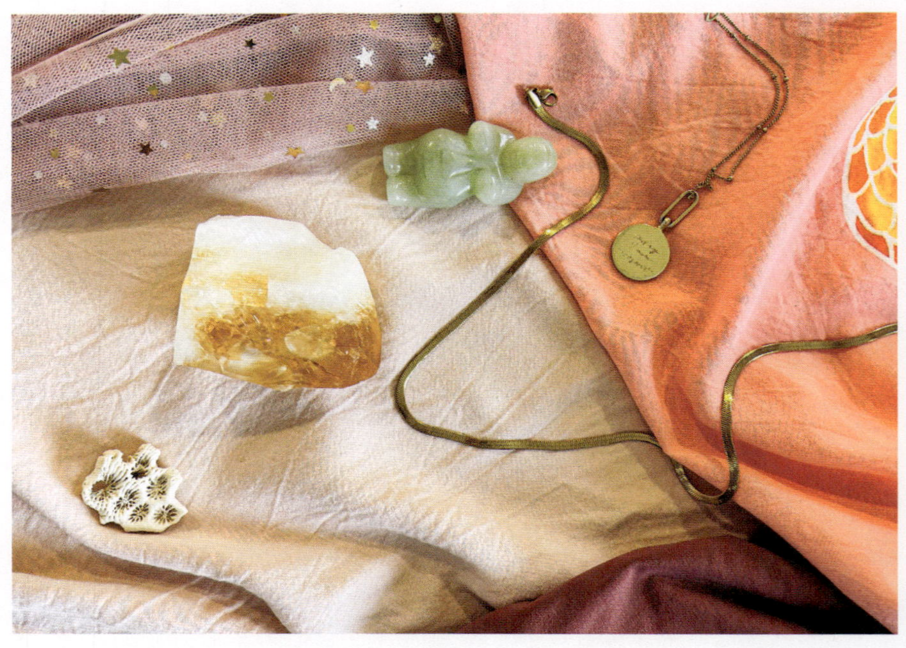

Palette #2

Coral is one of my favourite colours. This palette celebrates and elevates it with cool mauves, soft greens and warm peaches. See the inspiration come to life overleaf.

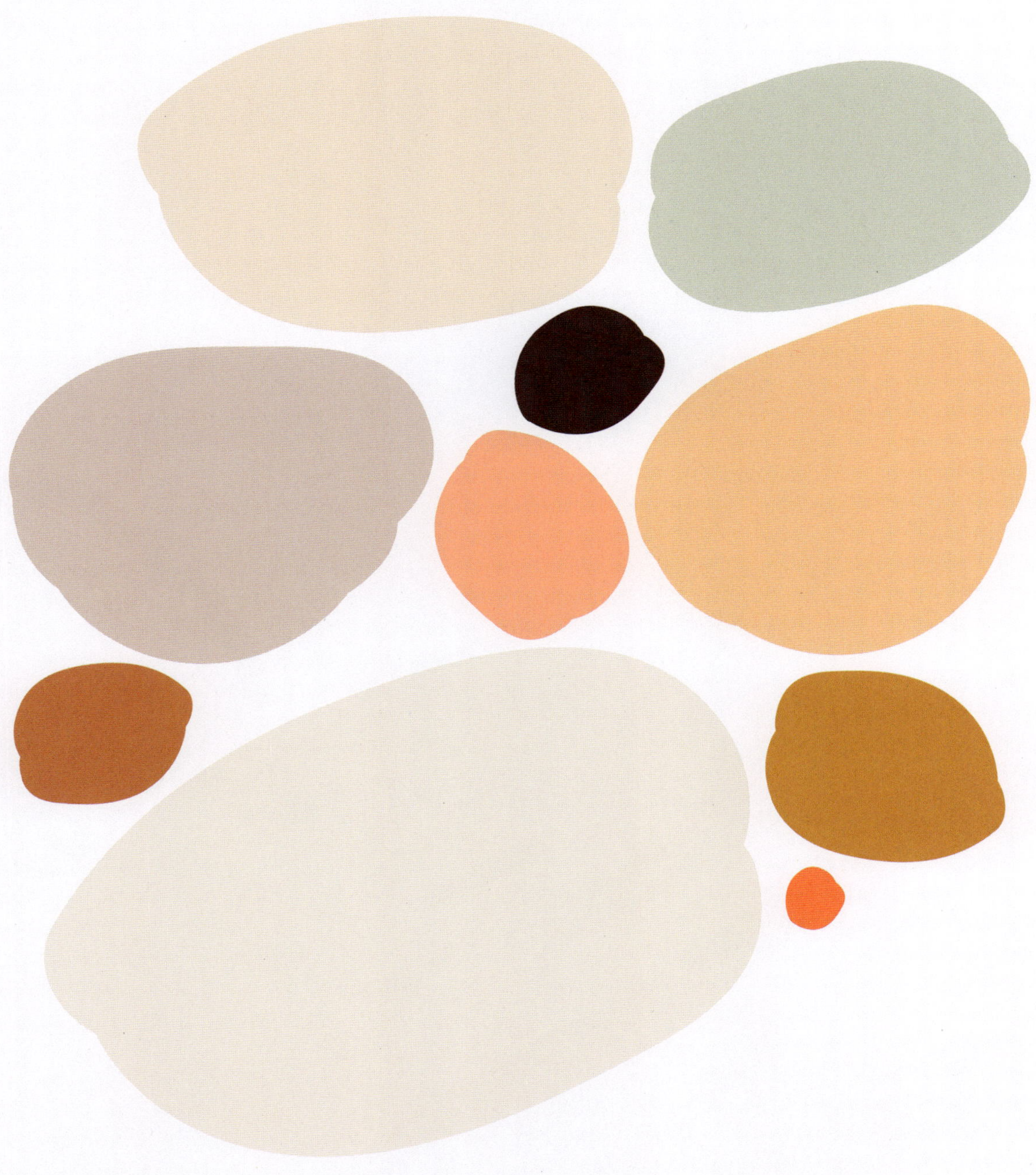

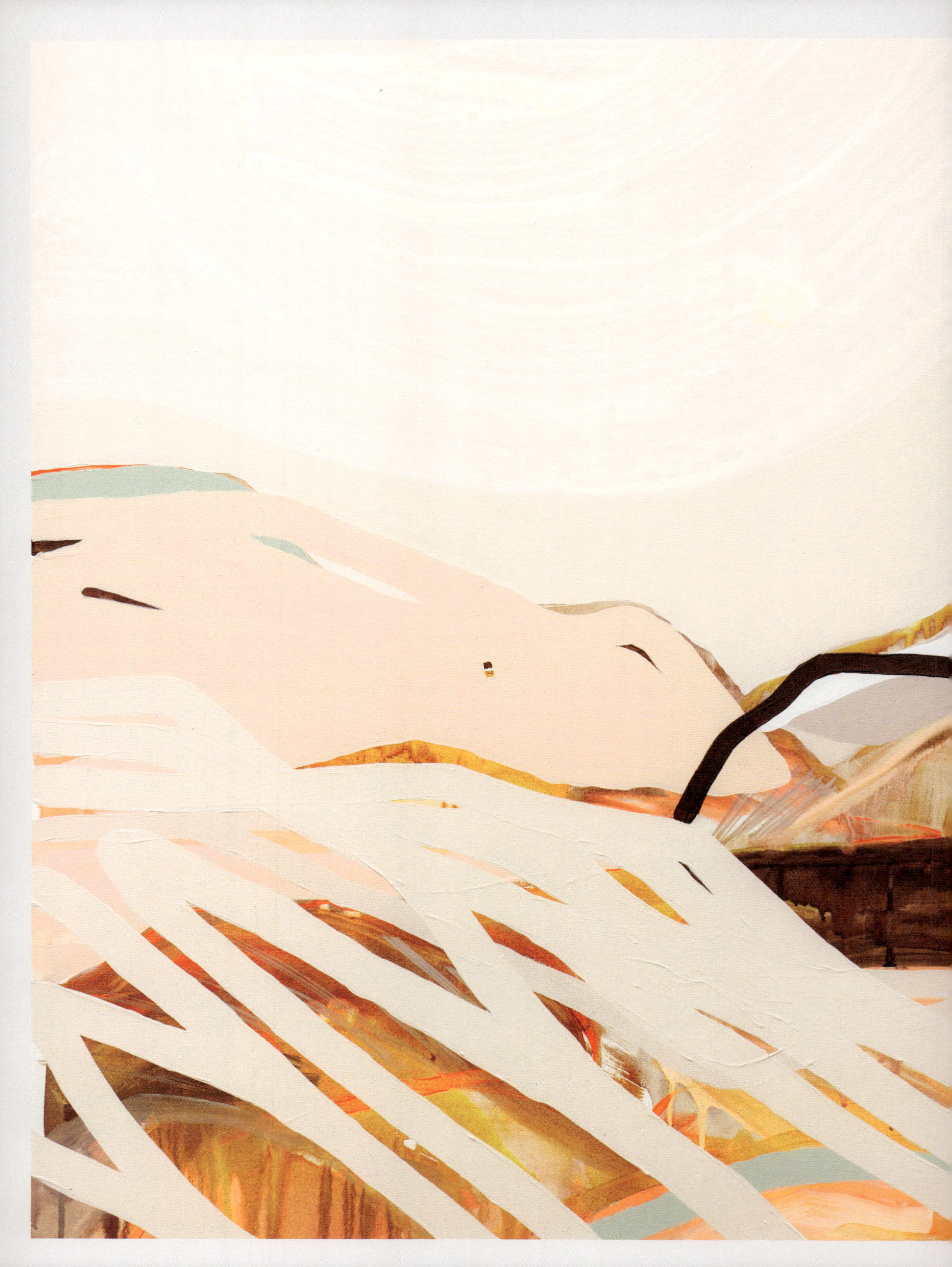

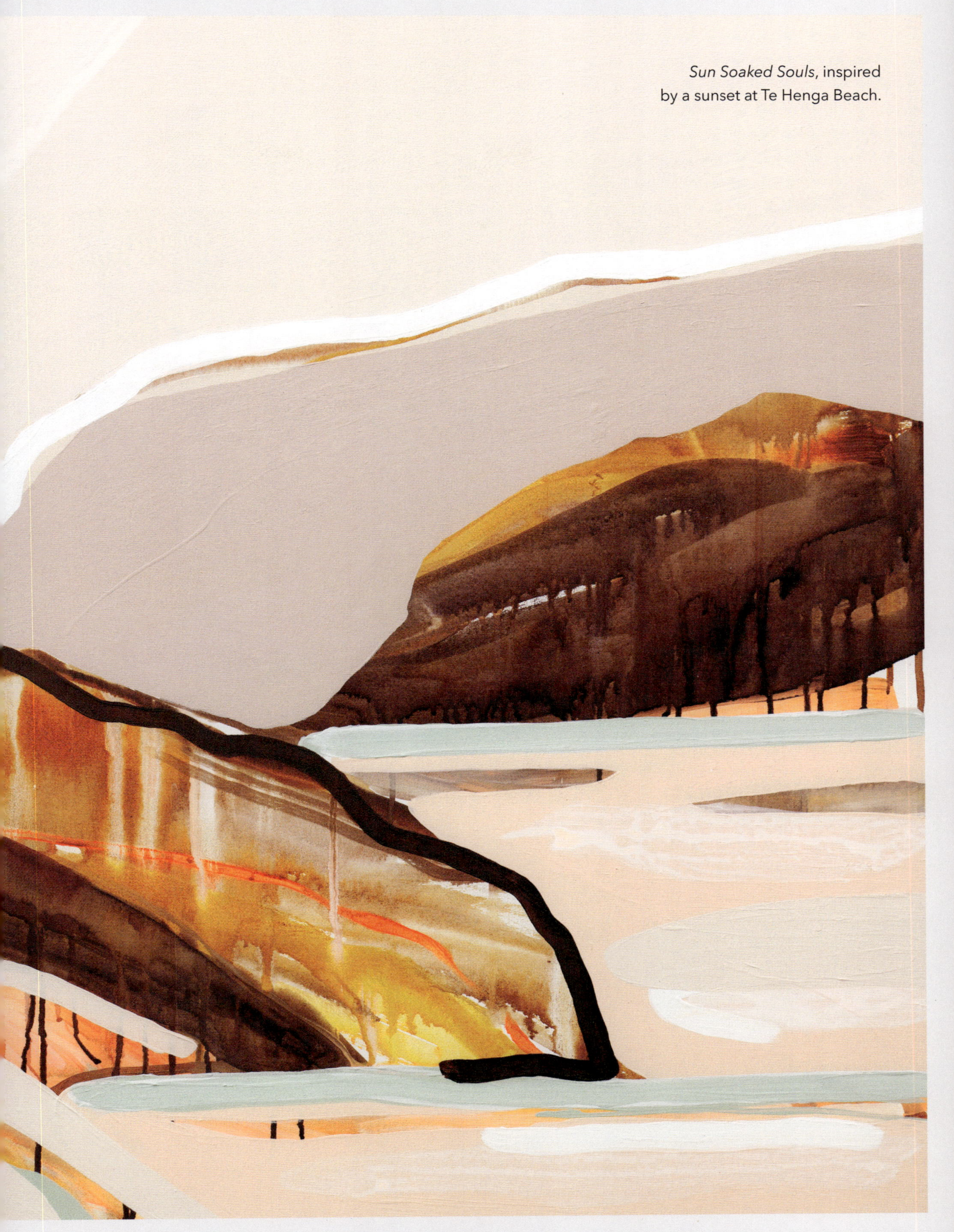

Sun Soaked Souls, inspired by a sunset at Te Henga Beach.

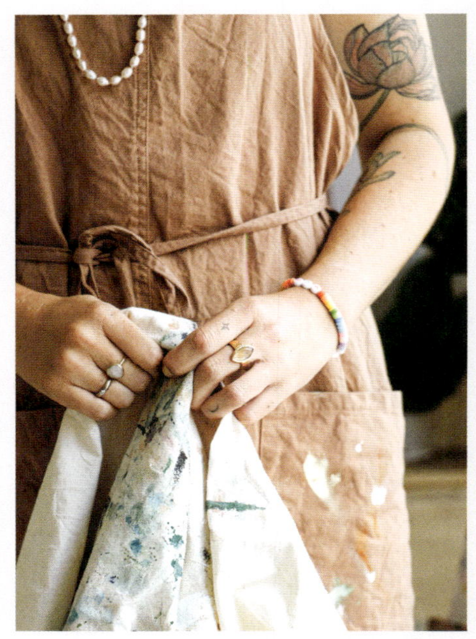

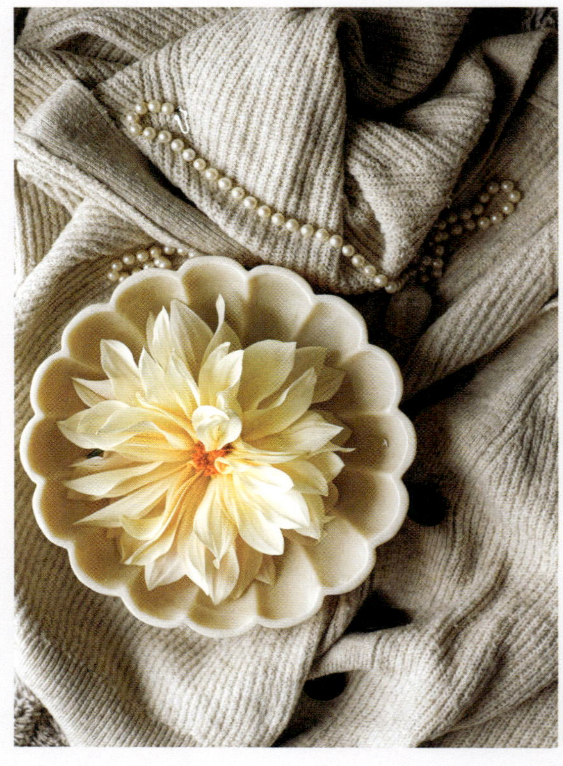

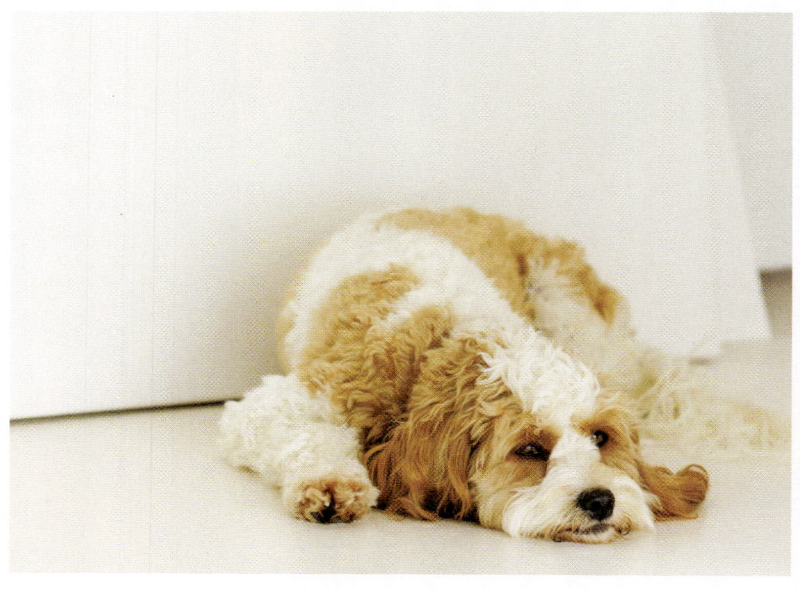

Palette #3

This warm, neutral palette feels like home. Soft tones of blush and beige come to life with a little ochre and a cool grey. See overleaf how this palette translates into an artwork.

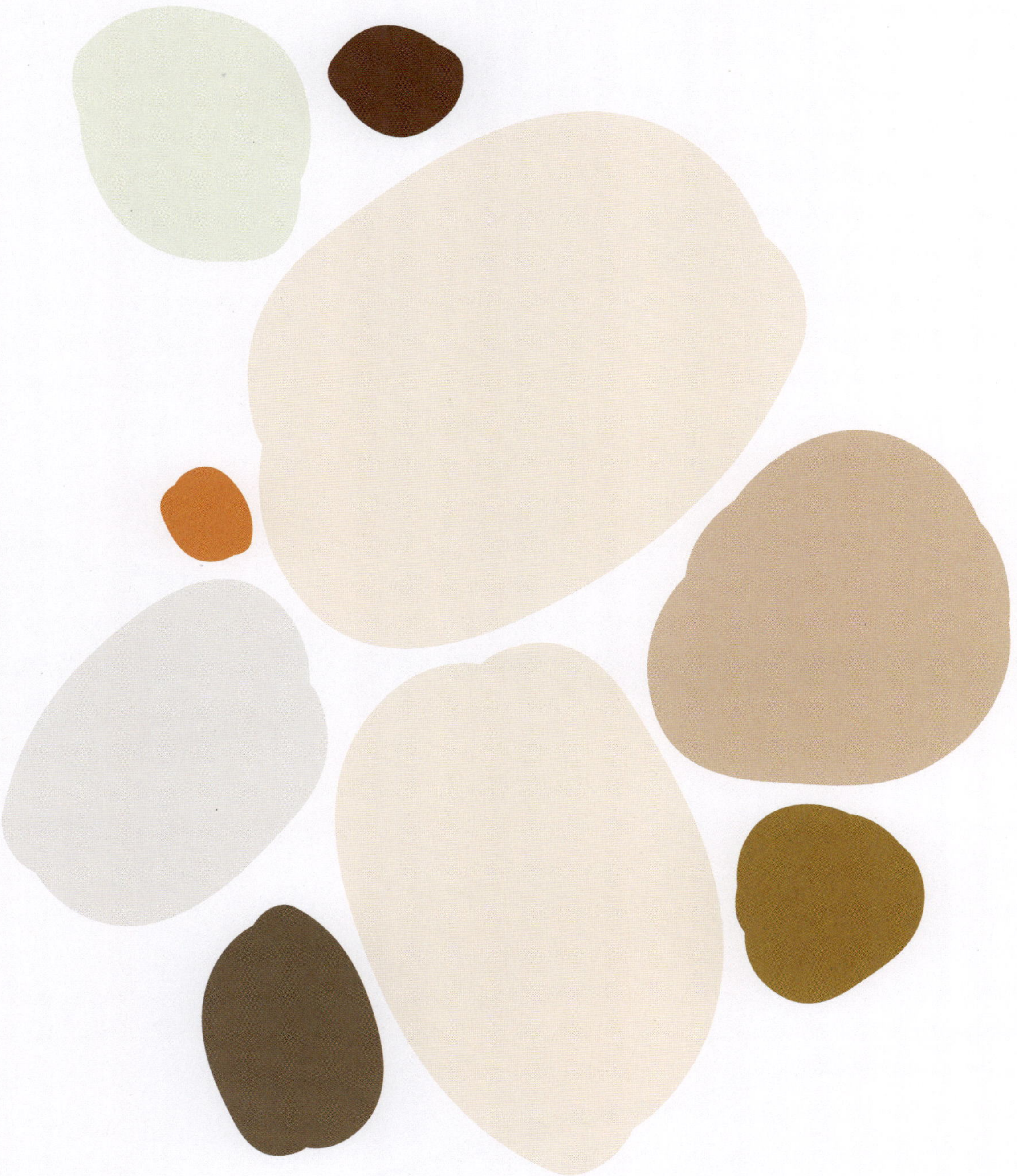

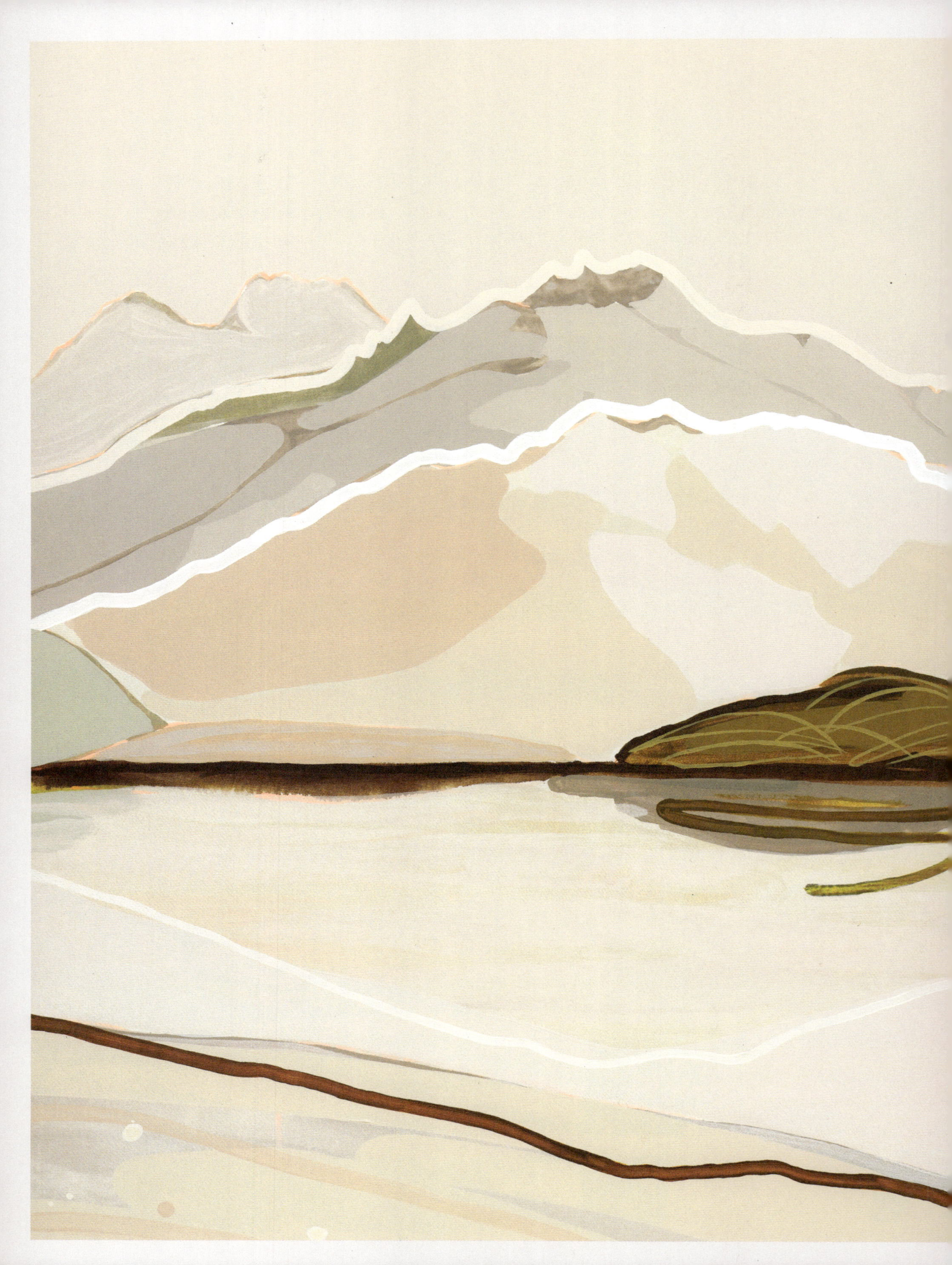

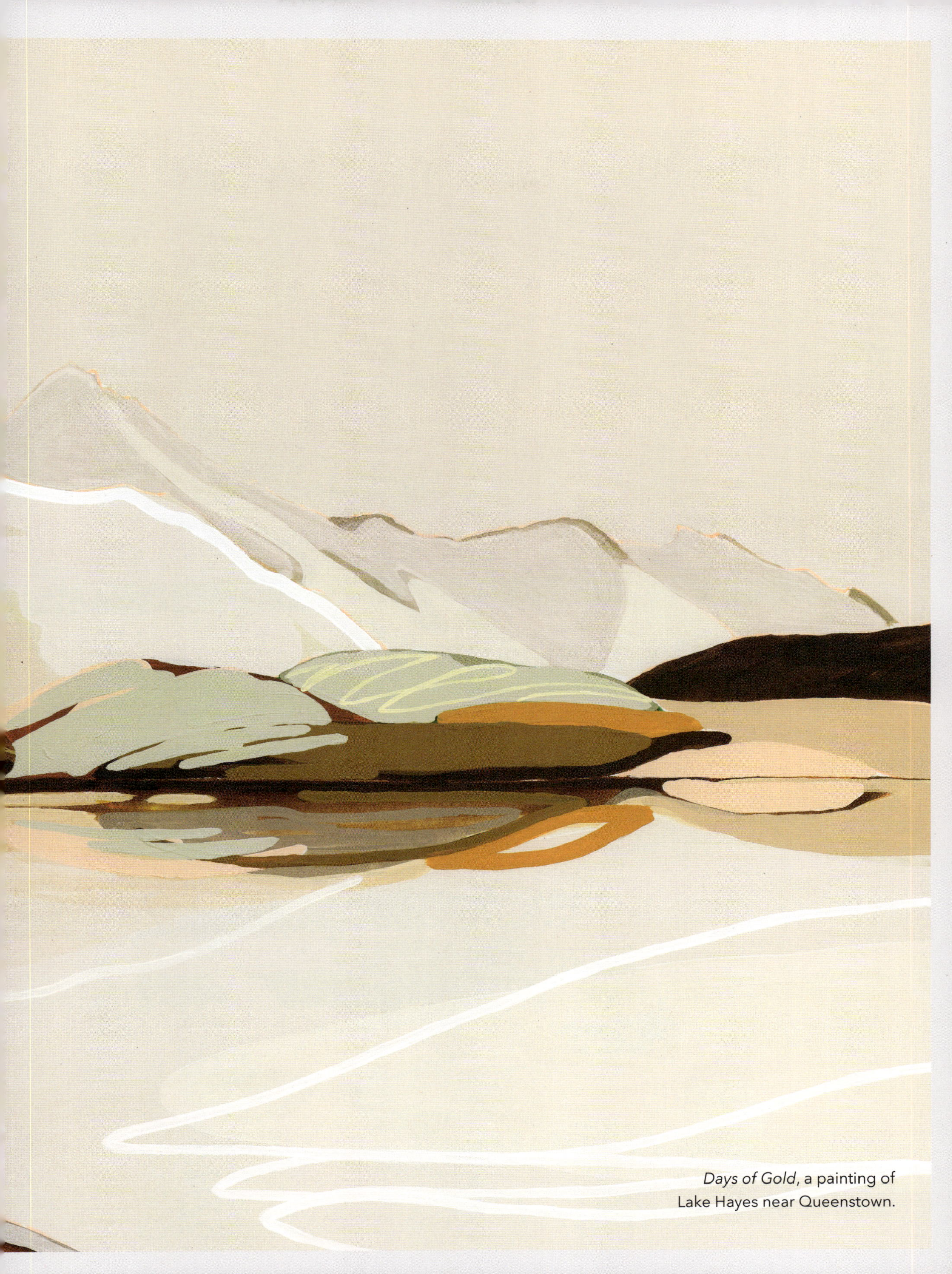

Days of Gold, a painting of
Lake Hayes near Queenstown.

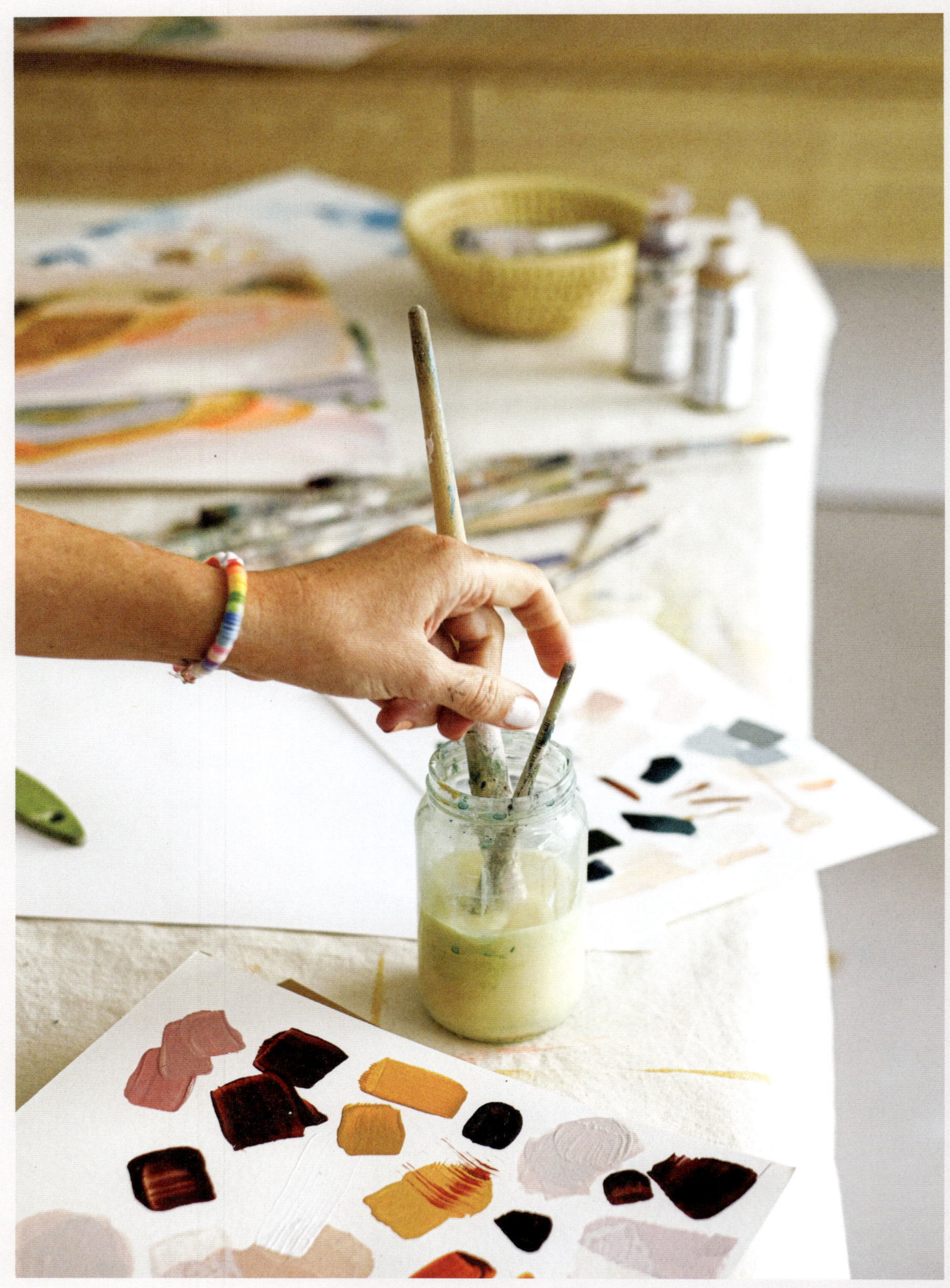

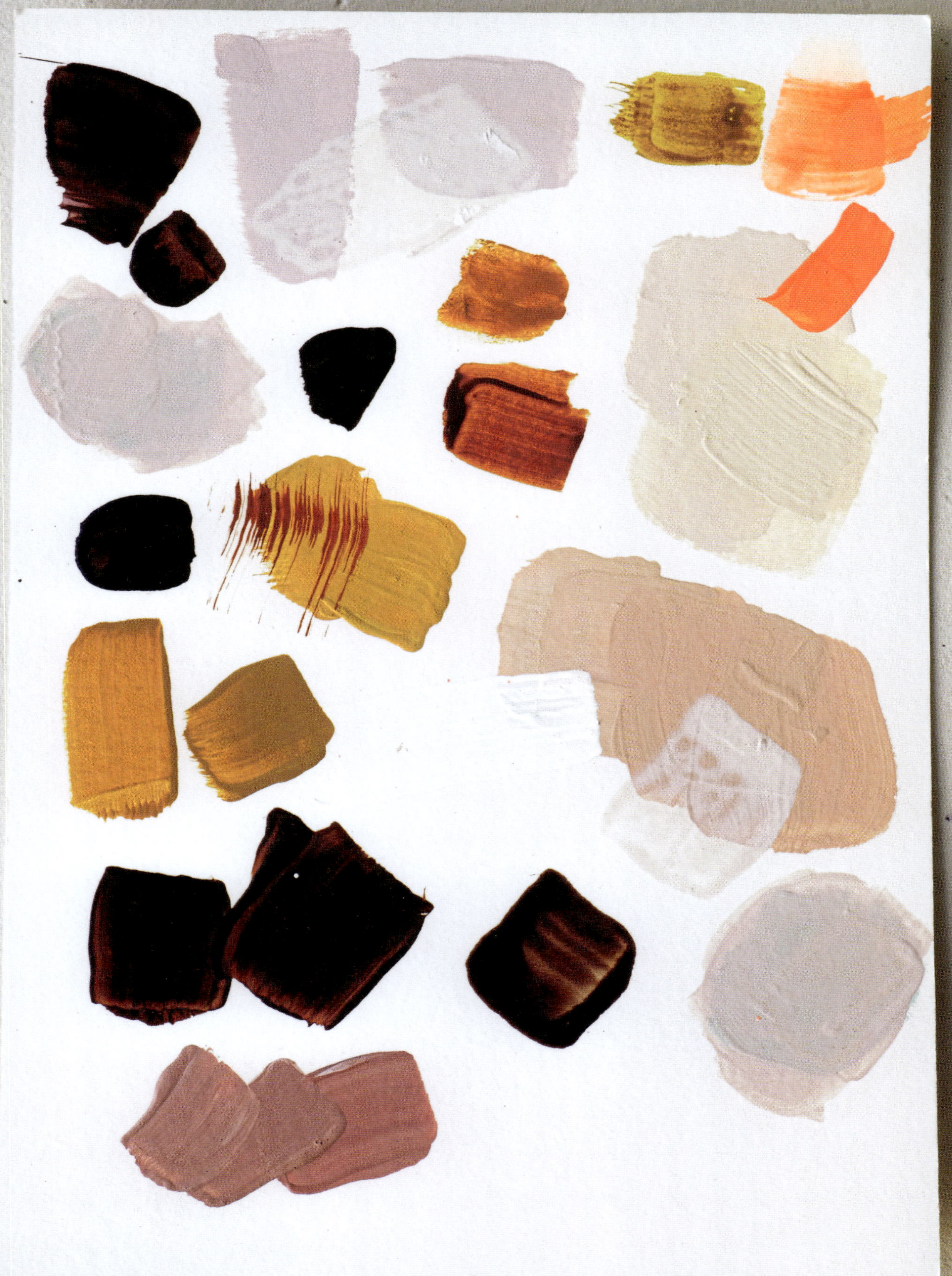

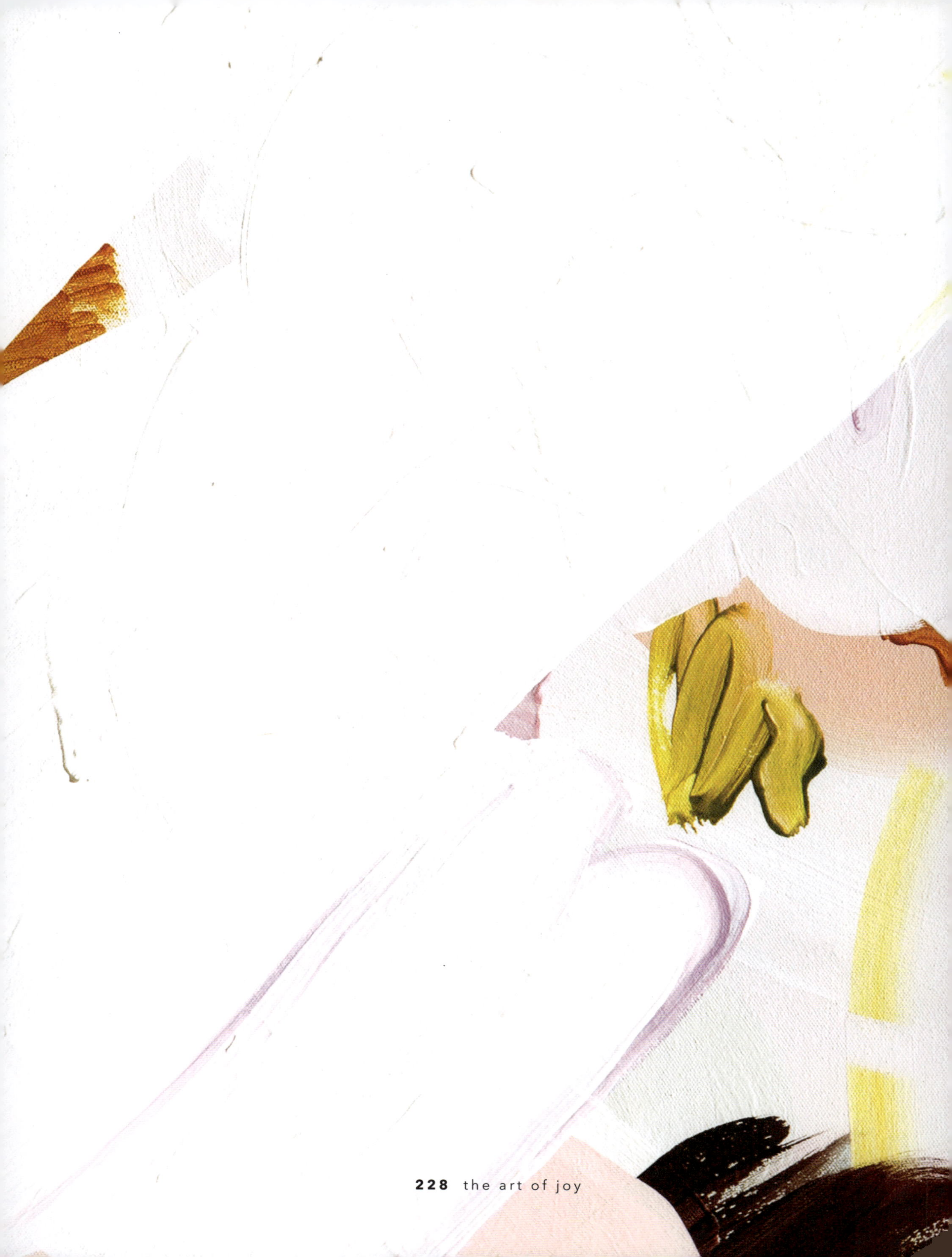

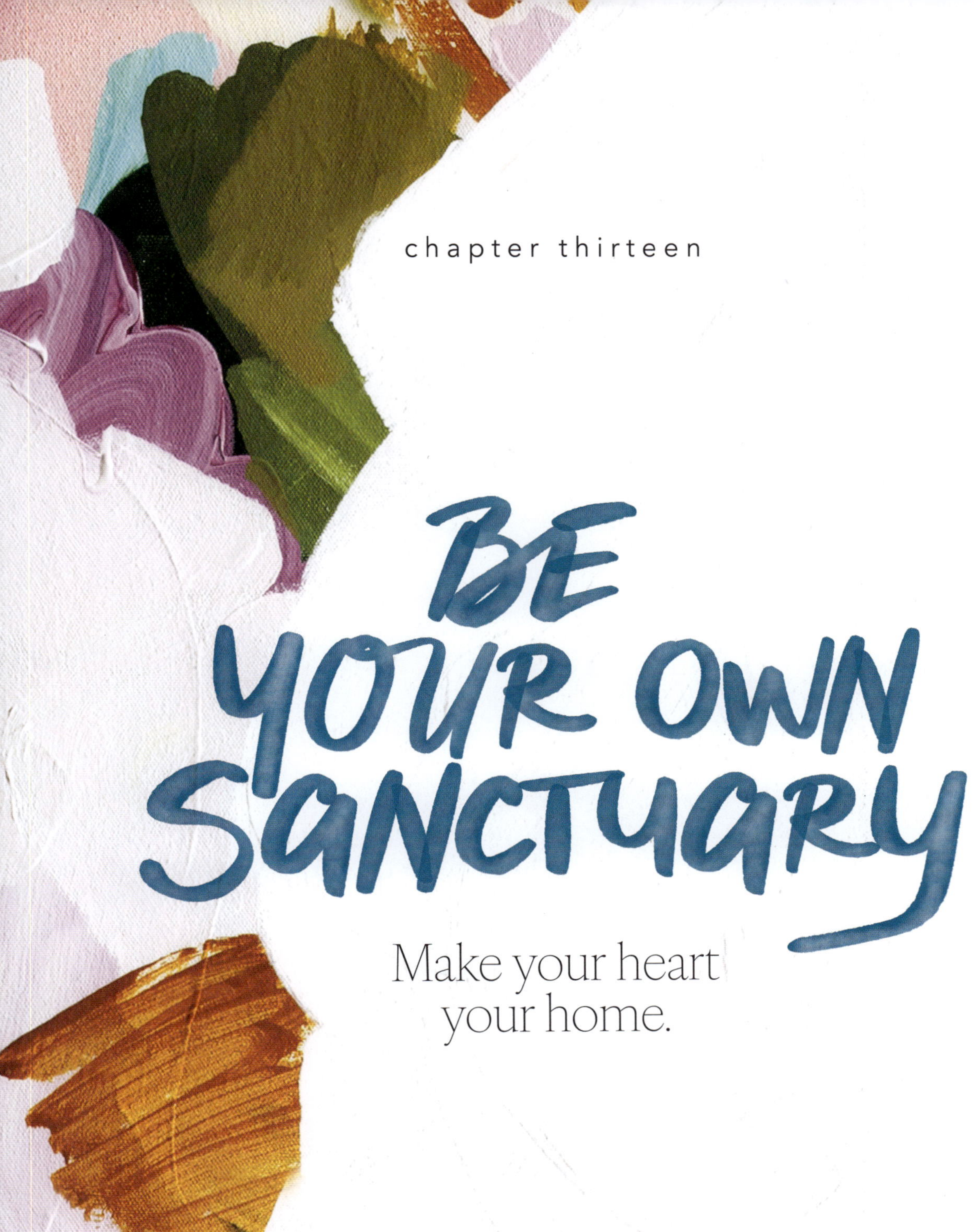

chapter thirteen

BE YOUR OWN SANCTUARY

Make your heart
your home.

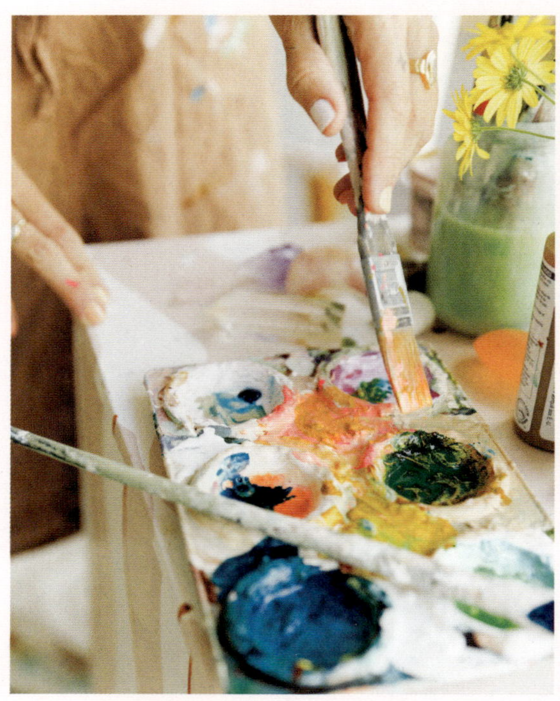

We have so many outward-focused labels that define us by how we relate to others – what we *do* for others. Mother, sister, manager, friend. With all of these roles, we often need to remember to think of ourselves. We've been raised to believe that thinking of ourselves is selfish, that being a mother or an **insert your job title here** should be fulfilling enough to fill our cups. But we forget to think of ourselves as *self*. Nurturing a connection to yourself, a sense of who you are, what you love and what you need, is a central part of this joy collage we're creating.

Connecting to ourselves can feel uncomfortable at first, it feels vulnerable and raw, so I suggest going into it with a softness and a feeling of self-compassion. Don't judge yourself or berate yourself for not being more in touch already. Speak to yourself like you would to a small child – with kindness, patience and care. The journey of connecting to the Self doesn't need to be rushed. Go at a pace that feels soft and healing to you.

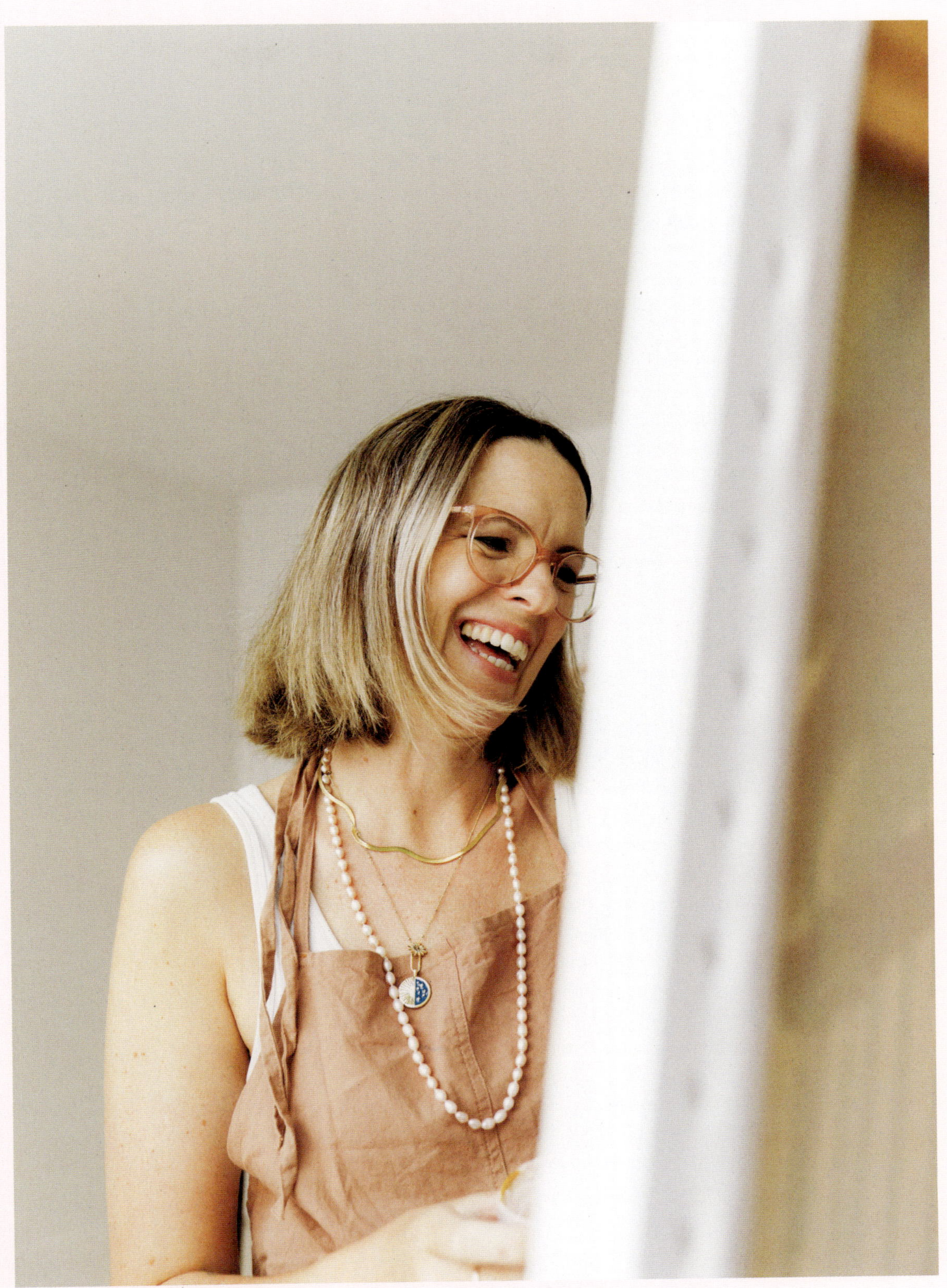

How do we find our 'Self'

The first step in this journey is to work out who your 'Self' is. Our mind chatter is made up of so many parts, and not all of them are our truest, wisest selves.

It is helpful to view these selves through the lens of Internal Family Systems (also known as IFS). This incredible framework, developed by Dr Richard Schwartz, explains that inside of us, we have many 'parts'; our personalities contain various versions of ourselves. These are often exiled versions of our younger selves that have developed to protect us from emotional danger. They act out, usually without us realising when certain trigger events happen. Underneath all of these 'parts', there is always a calm, wise, loving sense of self – The capital 'S' Self. The Self represents our truest nature, with all our different 'parts' separate. Picture your Self in the centre, and all the other parts moving in and out of frame when needed (see opposite).

I've done some 'parts work' (the term that IFS uses for communicating with the other aspects of ourselves), with my wonderful life coach and with my therapist, and discovered a part of me that comes in when I feel unseen, unnoticed … invisible. She's a six-year-old me, trying her best to be the cutest, most interesting child in a chaotic house full of older siblings. She acts up to be noticed, to feel the love and attention of the adults in her vicinity. She feels hurt when her older sisters don't allow her into their secret club at the top of the garden. She easily switches to victim mode when she feels ignored or excluded.

This part of me shows up in my adult life; she makes me act in ways that feel beyond my control – such as trying to get attention, and feeling devastated when it doesn't come. When I connect with her, I can feel her sadness and loneliness. I speak to her, I sit in an imaginary sandpit with her and make fairy villages out of flowers, acorns and leaves. All she needs is for me to be with her, in my imagination, to feel seen and understood for a few minutes. The me that is spending time with her is my Self.

You will recognise your authentic Self because it's ever-present and always feels like a wise and loving presence. If it doesn't feel like that, you're dealing with a different part that probably needs your love and care.

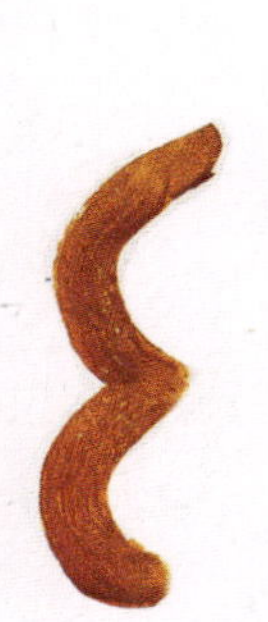

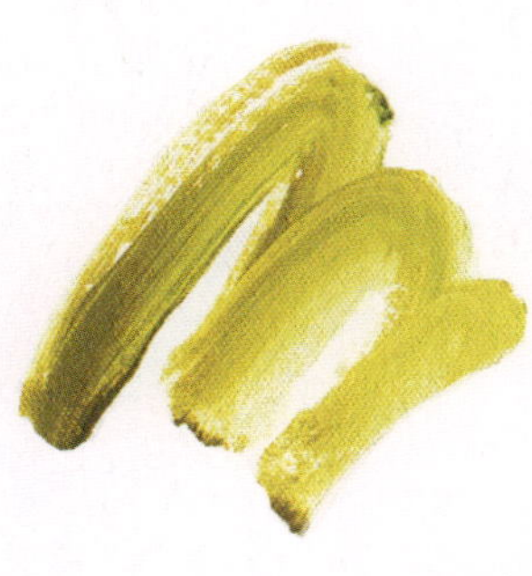

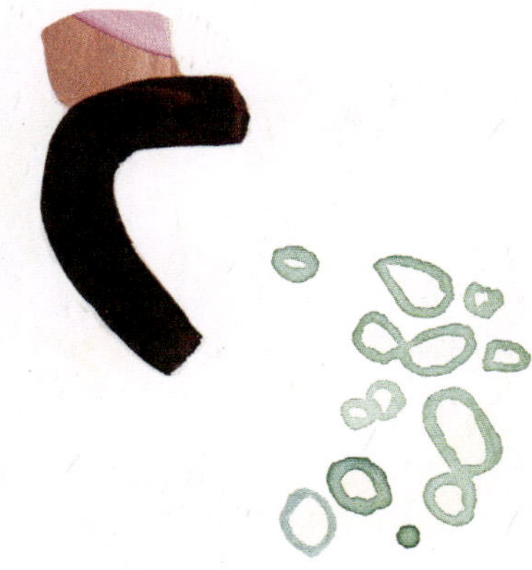

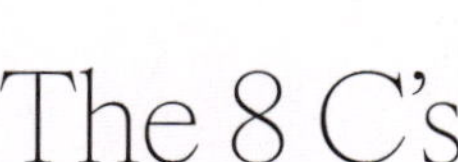

The 8 C's

Fundamentally, the Self represents our authentic identity, distinct from all of our individual parts. It is defined by the eight core qualities identified by IFS. These qualities are the Self's hallmark and help us recognise it over our exiled 'parts'.

1 Compassion

The ability to meet yourself and others with kindness, especially during difficult moments.

2 Curiosity

An open-hearted desire to understand what's really going on without rushing to judge or fix.

3 Clarity

Seeing situations and inner experiences with honesty and calmness, free from distortion.

4 Creativity

A willingness to explore, express, and imagine from a place of authenticity and freedom.

5 Calm

A grounded inner steadiness, even in the middle of emotional storms.

6 Confidence

Trusting in your own goodness and inner resources, no matter what you're facing.

7 Courage

The strength to meet discomfort, tell the truth, and act in alignment with your values.

8 Connectedness

A felt sense of belonging – to yourself, to others, and to something greater.

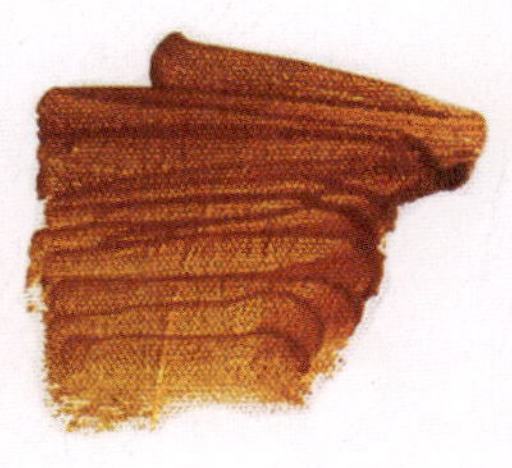

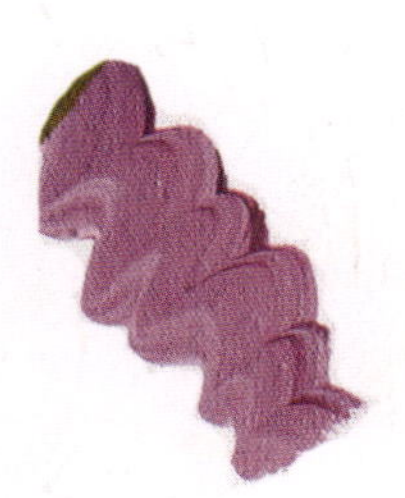

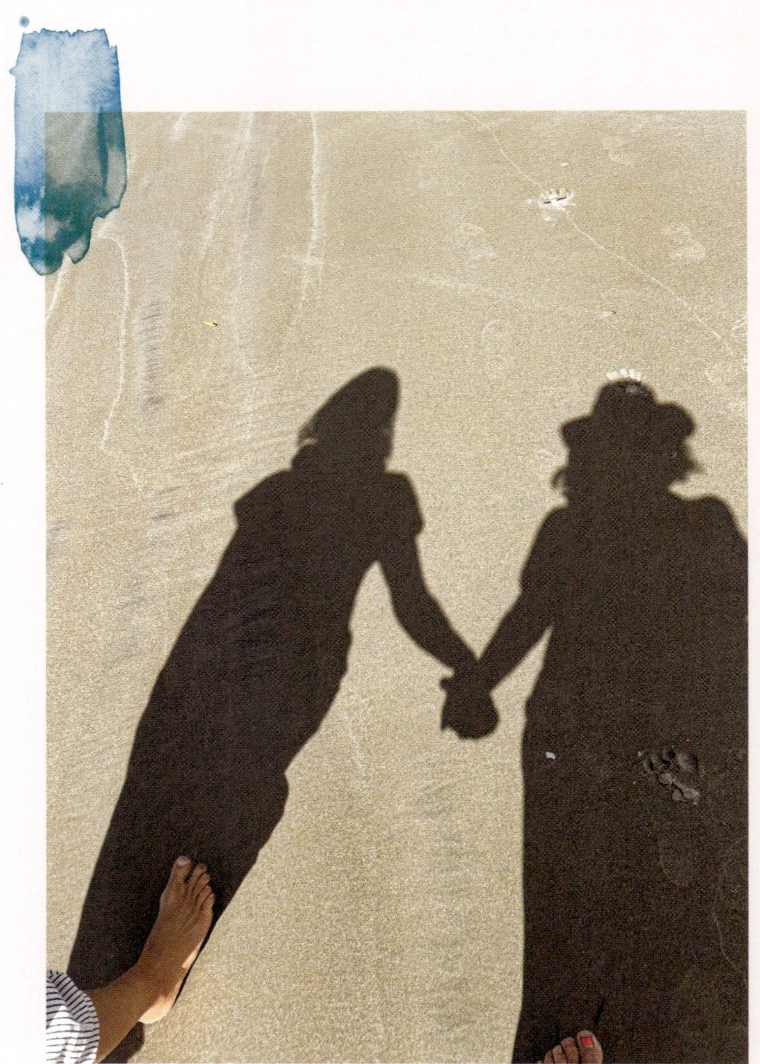

IT'S A LONG JOURNEY, BUT IF WE AIM TO WALK CLOSER TO WHO WE REALLY ARE, I THINK IT'S REWARDING.

Often, it feels like our parts are running the show. Sometimes they are! They step in with traits such as perfectionism and overworking. Some parts express hurt versions of our younger selves and make us easily triggered.

Internal Family Systems is a powerful framework and wonderful tool. If you feel called to, I urge you to look into it. There is a lot of information on podcasts and in books to get you started. I have listened to a few good ones on *We Can Do Hard Things* and one on *The Tim Ferriss Show*.

What good comes from turning to the Self?

Connecting to the Self is a tool for a more joyful, authentic life. Many of us live an entire life on autopilot. The programming of society and the big and small traumas of our upbringing and daily existence steer the ship. Society tells women that they need to get married and have children, it tells men that they need to be strong and never show emotions – and it forms so many toxic and harmful patterns in our lives that are sometimes hard to recognise.

I spent my teens and twenties convinced that my worth as a female came from the attention of boys and men. The purpose and drive of my personal life was to find a husband and have a family. I didn't even realise that this was conditioning; it felt like something I actually wanted – because of the stories I'd been told by society up until that point. I did find a husband and have a family. He was a good man, and a wonderful father – all of the things that one should look for in a life partner. But I realised in my early forties that my heart wasn't happy. My autopilot had taken me down a road that wasn't my truest, most authentic self.

Realising this was devastating and difficult. I was in an internal conflict for the longest time. Do I do my duty as a good person, a good girl, and stay in a place that wasn't right for my heart … or do I move on in search of my truth?

During this period, I read *Untamed* by Glennon Doyle. Strangely, I had owned the book for quite some time before opening its pages. I had a real gut feeling that there was truth in there – my truth – and that it would lead me down a path that scared me stiff. I remember saying to my girlfriends at the end of a Friday lunch (that we call Book Club to mask that it's an excuse to catch up and drink prosecco), 'I haven't read *Untamed* yet – I'm scared that it will make me leave my husband and become a lesbian.' Well, I did. And although the book didn't 'make' me do it – it did give me the courage I needed to make the decisions I knew were necessary to be true to myself.

Glennon (another person I refer to by first name because in my mind she's my bestie – please listen to her podcast, it will change your life) speaks about listening to your inner knowing – to the Self – to create a more authentic life.

I did. And for a while it was hell. Leaving a good man, 'breaking up' my family, and leaving a trail of devastation behind me did not feel like joy for quite some time. By the time I moved into my new home the feeling of truth, authenticity, and being fully in my own energy made sense of it all. I had done the hard thing, but it was the true thing. The realisations and developments that came afterwards have given me more joy than I knew was possible when I was living on autopilot.

I realise that this story might not encourage you to want to listen to your Self! It sounds scary. You can tune in for smaller things, less scary things, without upending your entire life. Maybe your Self will suggest doing more yoga or dancing in the rain. But every now and then a life does need to be flipped upside down to make sense of it, and a connection to yourself can give you the strength and courage to do that.

This process leads to the discovery of your unique way of living, your connection to your own life – rather than the script that was written by every other outside influence.

The Self as a refuge

It's very easy to become swept up in the chaos of daily life. As you have read so far, my joy practices often find junctures to come back into the present, or the body, to move away from the anxiousness and chatter inside our minds.

Coming back to the Self is a beautiful way to connect with the more loving, joyful aspects of life. A few moments a day of putting your hand on your heart and checking in with how you feel or what you need can remind us that there is more. That we're connected to a flow of love that's always available to access.

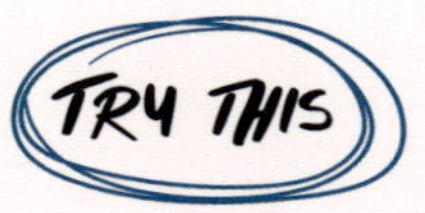

In the morning, during the few moments after you wake up (your eyes might still be closed), put your hand on your heart, take a deep breath, and ask yourself: 'What do you need today, my love?' Then listen.

Your Self will tell you what it needs – maybe a hug, or a slightly slower day than usual. Maybe it'll encourage you to spend a few minutes in nature, it might surprise you with a random request – stay open and curious; it could be the start of an exciting new path. By asking yourself, lovingly, what you need, you start connecting with the inner wisdom of your Self, and see your own needs as important.

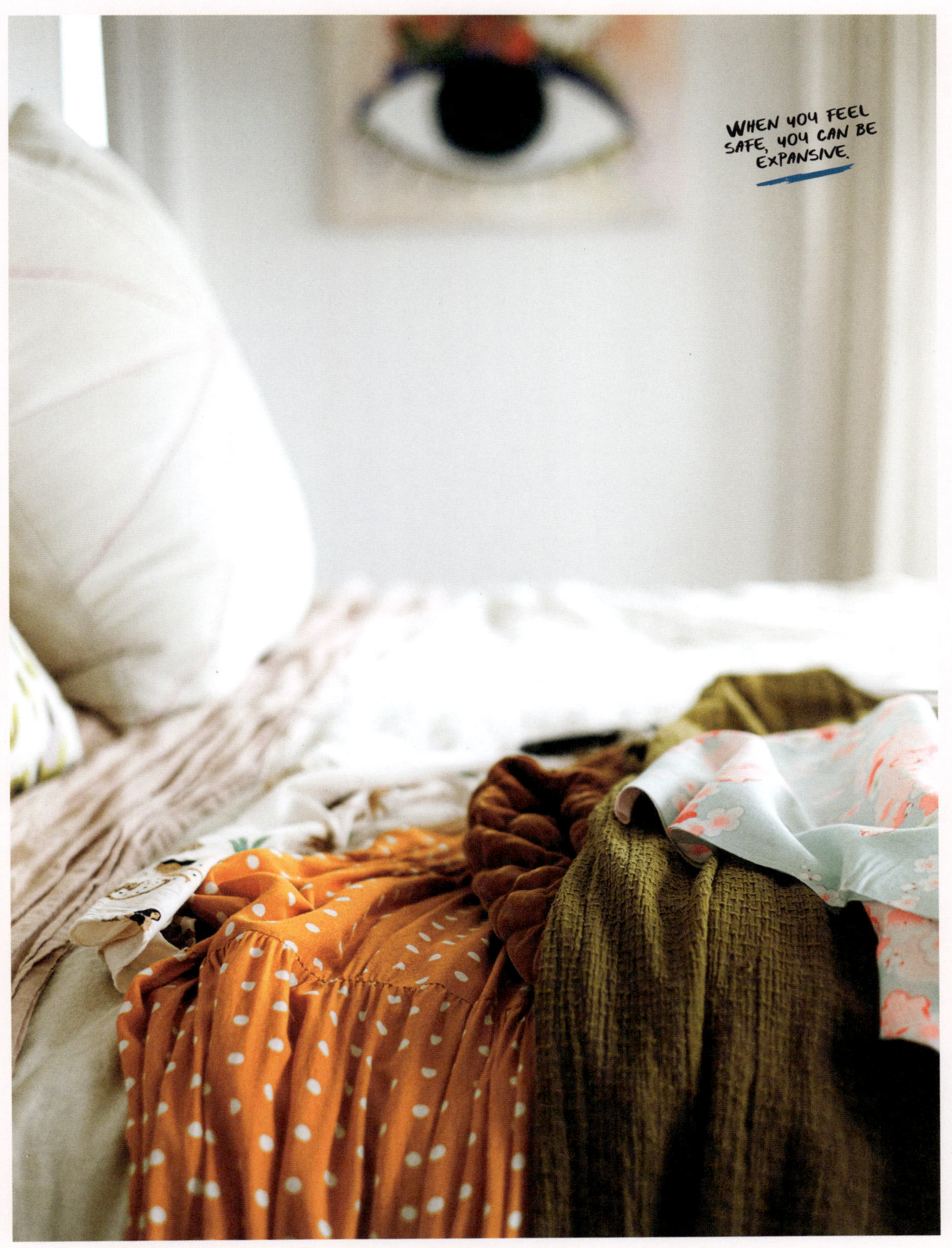
WHEN YOU FEEL SAFE, YOU CAN BE EXPANSIVE.

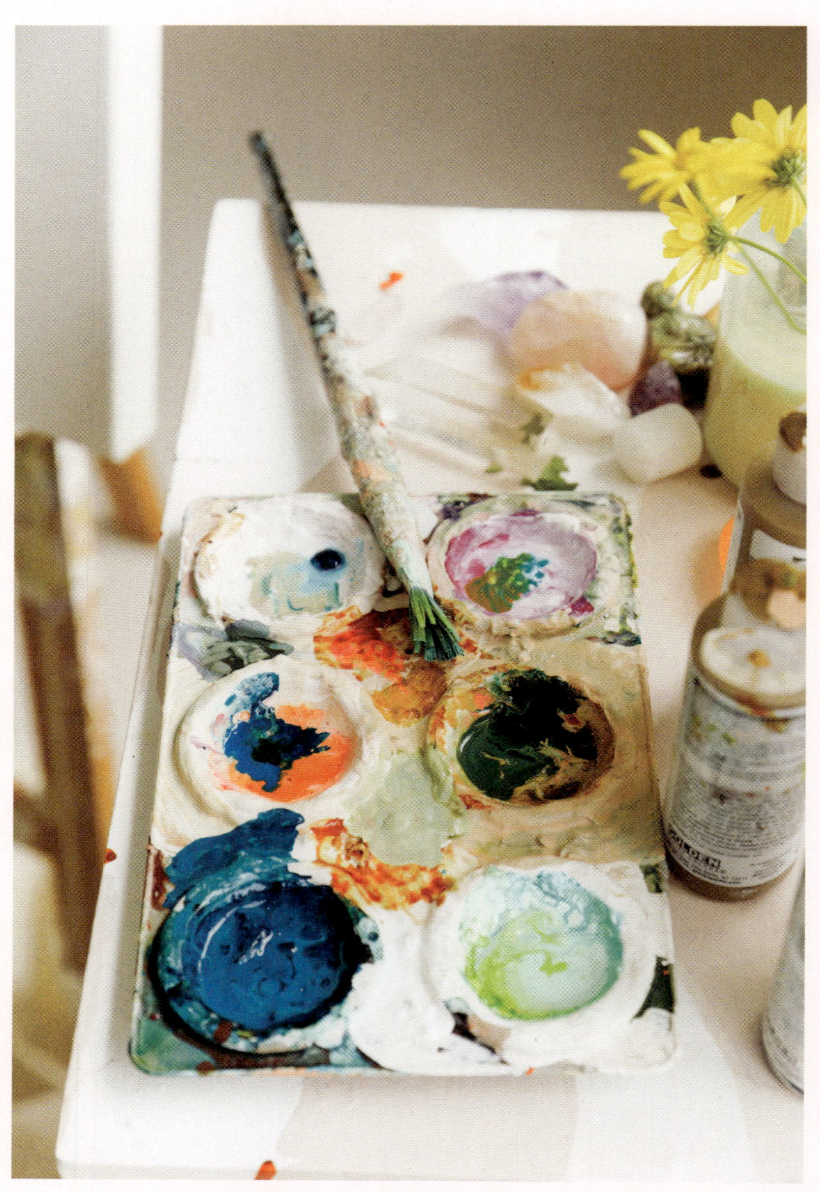

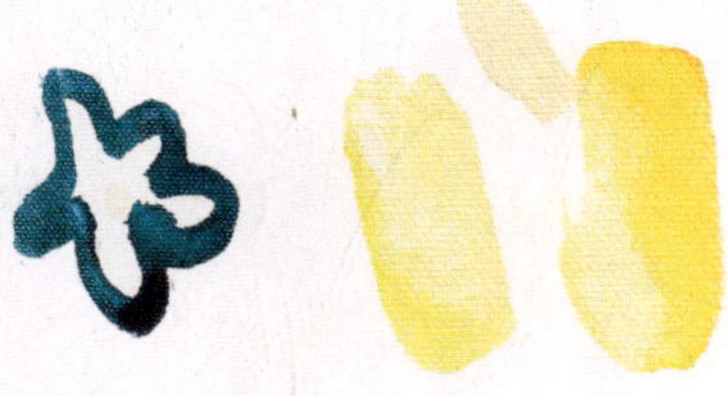

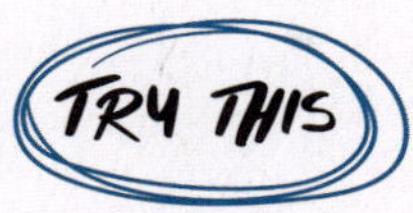

Tune into your truth

We're so used to looking outward for answers that it can feel unfamiliar to pause and check in with ourselves. This little practice is about creating a soft space to reconnect with your inner wisdom.

1 Get quiet

Find a few minutes where you won't be interrupted. Sit somewhere peaceful, place one or both hands on your heart, and close your eyes. Take a few slow breaths to settle.

2 Ask gently

What do I need right now?
Or
What would feel most supportive today?

3 Listen

Notice what comes up. It might be a word, a feeling, an image, or just a quiet knowing. Trust whatever arrives, even if it's small or subtle.

You don't have to act on it perfectly, but the more you practise asking and listening without judgement, the more attuned you'll become to your inner wisdom. Over time, this simple check-in can become one of your most powerful tools for choosing joy and living with intention.

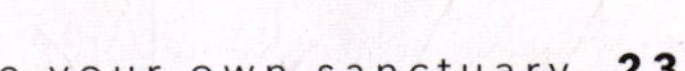

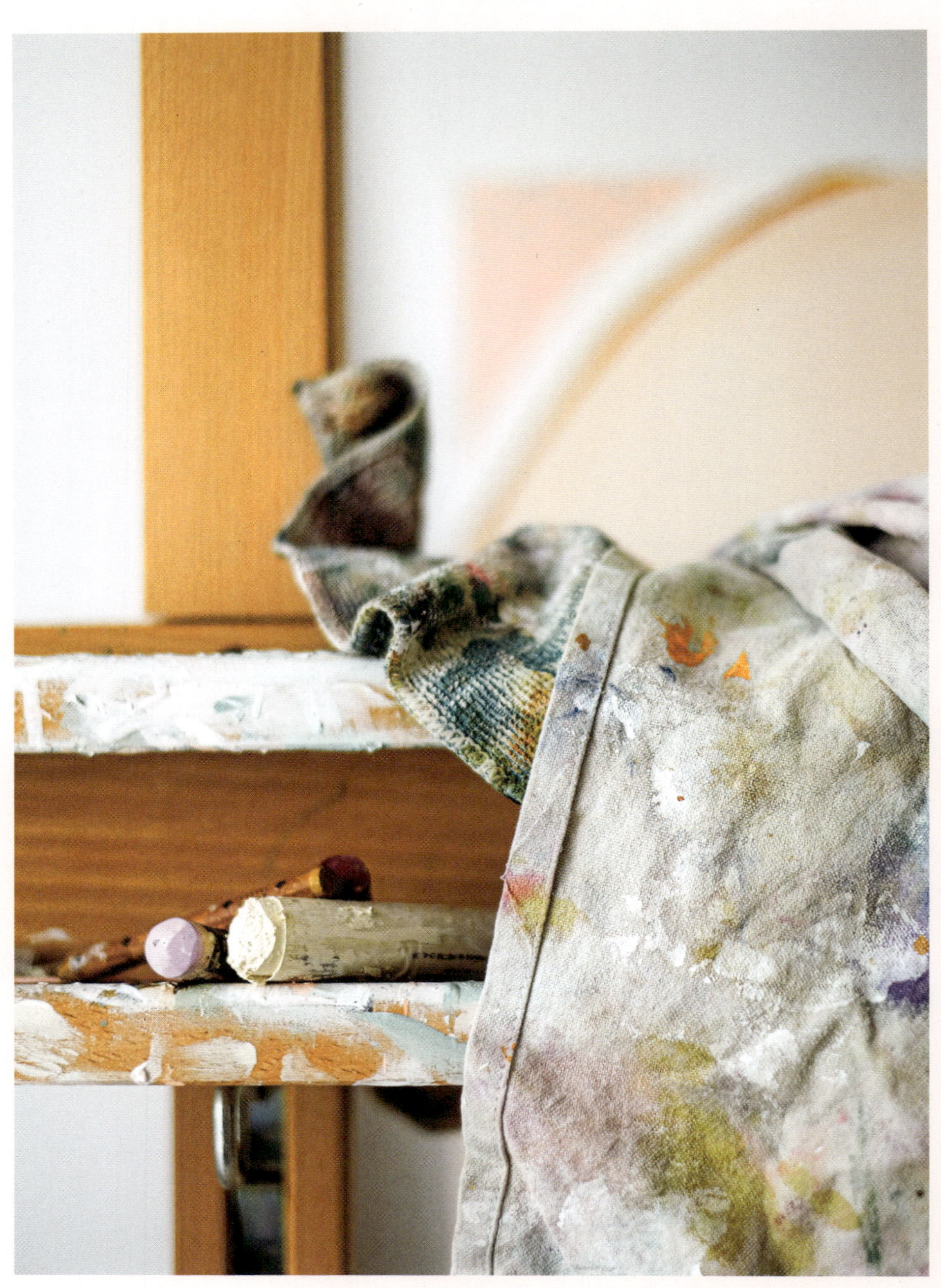

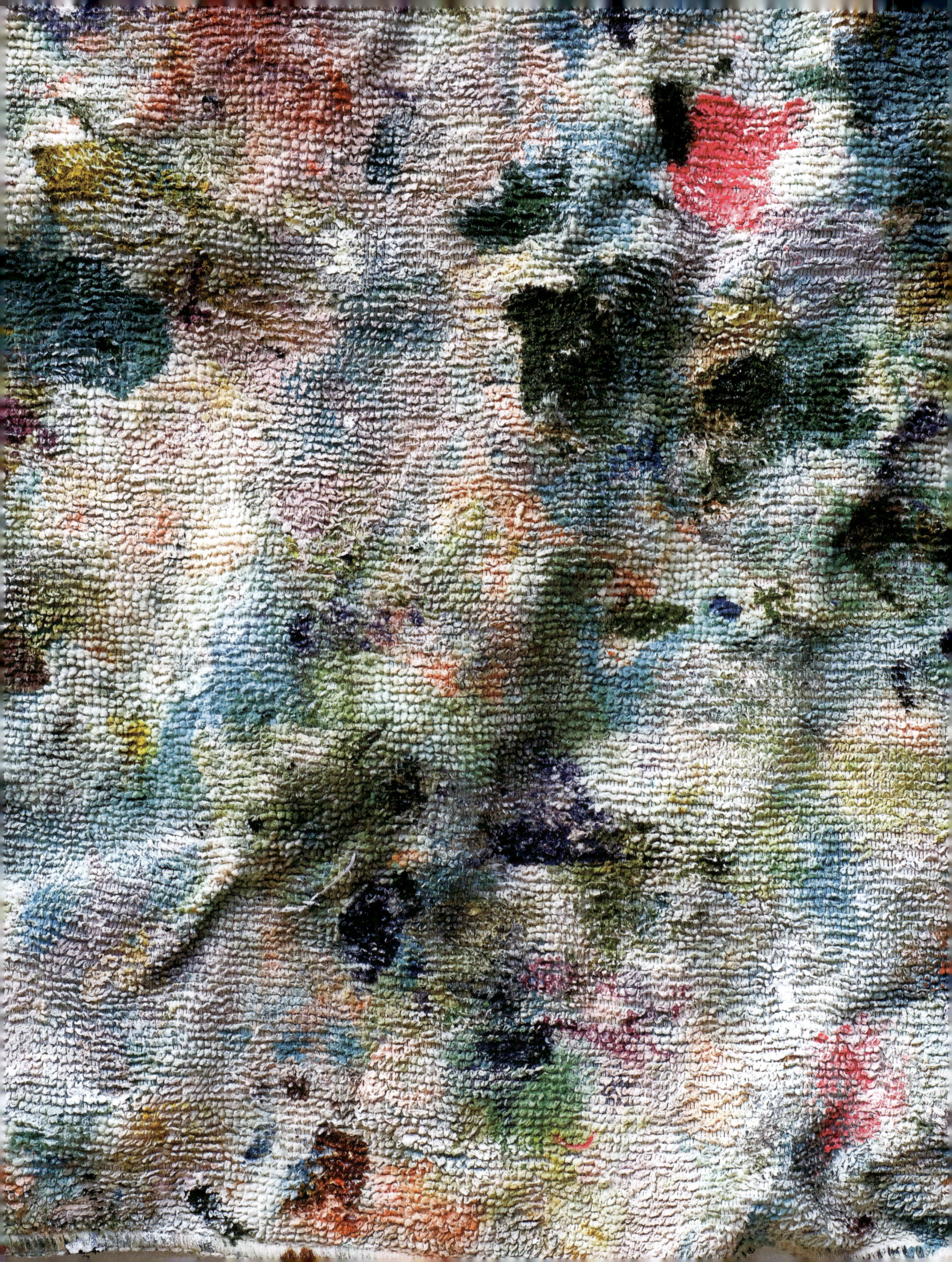

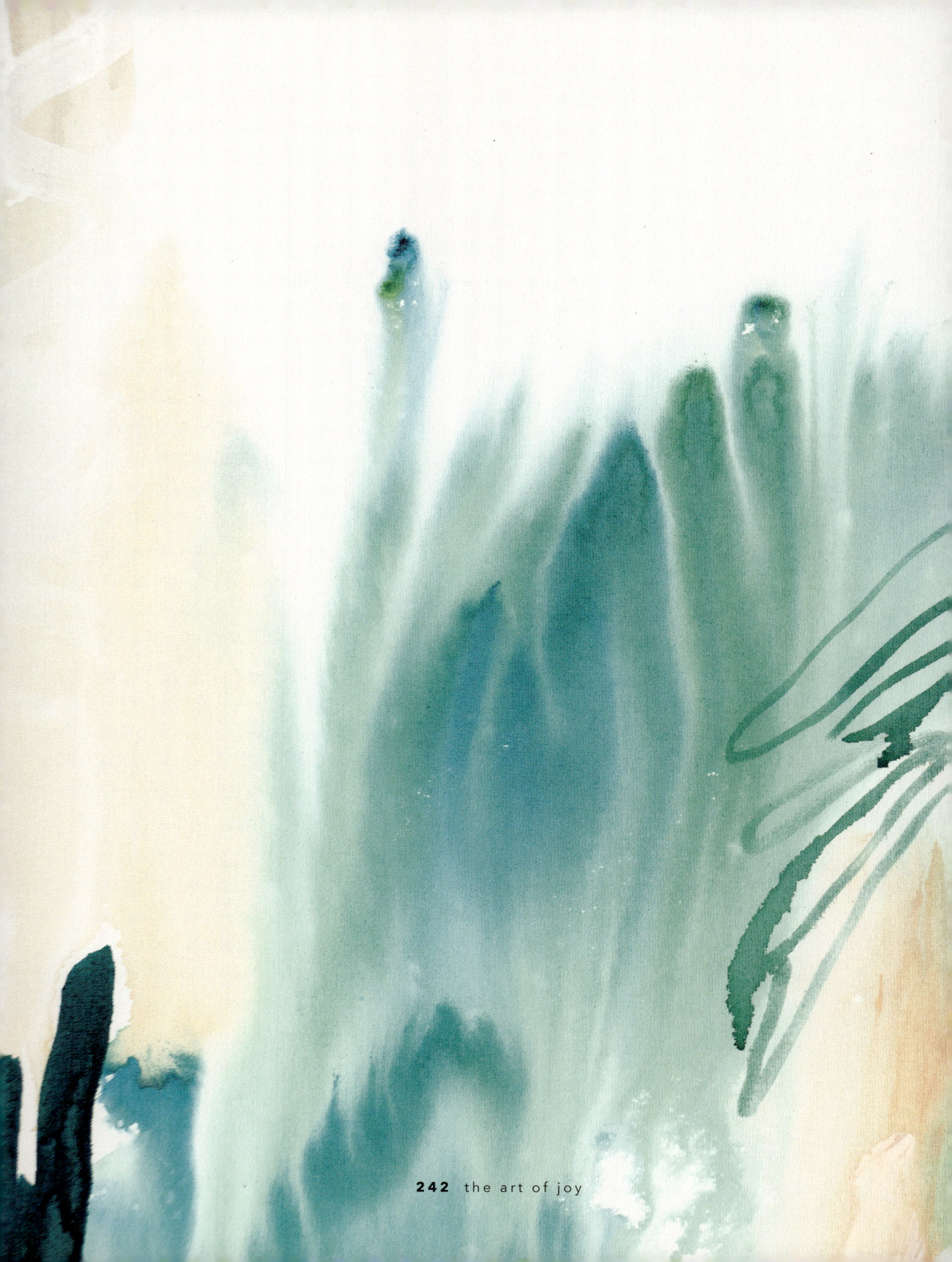

chapter fourteen

A JOYFUL CLOSING

Stand in awe.

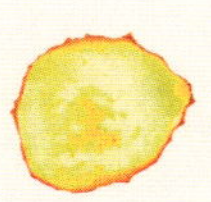

It's funny how things develop, how a creative child from South Africa with her head high in the clouds and her heart on her sleeve can find herself here. I'm in my mid-forties, in the tiny island country of New Zealand, so far away from everyone that it sometimes gets left off world maps. I'm a successful artist and mentor. I have a beautiful daughter, the most wonderful friends and a newly discovered sexuality. And here I am, writing the closing chapter of a book about joy.

The life I'm currently living is thousands of miles (physically and conceptually) from anything I could have dreamed of. Although I knew I would be an artist as a very young child, the older me discounted that as whimsy. I think this is an appropriate moment to find the thread that has led me here – what force, at the essence of my being, has allowed all of this to happen and propelled it forward?

It would really sum things up nicely if I could say it was *joy* – after all, that is the whole point of this endeavour. But joy is the product, not the cause. I'd say that the magical thread that has woven through this extraordinary life is awe.

I regularly allow myself to be bowled over by everyday beauty, and in doing so, the wonder of all things possible lights up in my belly. That sublime feeling of awe, which is much easier to access than you might think, has such a distinct tone. I feel like I could laugh and weep at once. Awe reminds me that the world is conspiring to make things magical, and some of that magic is here for me – so why not seek it out and make it mine?

We think of awe as the feeling we get at the mountaintop, with a sunset and a perfectly shaped flock of birds flying overhead. That is, indeed, awe. But awe is everywhere – whether you zoom out (think of the billions of stars in the night sky) or zoom in (the detailed network of veins on a single leaf). Or if you stay right where you are, with your hand on your chest and focus on the thought of your heart beating 60 to 100 times every minute of your entire life.

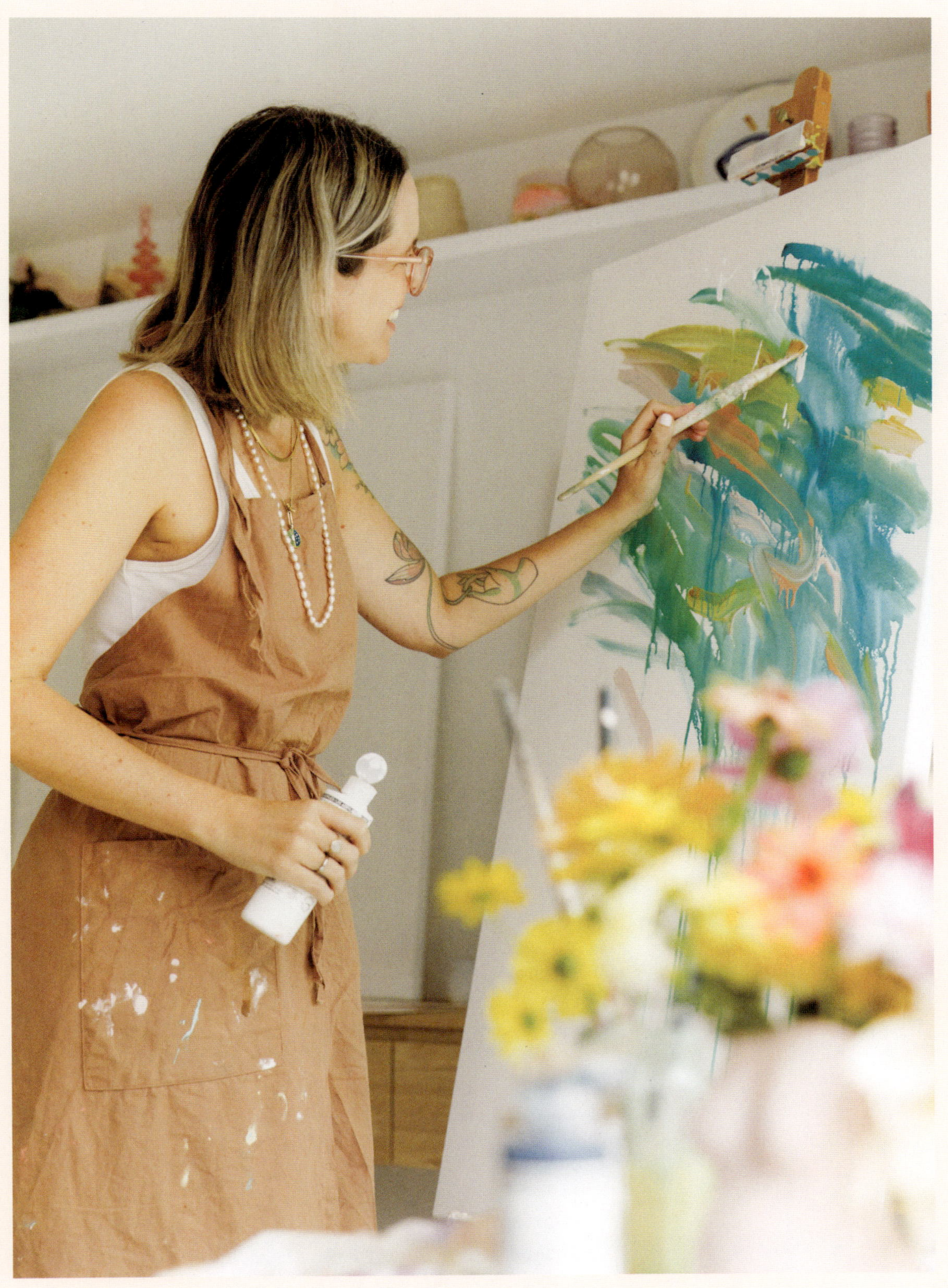

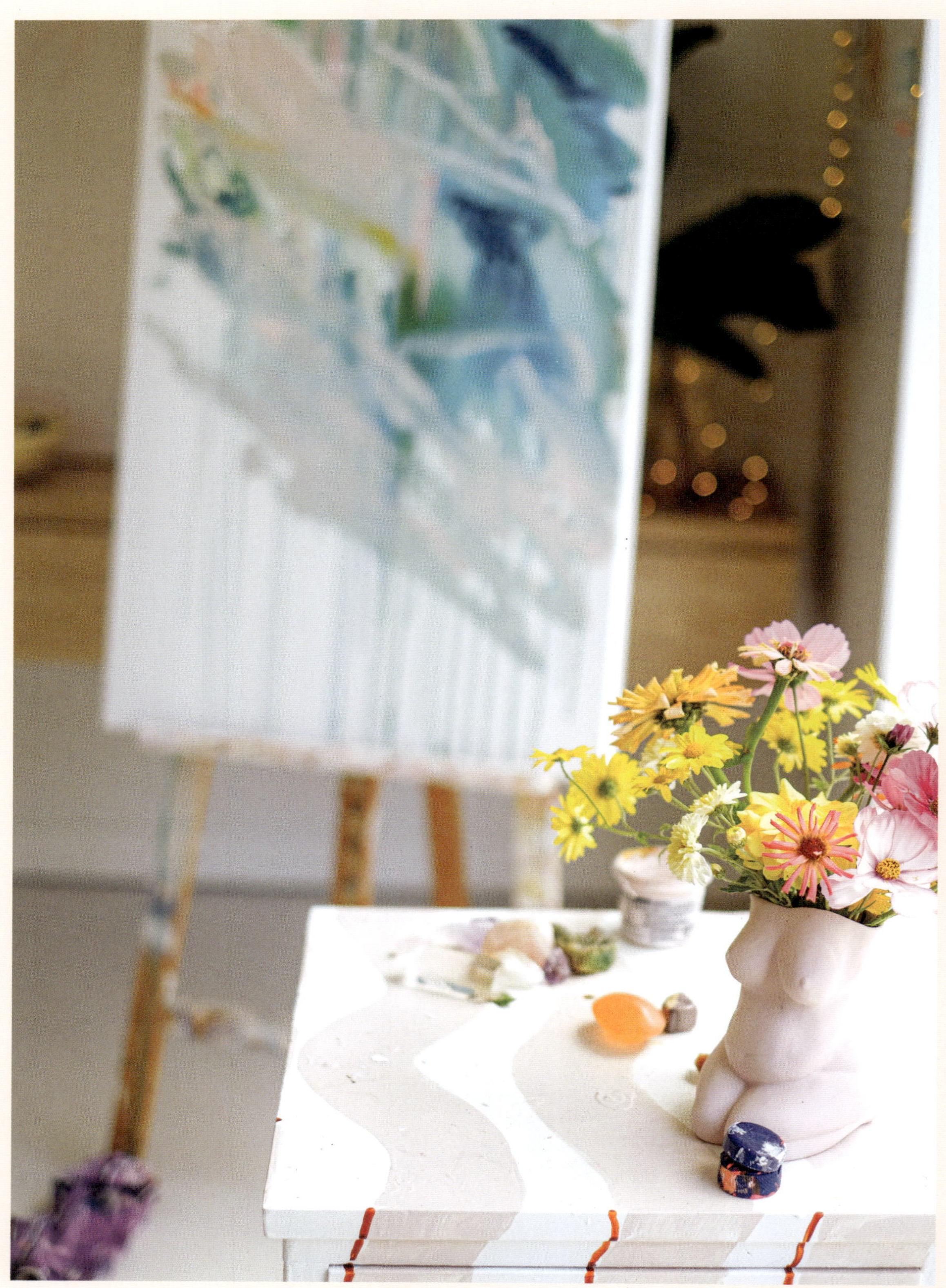

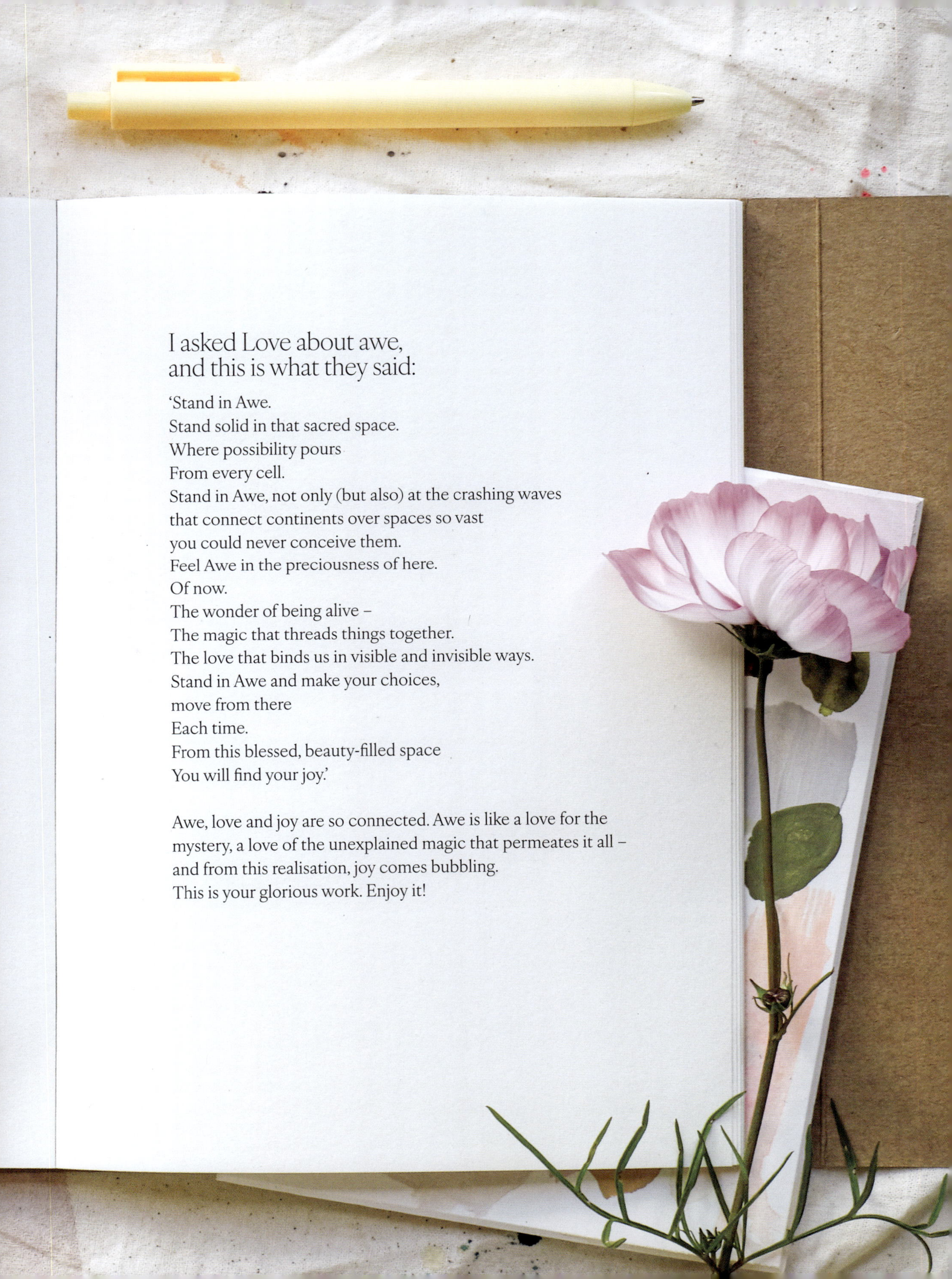

I asked Love about awe, and this is what they said:

'Stand in Awe.
Stand solid in that sacred space.
Where possibility pours
From every cell.
Stand in Awe, not only (but also) at the crashing waves
that connect continents over spaces so vast
you could never conceive them.
Feel Awe in the preciousness of here.
Of now.
The wonder of being alive –
The magic that threads things together.
The love that binds us in visible and invisible ways.
Stand in Awe and make your choices,
move from there
Each time.
From this blessed, beauty-filled space
You will find your joy.'

Awe, love and joy are so connected. Awe is like a love for the mystery, a love of the unexplained magic that permeates it all – and from this realisation, joy comes bubbling.
This is your glorious work. Enjoy it!

I hope that you find your own road to joy. Take anything and everything you want from this book and try what excites you. Prioritise wonder and awe. Prioritise a juicier, more exciting life.

You're here to live, play, create and connect, so go out and do it.

xx

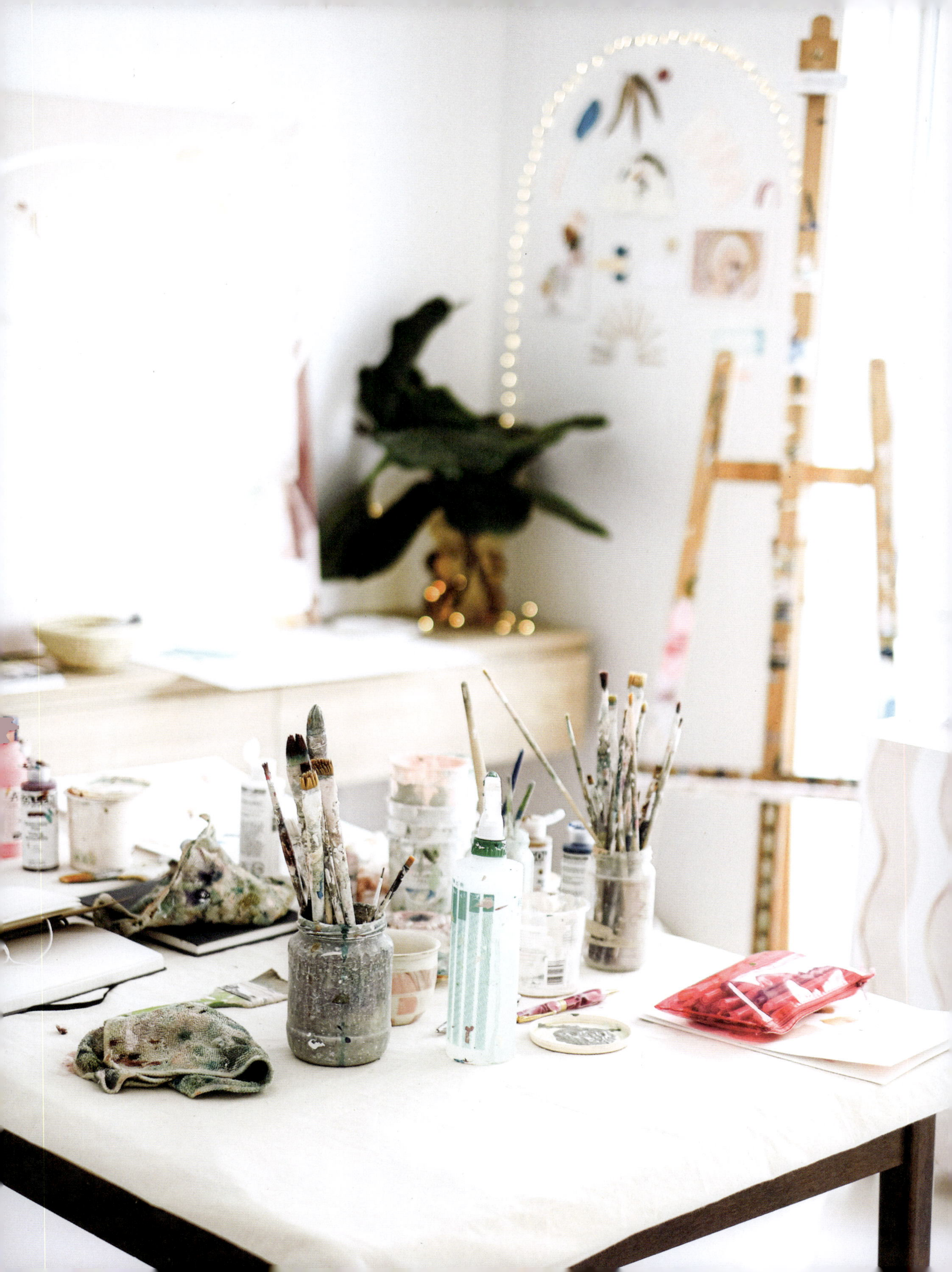

My joy references

Where can you go to fill your mind and heart with all of this info?

Podcasts

Bewildered with Martha Beck and Rowan Mangan
Everything Happens with Kate Bowler
Good Life Project with Jonathan Fields
On Being with Krista Tippett
Oprah's Super Soul
Pulling the Thread with Elise Loehnen
The Tim Ferriss Show
Unlocking Us with Brené Brown
We Can Do Hard Things with Glennon Doyle, Abby Wambach and Amanda Doyle

Books

A Beginner's Guide to the Universe by Mike Dooley
Big Magic by Elizabeth Gilbert
The Book of Delights by Ross Gay
The Creative Act by Rick Rubin
Eat, Pray, Love by Elizabeth Gilbert
Untamed by Glennon Doyle
The Untethered Soul by Michael A. Singer
Any by Mary Oliver
Any by Rumi

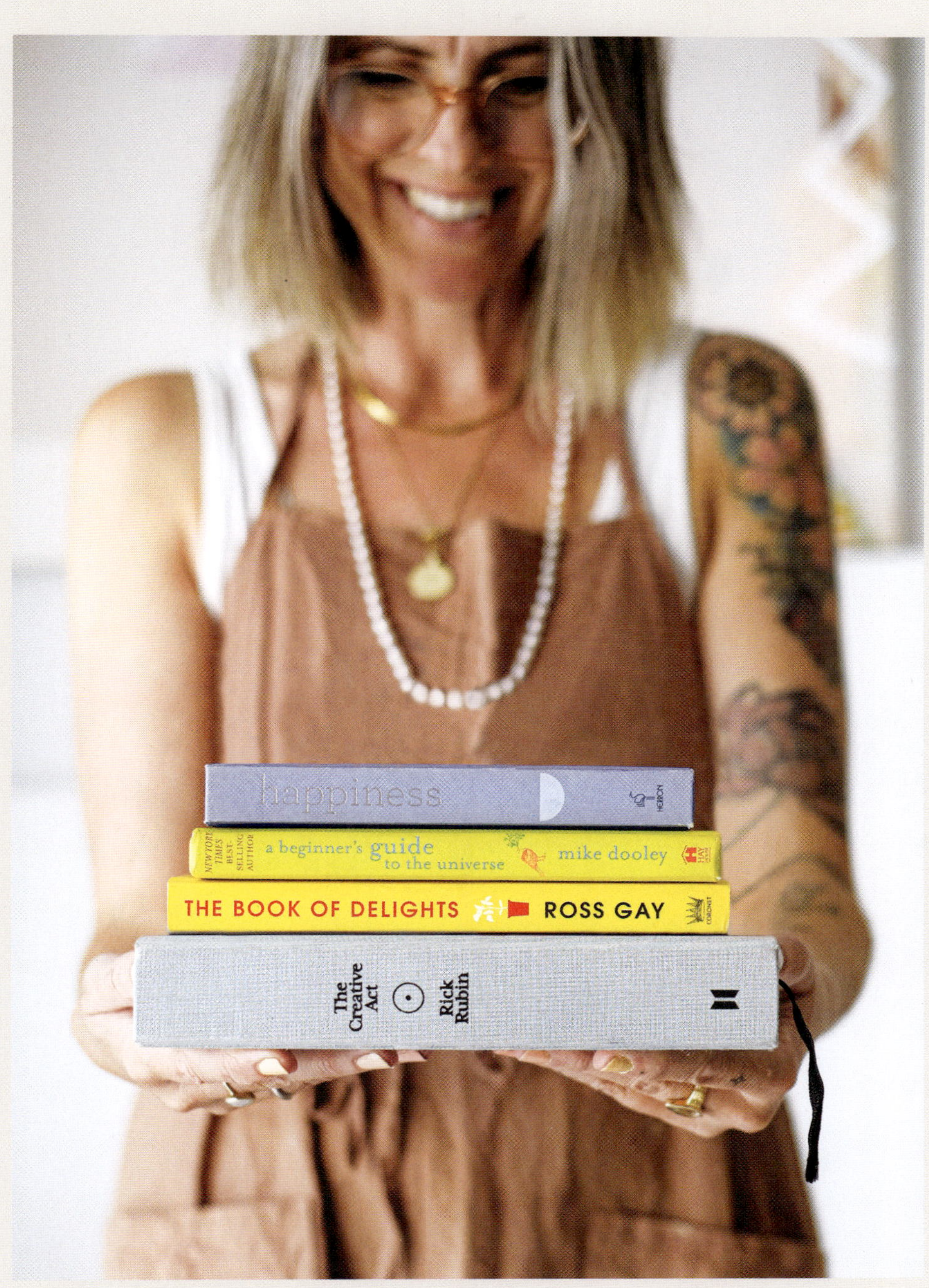
happiness
NEW YORK TIMES BEST-SELLING AUTHOR
a beginner's guide to the universe
mike dooley
THE BOOK OF DELIGHTS
ROSS GAY
The Creative Act
Rick Rubin

Bibliography

Achor, Shawn. *The Happiness Advantage: The Seven Principles of Positive Psychology That Fuel Success and Performance at Work.* Virgin, 2011.

Beck, Martha. *The Gathering Room.* Podcast. 2020–present.

Blondin, Sarah. *Live Awake.* Insight Timer. 2015–present.

Brown, Brené. *Daring Greatly: How the Courage to Be Vulnerable Transforms the Way We Live, Love, Parent, and Lead.* Penguin Life, 2016.

Brown, Stuart, and Vaughan, Christopher. *Play: How It Shapes the Brain, Opens the Imagination, and Invigorates the Soul.* Avery, 2009.

Bryant, Fred, and Veroff, Joseph. *Savoring: A New Model of Positive Experience.* Psychology Press. 2006.

Cameron, Julia. *The Artist's Way: A Spiritual Path to Higher Creativity.* Souvenir Press, 2021.

Chapman, Gary. *The 5 Love Languages: The Secret to Love That Lasts.* Jaico Book Distributors, 2008.

Doyle, Glennon. *We Can Do Hard Things.* Podcast. Cadence13, 2021–present.

Gay, Ross. *The Book of Delights: Essays.* Coronet, 2020.

Gilbert, Elizabeth. *Big Magic: Creative Living Beyond Fear.* Bloomsbury, 2016.

Parker, Priya. *The Art of Gathering: How We Meet and Why It Matters.* Penguin. 2019.

Singer, Michael A. *The Untethered Soul: The Journey Beyond Yourself.* New Harbinger Publications, 2007.

Zahn, R. et al., 'Gratitude has long lasting effects on the brain'. *Proceedings of the National Academy of Sciences, 104* (15), 6430-6435, 2007. https://doi.org/10.1073/pnas.0607061104

Index

My heartfelt thanks

It certainly takes a village to create a book, and I'm thankful to everyone who played a part in it – big or small.

A huge thanks to Tonia from Koa Press, for taking a chance on this passion project – it has been a wonder watching you bring it to life.

To Adrienne Pitts, it was a delight spending time with you, thank you for capturing the joy of my practice in such stunning images.

To Katie Bosher, thank you for taking this book to a whole new level – finding the gems and making them shine. Your insight and understanding of the topic of joy is invaluable.

To Lucinda Diack and Belinda O'Keefe for making sense of my ramblings, without ever losing my sometimes quirky voice.

To my magical daughter, Mila. You teach me daily to be the best version of myself that I can, I am the luckiest mum in the world and I love you to pieces.
To Hayley and Keah for helping with photography (and life). It is lovely being shown through the eyes of people who know me so well.
To Sarah, thank you for your light and for being my biggest cheerleader.

A warm thanks to Mom, Ant, Debs, and Kerry … even though you're not with us, you were with me on this writing journey, my original writing mentor … Dad and Wendy (and your wonderful clan). Family, although complicated, means more and more to me as I get older.

So much of my joy-filled worldview has been inspired by the podcasts and books I consume. A disproportionate amount of that inspiration comes from a group of women: Liz Gilbert, Glennon Doyle, Abby Wambach, Amanda Doyle, Martha Beck, and Rowan Mangan. These women speak their truth, open their hearts and make sense of the mess and beauty of being alive (also a group of women who have inspired me to come out as queer so late in life).

And of course Peaches and Bean, my little furry balls of joy. Life without you would be easier, but so, so much duller.

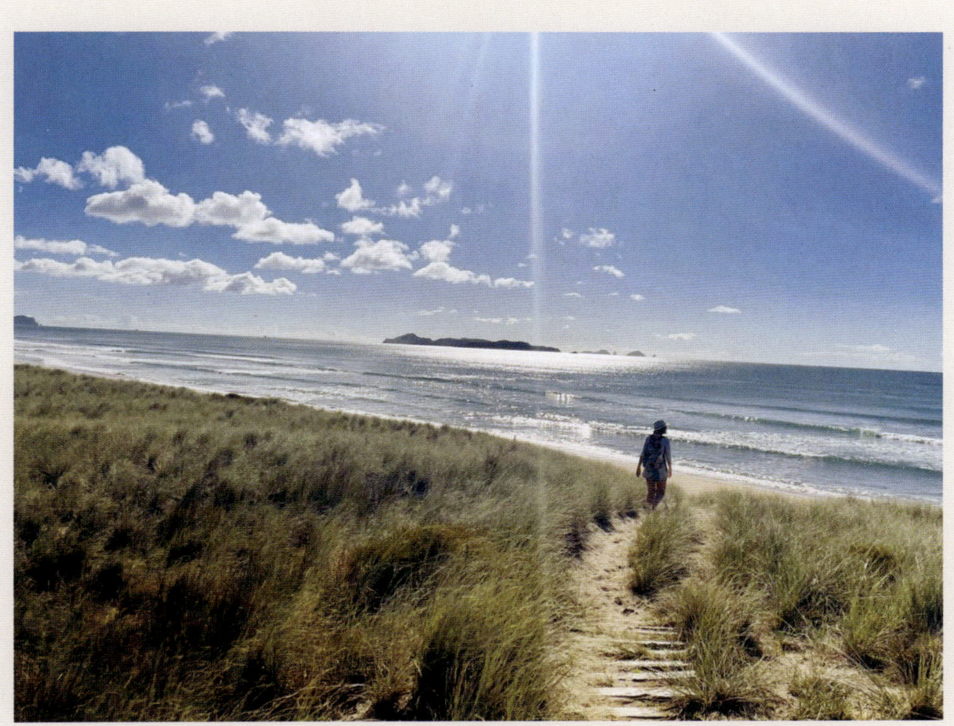

WE GET TO CHOOSE OUR OWN ADVENTURE - WHAT PATH ARE YOU CHOOSING?

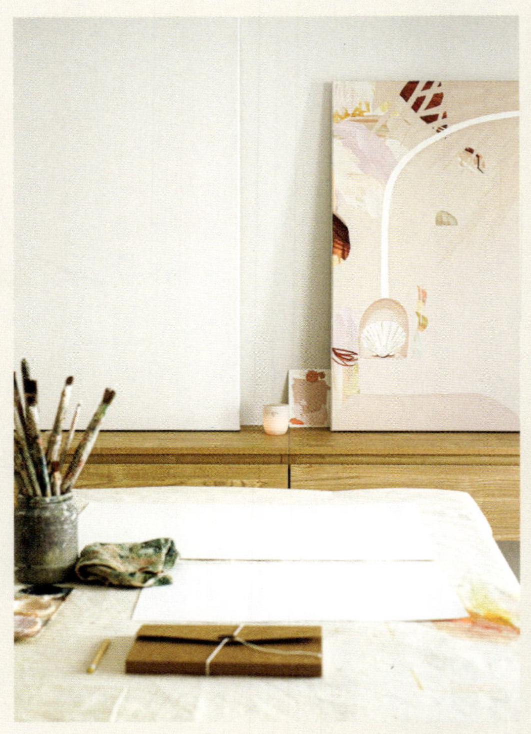

Published in 2025 by Koa Press Limited.
www.koapress.co.nz
@koapress

The Art of Joy
ISBN 978-0-473-69973-4

10 9 8 7 6 5 4 3 2 1

Publisher and Director: Tonia Shuttleworth
Editors: Lucinda Diack & Katie Bosher
Proofreader: Belinda O'Keefe
Designer: Tonia Shuttleworth
Photographers: Adrienne Pitts @hellopoe (pages 6, 13, 21, 28, 70, 72, 74, 103, 116, 117, 155, 161, 165, 205, 222, 230, 231, 238, 245 & back cover), Jen Sievers @jensievers_art & Tonia Shuttleworth @toniashuttleworth

A catalogue record of this book is available from the National Library of New Zealand.

Printed in China by 1010 Printing.